F JUNG
May 20, 1980

An Atlas of Artifacts

An Atlas of Artifacts
Encountered in the Preparation of Microscopic Tissue Sections

By

SAMUEL WESLEY THOMPSON, D.V.M., M.S.

Diplomate of the American College of Veterinary Pathologists
Manager of Pathology
Subdivision of Toxicology and Pathology
Research Department
CIBA-GEIGY Pharmaceuticals Division
CIBA-GEIGY Corporation
Summit, New Jersey

and

LEE G. LUNA, D.Lit., H.T. (ASCP)

Chief of the Histopathology Laboratories
Armed Forces Institute of Pathology
Washington, D.C.

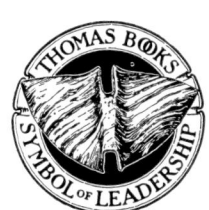

CHARLES   C   THOMAS   •   PUBLISHER
Springfield   •   Illinois   •   U.S.A.

Published and Distributed Throughout the World by
CHARLES C THOMAS • PUBLISHER
Bannerstone House
301-327 East Lawrence Avenue, Springfield, Illinois, U.S.A.

This book is protected by copyright. No part of it may be reproduced in any manner without written permission from the publisher.

© *1978, by* CHARLES C THOMAS • PUBLISHER
ISBN 0-398-03624-1
Library of Congress Catalog Card Number: 76-44848

With THOMAS BOOKS careful attention is given to all details of manufacturing and design. It is the Publisher's desire to present books that are satisfactory as to their physical qualities and artistic possibilities and appropriate for their particular use. THOMAS BOOKS will be true to those laws of quality that assure a good name and good will.

Library of Congress Cataloging in Publication Data

Thompson, Samuel Wesley.
   An atlas of artifacts encountered in the preparation of microscopic tissue sections.

   Bibliography: p.
   Includes indexes.
   1. Histology, Pathological—Atlases. 2. Histology—Atlases. I. Luna, Lee G., joint author. II. Title. III. Title: Artifacts encountered in the preparation of microscopic tissue sections. [DNLM: 1. Histological technics—Atlases. QA517 T476a]
RB33.T48   611'.018'028   76-44848
ISBN 0-398-03624-1

Printed in the United States of America

To
Elson B. Helwig, M.D.

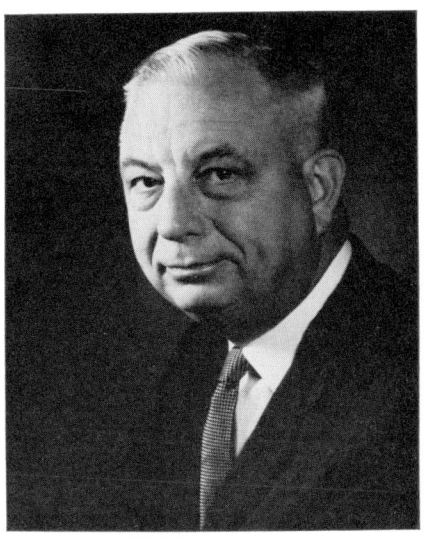

Doctor Elson B. Helwig was born in Pierceton, Indiana on March 5, 1907. He received the Bachelor of Science degree from the Indiana University in 1930 and a Medical Degree in 1932 from the Indiana University Medical School, Indianapolis, Indiana. Following graduation, he interned at City Hospital, Indianapolis from 1932 to 1933 followed by residencies from 1933 to 1936 at City Hospital, Indianapolis Institute of Pathology, Western Reserve University, Cleveland City Hospital, Cleveland. From 1936 to 1939 he served as assistant pathologist at the New England Deaconess Hospital, Boston, and was certified by the American Board of Pathology in 1939.

During World War II (1942-1946) Doctor Helwig served as a physician in the United States Army. His assignments included the Army Medical Museum; Chief of Laboratory Service, Bruns General Hospital; Chief of Pathology and Executive Officer, 18th Medical General Laboratory, Pacific Ocean areas. Upon separation from active duty, he served in the Army Reserves from 1946 to 1967 where he attained the rank of Colonel. From 1946 to the present, Doctor Helwig has served at the Armed Forces Institute of Pathology, first as senior pathologist from 1946 to 1947; then as Chief of Dermal and Gastrointestinal Pathology from 1947 to the present time. He served as Chief, Division of Pathology from 1955 to 1959, at which time the name of the Division was changed to Department of Pathology. In 1975 the Department's name was again changed to Center for Advanced Pathology and remained under his direction. In addition, he has served as Associate Director for Consultation, Armed Forces Institute of Pathology from 1963 to the present time.

Doctor Helwig holds membership in eighteen medical societies including the American Association of Pathologists and Bacteriologists, American Society of Clinical Pathologists, American Medical Society, American Academy of Dermatology, and International Academy of Pathology. He has also been honored with honorary memberships in the Sociedad Columbiana de Patologica, Atlantic Dermatologic Society, Ontario Association of Pathologists, Michigan Society of Pathology and La Societe Trancaise de Dermatologie de Syphiligrahie. His teaching associations and appointments with professional schools since 1933 have included Indiana University, Western Reserve, Washington University, George Washington University, Temple University, Walter Reed General Hospital, and the Skin and Cancer Hospital in Philadelphia.

Over thirty-five awards and honors have been bestowed upon Doctor Helwig during his career, including awards for scientific presentations, exhibits, essay contests for research, achievement in dermatologic medicine, recognition for achievements and devotion, as well as numerous awards for Outstanding and Sustained Superior Performance, the Department of the Army Exceptional Civilian Service Award, and the Department of Defense Distinguished Civilian Service Award. He was a nominee for the Department of the Army's Rockefeller Public Service Award. A most outstanding tribute paid Doctor Helwig for his significant contribution to mankind took place in 1966 when he was awarded the President's Award for Distinguished Federal Civilian Service. He is the second physician to have received this most prestigious award which was presented to him by the late President of the United States, Lyndon B. Johnson.

Doctor Helwig has authored or coauthored over 130 scientific papers and two books and has prepared five syllabuses on Dermal Pathology and Gastrointestinal Pathology. He has given more than 100 lectures and short courses on skin and gastrointestinal pathology in the United States, New Zealand, Japan, Europe, South America, Mexico, and Canada. He has been a member of numerous panels at scientific meetings.

It is with great pleasure that I dedicate this book to Doctor Helwig, an outstanding physician, and wise counsellor.–Lee G. Luna

Preface

*W*HAT ONE MAY SEE upon the microscopic examination of tissue sections of specimens of animal tissues is not always related to the normal histology or pathology of the tissue in question. Defects or abnormalities in tissue sections may result from faulty processing of the tissue specimens. These we shall refer to as artifacts. Some artifacts are readily distinguishable from normal or pathologic tissue components and some are difficult to distinguish from such entities.

With the aid of black and white photographs and selected color photographs, we have endeavored to illustrate several hundred of the artifacts which are most frequently encountered in the preparation of microscopic tissue sections as well as several of the rare types of artifacts. In our consideration of artifacts, we have approached the subject in the same sequence, as set forth in the Contents, that is routinely employed in the collection, fixation, and processing of tissue specimens to completed tissue sections. The legends for the 500 illustrations presented within this text present a description of each artifact, its cause or causes, and methods for its prevention and/or correction.

The purpose of our endeavor is to bring to the awareness of pathologists, histologists, morphologists, and technologists the variety of artifacts that may interfere or obscure in the interpretation of microscopic tissue sections. By providing reliable information on their probable individual or cooperative role in the production of such artifacts and the techniques necessary to avoid their occurrence it is hoped that this text will assist those readers who are responsible for quality control within histology and histopathology laboratories.

As general references for the information presented within this text, unless otherwise stated, we have routinely utilized the *Manual of Histologic Staining Methods of the Armed Forces Institute of Pathology* (3rd Edition, Lee G. Luna, Editor, New York, McGraw-Hill Book Company, 1968, 258 pp.) and Thompson, S. W., *Selected Histochemical and Histopathological Methods* (Springfield, Thomas, 1966, 1639 pp.). The information presented in the legends for the figures of this atlas constitutes a revision and/or addition to information set forth on this subject area in the latter text. All photographs within the text which are identified by an Armed Forces Institute of Pathology

Negative Number are authorized and approved for publication herein by The Director, Armed Forces Institute of Pathology, Washington, D.C.

SAMUEL W. THOMPSON
LEE G. LUNA

Acknowledgments

THE DATA PRESENTED in this text is largely derived from investigations carried out in the authors' laboratories. To this body of data we have been privileged to add contributions (as cited in appropriate figure legends) furnished by the following investigators: James Robert Maitland Innes, D.Sc., Ph.D., M.R.C.V.S., Sc.D. (Contab), F.R.C. Path., Washington, D.C. (deceased); Wayne Kampa, H.T. (ASCP), Mayo Clinic, Rochester, Minnesota; JoAnn R. Matthews, B.A., M.S., and Lawrence E. Schellhammer, B.S., H.T. (ASCP), Pathology Department, CIBA-GEIGY Pharmaceuticals Division, Summit, New Jersey; Fred Sigler, D.V.M., M.S., Norwich Pharmacal Company, Norwich, New York, and William L. Wooding, D.V.M., M.S., Lederle Laboratories, Pearl River, New York.

A number of colleagues have assisted the authors in the preparation of many of the photographs presented throughout the text. We are most grateful to the assistance provided by JoAnn R. Matthews, Lawrence E. Schellhammer, Bart Wanger, Chief-Research Laboratory and Charles West, H.M.C., U.S.N., Administrator, Histopathology Laboratories, Armed Forces Institute of Pathology, Washington, D.C., and William L. Wooding. Technical assistance in photography was provided by Charles E. Edwards and Luther Duckett, Department of Photomicrography, Armed Forces Institute of Pathology, Washington, D.C. and Mr. Dwight Faulkner of the Photography Laboratory, Research Department, CIBA-GEIGY Pharmaceuticals Division, Summit, New Jersey. Appreciation is expressed to Joanne Errante and Roberta Mosedale who typed portions of the draft manuscript and to Barbara Jean Thompson who typed the final version of the entire manuscript.

S.W.T.
L.G.L.

Contents

	Page
Dedication	v
Preface	vii
Acknowledgments	ix

Chapter

		Page
I	Artifacts Resulting from Antemortem Procedures	3
II	Artifacts Resulting from Necropsy Procedures	13
III	Artifacts Resulting from Fixation Procedures	22
IV	Artifacts Resulting from Processing Procedures	63
V	Artifacts Resulting from Embedding Procedures	85
VI	Artifacts Resulting from Microtomy Procedures	91
VII	Artifacts Resulting from the Mounting of Tissue Sections on Glass Slides	107
VIII	Artifacts Encountered in Staining Procedures	120
IX	Artifacts Resulting from Coverslipping Procedures	163

Index 177

An Atlas of Artifacts

I

Artifacts Resulting from Antemortem Procedures

INTRODUCTION

SEVERAL TYPES of artifacts which may be observed in microscopic tissue sections, and are not the fault of the histotechnologists, may have their origin in clinical procedures performed antemortem, or antemortem environmental factors. Examples of such antemortem artifacts included in this chapter are:

> Talcum powder
> Suture material
> Thermal dehydration
> Chemical dehydration
> Carbon particles
> Surgical gauze
> Parched earth effect

Figure 1. *Talcum Powder in a Skin Biopsy.* In this tissue section of a skin biopsy from a human being, as observed by partial polarization, birefringent crystals are present. This artifact results from contamination of the surgical (biopsy) site by the surgeon. The crystals are starch and hydrous magnesium silicate, commonly known as talcum powder. The talcum powder was derived, most probably, from the surgeon's gloves. (H&E, partially polarized light, ×350) (AFIP Negative No. 72-5343)

Figure 2. *Suture Material.* This artifact is suture material that was left in a biopsy specimen of muscle tissue of a human being by the surgeon at the time the specimen was placed in the fixative. At the time the tissue section is cut (see also Chapters II and VI) the suture material, being harder than the surrounding tissue, is pushed ahead of the microtome knife and results in shattering of the tissue adjacent to the site of localization of the suture material. (H&E, ×70) (AFIP Negative No. 71-11702)

Figure 3. *Suture Material.* This is the same tissue section as depicted in Figure 2 as observed by means of partial polarization. The particles of suture material are anisotropic. Such artifacts can be avoided if the suture material is removed from the tissue specimen prior to being placed in the fixative. (H&E, partial polarization, ×70) (AFIP Negative No. 71-11702)

Figure 4. *Thermal Dehydration.* The tissue section is a skin biopsy from a human being which was removed by a thermal knife. The peripheral tissues at the base of the biopsy are literally cooked resulting in dehydration due to heat and coagulation of protein tissue components. The vacuolation of the stroma of the biopsy is a result of the rapid removal of fluid from the tissue by the application of heat and the densely stained interstitial tissue results from dehydration and coagulation of protein. (H&E, ×195) (AFIP Negative No. 72-3899)

Figure 5. *Thermal Dehydration.* This specimen is a skin biopsy from a human being which was removed by a thermal knife (see also Figure 4). The large, densely stained area of material within the lumen of a blood vessel, seen in the upper right quarter of the field, resulted from the coagulation of protein by the application of heat. Note the vacuolation of the stroma. (H&E, ×195) (AFIP Negative No. 72-3898)

Figure 6. *Thermal Dehydration.* Another skin biopsy which was removed by a thermal knife from a human being is depicted (see also Figures 4 and 5). In the field shown at the right, which is stained with hematoxylin and eosin, the dark-stained area at the edge of the biopsy is the result of hyperacidophilia resulting from the coagulation of protein tissue components by the application of heat. If this burned (cooked) area of the tissue section is stained by means of a modified Verhoeff's elastica stain, as seen in the field at the left, the hyperacidophilic coagulated protein will stain in the same fashion as elastic fibers. Note the vacuolation of the stroma. (H&E and Verhoeff's elastica stain, ×60) (AFIP Negative No. 71-7858)

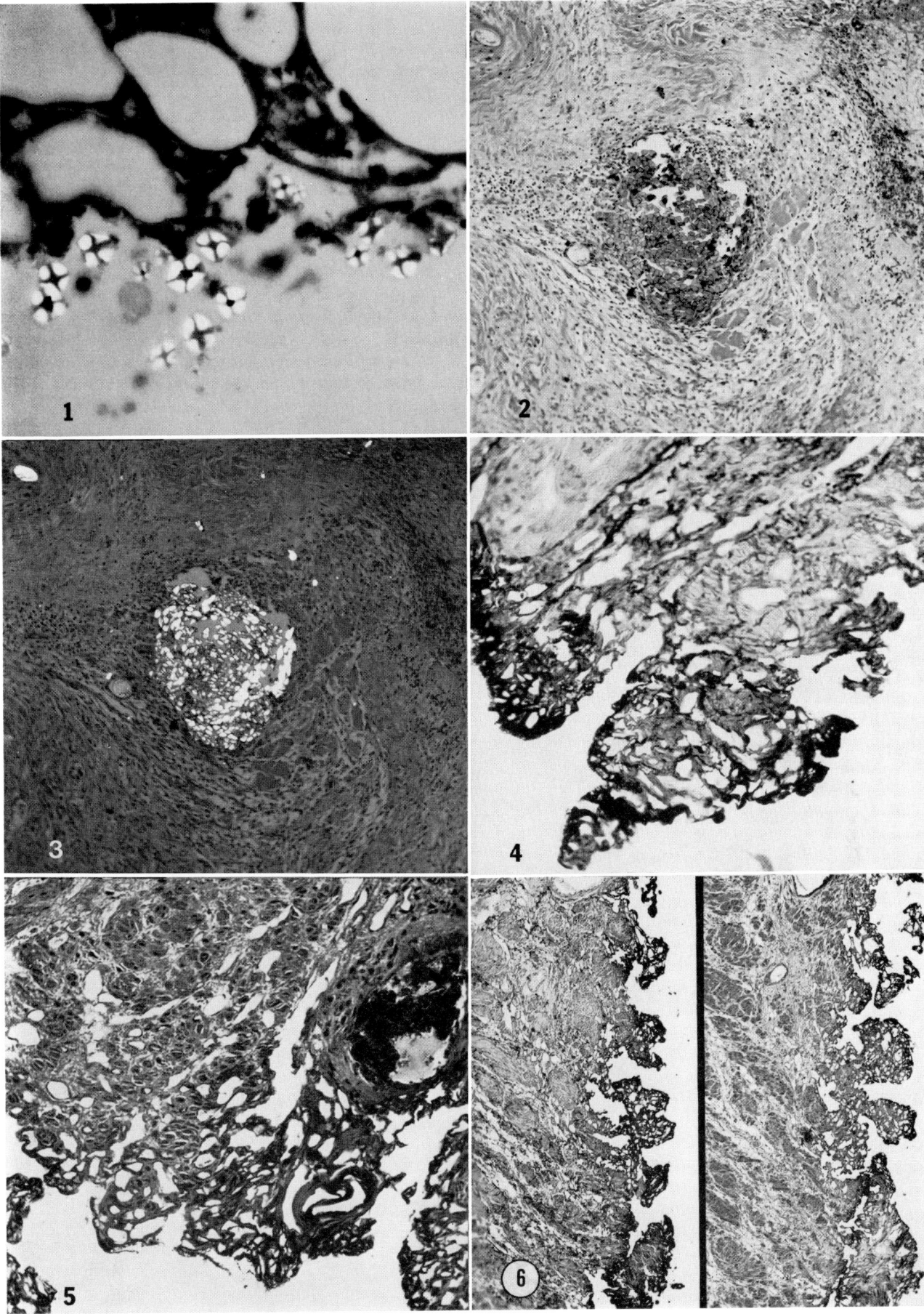

Figure 7. *Thermal Dehydration*. This is a paraffin-embedded tissue section of a specimen of the uterus of a human being which was removed surgically with a thermal knife. The dark stained area is burned tissue as demonstrated by the modified Verhoeff's elastica stain of Hinshaw, J. R. and Pearse, H. E. (*Surg Gyn Obstet, 103:*726-730, 1956) (see also Chapter IV). This staining technique clearly delineates between burned (dark-stained) and normal (light-stained) areas of the tissue section. (modified Verhoeff's elastica stain, ×35) (AFIP Negative No. 68-7459)

Figure 8. *Chemical Dehydration*. The paraffin-embedded tissue section depicted here was prepared from a surgical specimen of human skin. Lysol® was used to sterilize the instruments used for taking the biopsy and Lysol residues on the instruments produced chemical dehydration (burning) of the tissue prior to fixation (see also Figure 9). (H&E, ×100) (AFIP Negative No. 73-2911)

Figure 9. *Chemical Dehydration*. These three tissue sections are all taken from the same biopsy of human skin as depicted in Figure 8. The section at the right is stained by Masson's trichrome technique. The section at the top on the left is stained with alcian blue, and the duplicate section at the lower left of the photograph is stained by Van Gieson's elastica stain. The supposed lesion which prompted the use of these stains for the study of connective tissues is an artifact (chemical dehydration) caused by the effect of Lysol disinfectant on the biopsy specimen. (connective tissue stains, ×70)

Figure 10. *Carbon Particles*. The artifact depicted in this photomicrograph of a paraffin-embedded tissue section of a specimen of a human lung is inspired carbon dust. Note that the carbon particles have been phagocytized by alveolar lining cells and that there is no other reaction to the presence of the particulate matter. (H&E, ×150) (AFIP Negative No. 73-2910)

Figure 11. *Carbon Particles*. This is another field of view of the same tissue section as depicted in Figure 10 to demonstrate that the inhaled carbon particles (soot, smoke, dust) are present within the cytoplasm of septal cells which are free within alveolar lumina (see also Figure 12). (H&E, ×150) (AFIP Negative No. 73-2912)

Figure 12. *Carbon Particles*. This is a higher magnification of the central portion of the field of view depicted in Figure 11. Note the accumulation of carbon particles in the cytoplasm of free phagocytes within an alveolar lumen. To the author's knowledge, there is no satisfactory method for the specific histochemical identification of carbon. (H&E, ×615) (AFIP Negative No. 73-3269)

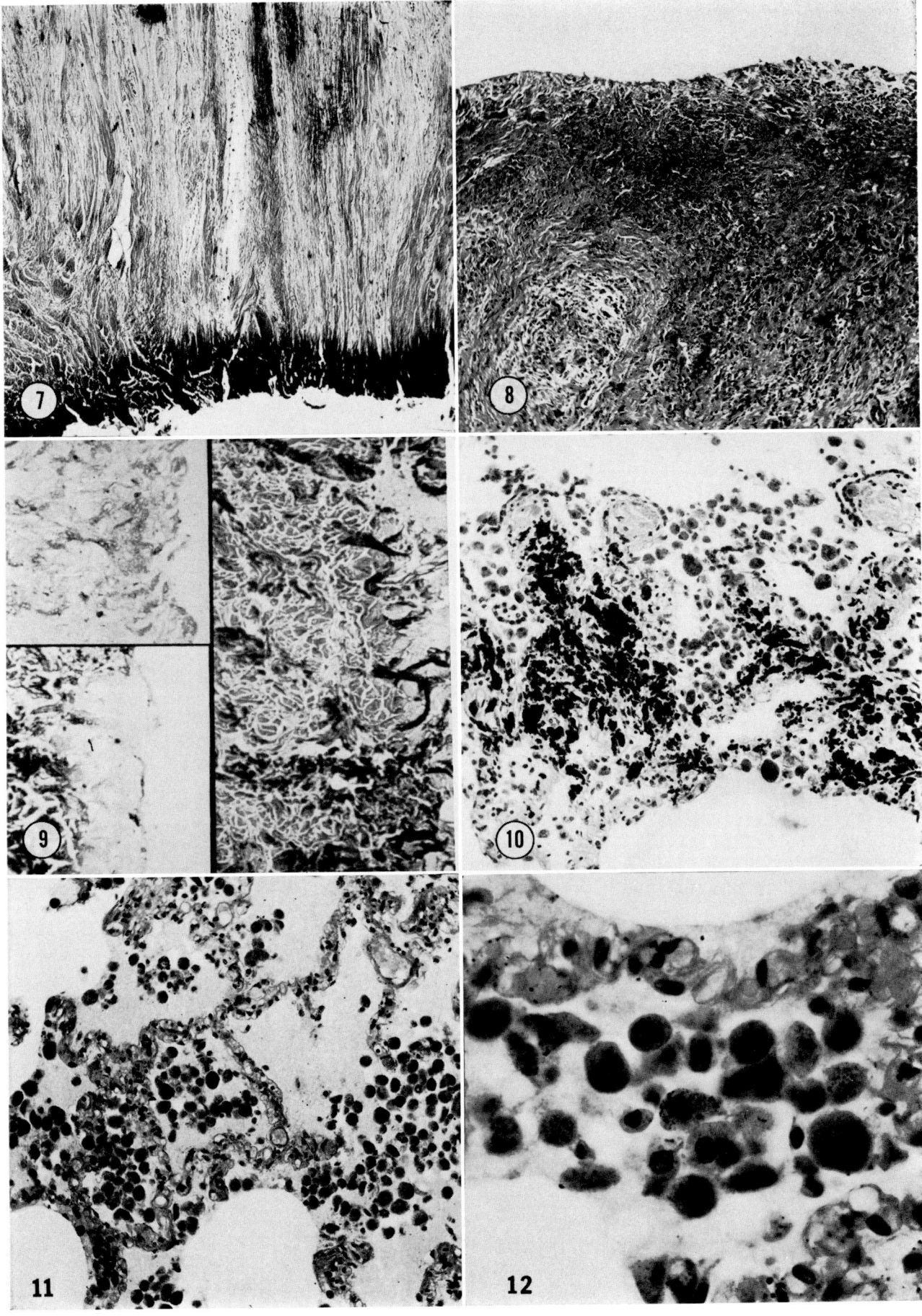

Figure 13. *Surgical Gauze.* The materials seen within round structures throughout this paraffin-embedded tissue section of a specimen of a human tissue mass are gauze fibers. This gauze was left in a patient during an operation. The patient subsequently complained of an additional growth of tissue in the general region of the original operation. A second operation was performed and a tissue mass was removed. Upon microscopic examination it was determined that the mass was a tissue reaction to a gauze pad which had unintentionally been left in the patient during the first operation. (H&E, ×80) (AFIP Negative No. 74-7733)

Figure 14. *Surgical Gauze.* This is a different field of view of a portion of the same tissue section depicted in Figure 13 as viewed by means of partial polariscopy. The gauze fibers are anisotropic. (H&E, ×80) (AFIP Negative No. 74-7735)

Figure 15. *Surgical Gauze.* This tissue section was prepared from the same paraffin-embedded specimen as depicted in Figures 13 and 14. It was stained with Giemsa stain which characteristically stains cotton fibers a bright green color. This staining technique served to confirm that the foreign material observed in Figure 13 was derived from cotton gauze pad fibers. (Giesma, ×80) (AFIP Negative No. 74-7734)

Figure 16. *Respirator-induced Artifact.* The parched-earth effect noted in this tissue section of a specimen of formalin-fixed human brain tissue resembles some of the artifacts which can be produced by faulty microtomy or mounting procedures (see Chapters VI and VII). However, the artifact depicted here resulted from the exposure of a dying human being to an artificial respirator. The brain substance became liquified and the artifact occurred during routine fixation and processing. Technically, there is nothing which can be done to correct or prevent this type of artifact. (H&E, ×3) (AFIP Negative No. 73-4919)

Figure 17. *Respirator-induced Artifact.* This is a higher magnification of a portion of the tissue section depicted in Figure 16. The pattern of the parched-earth effect which results from exposure of a dying person to an artificial respirator is linear which differs from that produced by excessive dehydration of the specimen which is characterized by a zig-zag pattern as described in Chapter VI. (H&E, ×80) (AFIP Negative No. 73-4917)

Figure 18. *Cracking of Tissue Structures.* This photograph depicts a paraffin-embedded tissue section of a specimen of human brain tissue which exhibits the parched-earth effect. The artifact resulted from the antemortem exposure of the patient to an artificial respirator (see also Figures 16 and 17). (H&E, ×12) (AFIP Negative No. 74-4461)

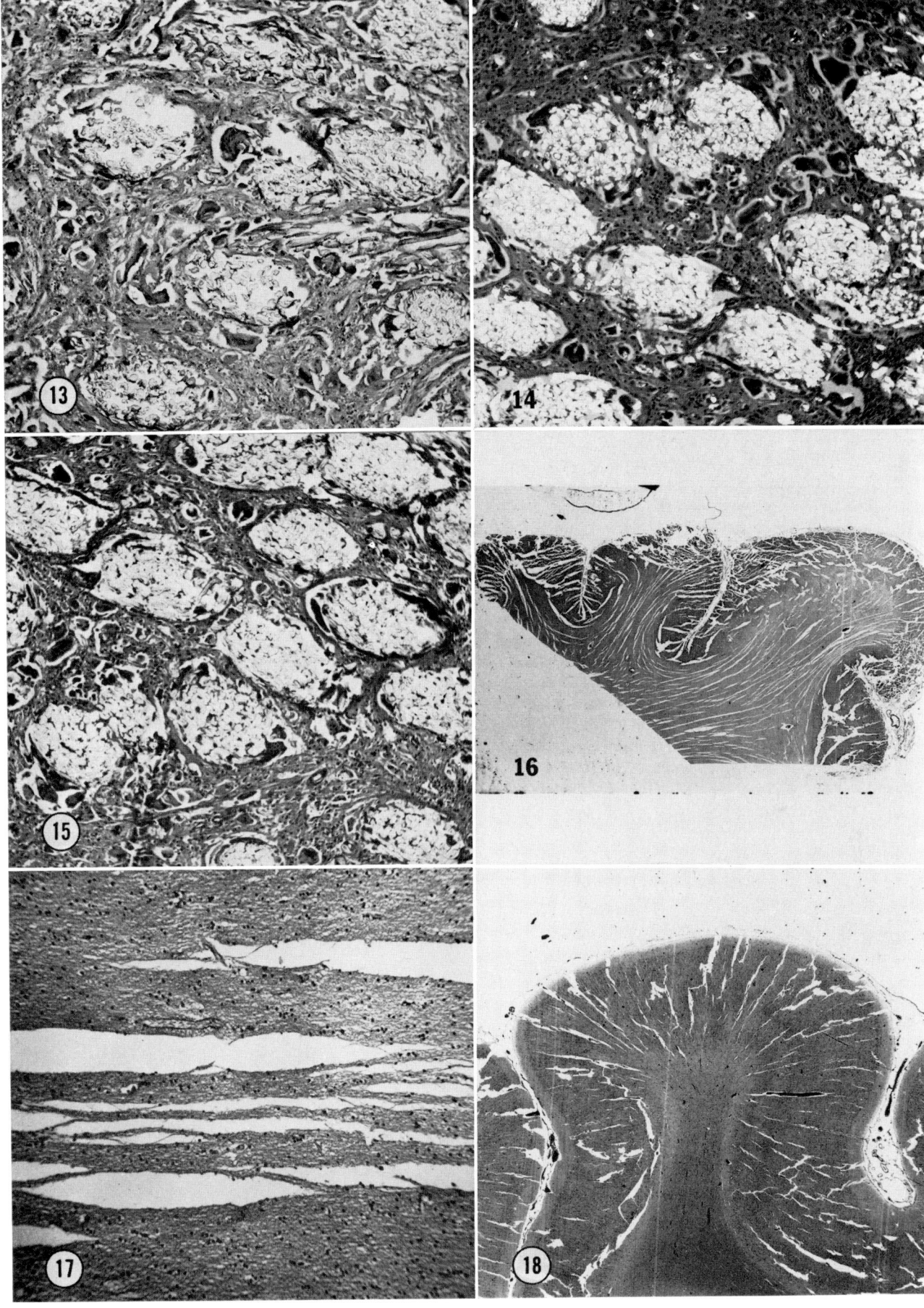

Figure 19. *Cracking of Tissue Structures.* This unstained, paraffin-embedded tissue section of human brain tissue was prepared from the same specimen as depicted in Figure 18. The parched-earth effect is very evident. However, it is not possible from this preparation to determine if the artifact was caused by antemortem treatment of the patient or faulty laboratory technique subsequent to paraffin embedding of the tissue specimen. (Unstained, ×12) (AFIP Negative No. 74-4460)

Figure 20. *Cracking of Tissue Structures.* This is the same field of view depicted in Figure 19 as viewed by means of partial polariscopy. The tissue section is unstained and has not been decerated. Note that the cracks contain paraffin embedding medium which is anisotropic. The presence of embedding medium within the cracks indicates that the artifact resulted from antemortem procedures performed prior to embedding of the tissue specimen. If the parched-earth effect had resulted from faulty microtomy or mounting procedures, the cracks would not contain embedding medium. (Unstained, ×12) (AFIP Negative No. 74-4459)

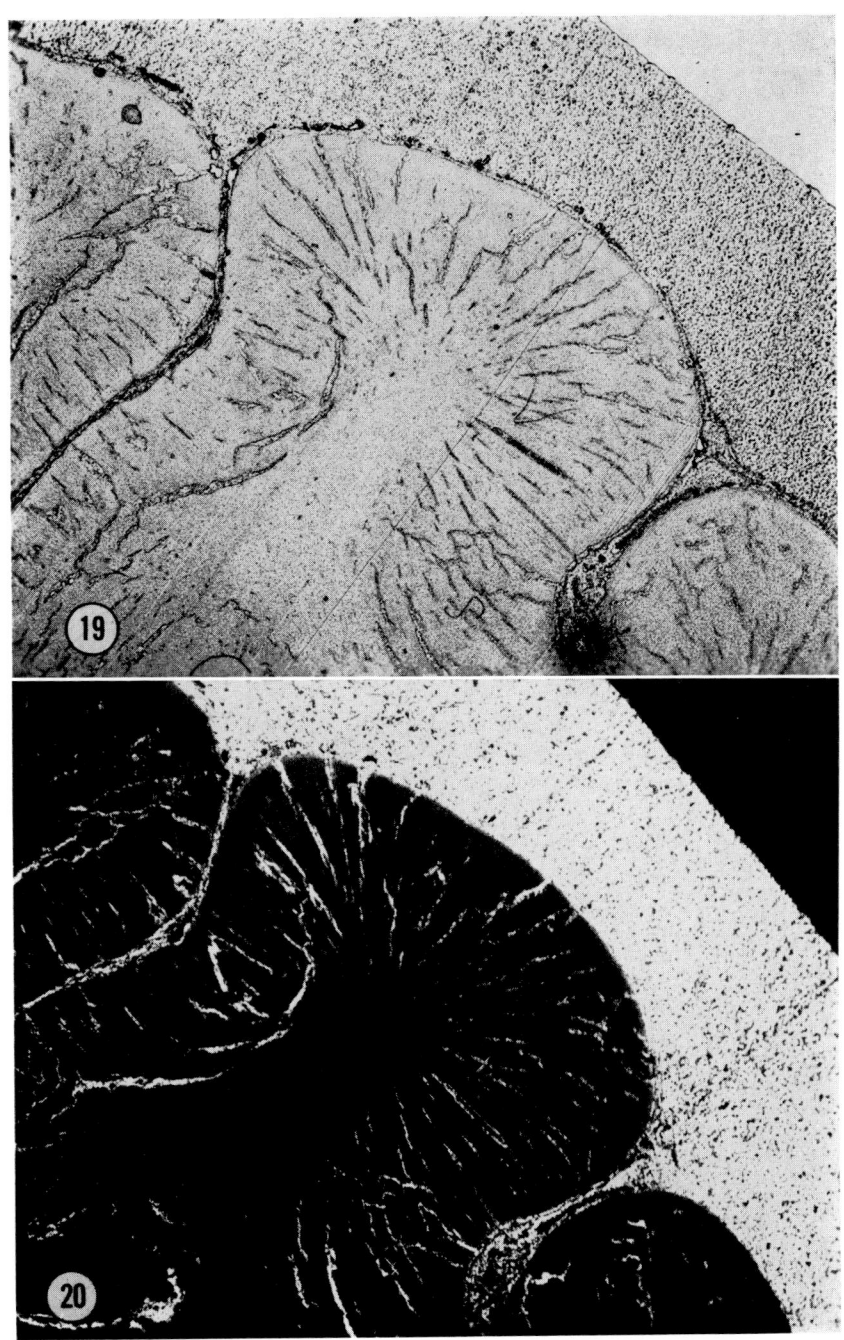

II

Artifacts Resulting from Necropsy Procedures

INTRODUCTION

NUMEROUS ARTIFACTS which are observed in microscopic tissue sections have their origin in procedures performed by the prosectors during necropsy procedures. In this chapter, the authors have emphasized those resulting from the freezing of unfixed gross tissue specimens in order to depict the resultant artifacts in a variety of different types of tissue. Examples of artifacts, resulting from necropsy procedures, included in this chapter are:

        Talcum powder
        Pressure effects
        Plant material
        Hair as contaminants
        Suture material
        Contamination with bone fragments
        Freezing artifacts

Figure 21. *Talcum Powder.* In this tissue section of a specimen of human skin, particles of talcum powder (starch and hydrous magnesium silicate) are present (see also Chapter I). This is a most common artifact and can result by contamination with dusting powder used in surgical gloves worn by the surgeon (Chapter I), or the prosector during the course of a necropsy or subsequent to the necropsy when the specimens are being trimmed for fixation or for processing subsequent to fixation (see Chapter IV). As seen within tissue sections, the classic appearance is a hexagonal crystal. The crystal stains grey with hematoxylin and eosin as seen in the left half of the figure. It is periodic acid-Schiff-positive and stains green with Geimsa-type preparations. By polariscopy, a Maltese cross is observed as seen in the right half of the figure. These crystals pose no particular problem but are objectionable if seen in large numbers. This is especially true if the slide is to be photographed or if polariscopy is required for the identification of other crystalline materials. This artifact cannot be removed from tissue sections, and little can be done about its presence after surgery, but particular care should be taken during macrosectioning to eliminate its introduction during this procedure. (H&E, without and with polariscopy, ×115) (AFIP Negative No. 67-2660)

Figure 22. *Pressure Effects.* The elongation of nuclear material observed in the central portion of this tissue section of a human necropsy specimen (tissue unknown) results from the fresh tissue specimen being squeezed excessively by either the surgeon or prosector prior to fixation. Such artifacts cannot be corrected during processing of the tissue specimen. However, they can be prevented by proper handling of fresh tissue specimens prior to fixation. (H&E, ×150) (AFIP Negative No. 73-2907)

Figure 23. *Plant Material.* A fragment of plant tissue which contaminated the gross specimen at the time of necropsy is depicted in this tissue section of the liver of a domestic animal. The plant tissue caused the tissue section to split due to the shrinking effects of the alcohols and xylene used in the staining procedure. (H&E, ×70) (AFIP Negative No. 73-4141)

Figure 24. *Plant Material.* This is the same tissue section as depicted in Figure 23 as viewed by partial polariscopy. Such plant material is anisotropic. (H&E, ×70) (AFIP Negative No. 73-4140)

Figure 25. *Hair as Contaminants.* This paraffin-embedded tissue section of a specimen of the thyroid gland and trachea of a rat was fixed in neutral buffered 10% formalin. It was contaminated with fragments of the animal's hair, by the prosector, at the time of necropsy and prior to fixation. Such surface contaminants frequently are not removed by washing the tissue specimens subsequent to fixation and prior to further processing. (H&E, ×40) (Contributed by Dr. W. L. Wooding)

Figure 26. *Hair as Contaminants.* This is a higher magnification of a portion of the tissue section depicted in Figure 25. The cross section of hair is more readily discerned on the surface of the specimen. Because of the frequency of such surface contaminants occurring during necropsy, fixed gross tissue specimens should be examined with a hand lens after washing. This is most readily accomplished immediately prior to trimming the gross specimen for tissue processing and infiltration. In this instance, the tissue specimen was embedded in such a fashion that the hair which had contaminated the specimen had its long axis presented at a right angle to the surface of the block which was presented to the microtome knife. Therefore, the hair was cut crosswise and although it was firmer than the adjacent tissue, it was not pushed into the tissue by the knife. However, if the orientation had been such that the hair had not had its long axis presented at a right angle to the surface of the block, the knife could have pushed it into the tissue and produced some shattering of the softer tissue much as depicted in Figure 27. The fact that the hair was not pushed into the tissue also indicates that a sharp knife was used for sectioning. A knife edge that was less than ultrasharp would have resulted in tearing of the tissue due to the pushing of the hair through the specimen. This is a good example of an artifact problem which can be prevented by the use of a sharp knife. (H&E, ×140) (Contributed by Dr. W. L. Wooding)

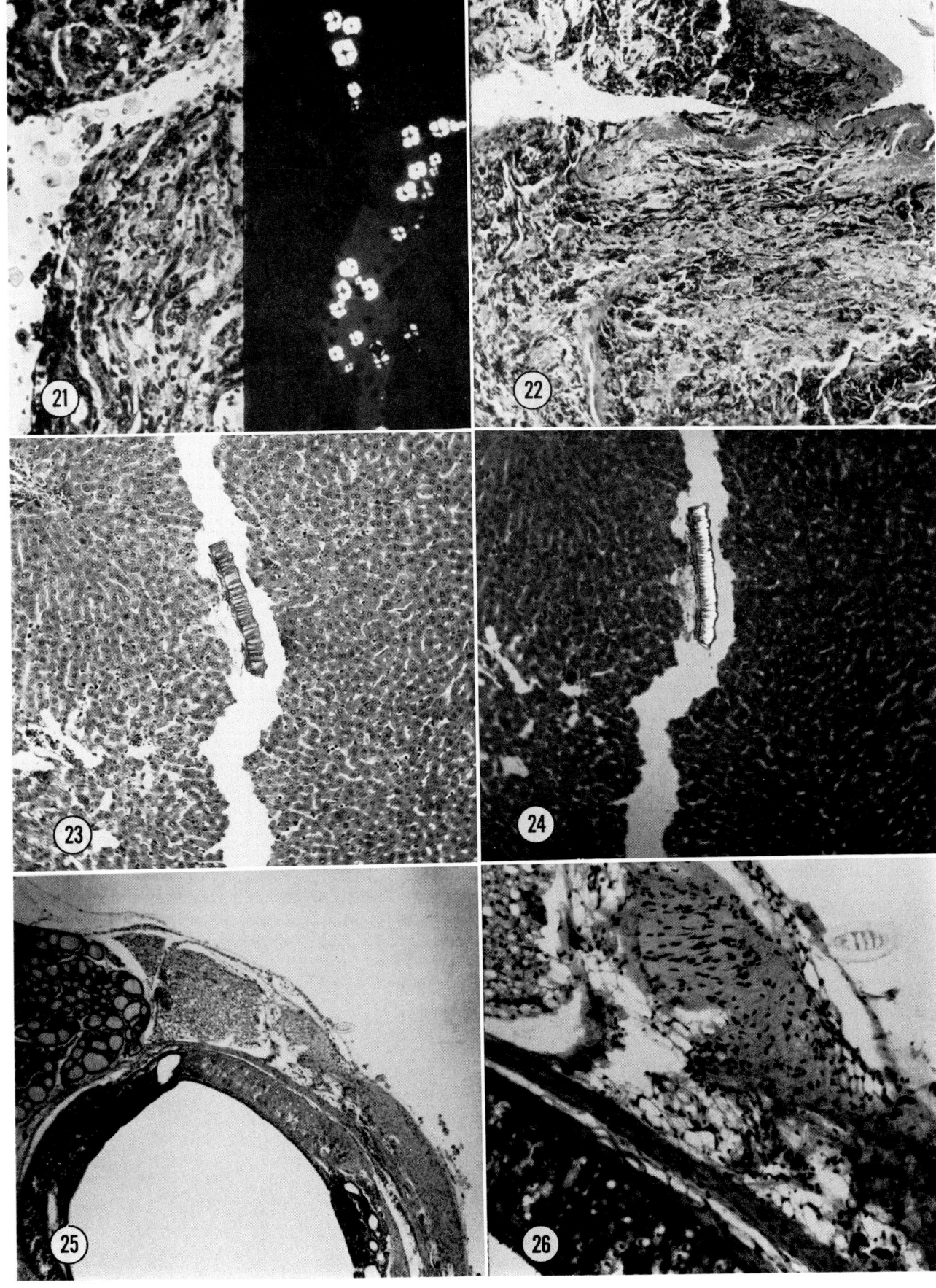

Figure 27. *Hair as Contaminants.* This figure illustrates a segment of a hair shaft embedded in the brain of a rat. The hair shaft was implanted in the tissue as a result of sloppy technique of the prosector. The hair shaft has caused the tissue section to split as it is cut on the microtome because of the fact that the hair is harder than the surrounding paraffin-infiltrated tissue and is pushed rather than being cut by the knife. The alternately light and dark stained areas of the adjacent tissue result from the vibration of the knife edge as it strikes the hair shaft so that the alternately thin and thick (wavy) zones of the tissue slice were produced. Also, notice the more pronounced knife line leading from the hair. (H&E, ×40) (Contributed by Dr. W. L. Wooding)

Figure 28. *Suture Material.* This artifact is suture material that was left in the gross tissue specimen by the prosector at the time the specimen was placed in the fixative. At the time that the tissue section is cut (see also Chapter I and VI) the suture material, being harder than the surrounding tissue, is pushed ahead of the microtome knife and results in shattering of the tissue adjacent to the site of localization of the suture material. The particles of the suture material are anisotropic. (H&E, ×35) (Contributed by Dr. W. L. Wooding)

Figure 29. *Contamination with Bone Fragments.* Not infrequently in the performance of necropsies of laboratory animals, fragments of bone are deeply impregnated within specimens of brain tissue because of carelessness on the part of the prosector in opening the cranium to remove the brain. This is a paraffin-embedded tissue section of a specimen of the cerebrum of a monkey. Fragments of bone were impregnated deep within the gross specimen at the time of necropsy. Such fragments of nondecalcified bone are extremely hard in comparison to the surrounding brain tissue. In addition to nicking the edge of the microtome knife, they are pushed through the tissue block or are moved laterally by the knife edge as it passes through the embedded tissue. As depicted here, the displacement of such fragments of bone causes much shattering and distortion of the tissue section. Irregularly spaced lines and grooves, which stain more intensely than surrounding tissue, are associated with the shattering and damage to the microtome knife. (H&E, ×26) (Contributed by Mr. L. E. Schellhammer)

Figure 30. *Contamination with Bone Fragments.* This is a higher magnification of a portion of the tissue section depicted in Figure 29. The shattering of the tissue resulting from such careless necropsy technique is more clearly depicted. (H&E, ×66) (Contributed by Mr. L. E. Schellhammer)

Figure 31. *Contamination with Bone Fragments.* This paraffin-embedded tissue section was obtained from another area of the brain of the same monkey as depicted in Figures 29 and 30. The gross specimen was deeply impregnated with fragments of bone during the necropsy procedure. Gaping holes are seen within the finished tissue section resulting from fragments of bone which were pushed completely out of the section by the microtome knife. Irregularly spaced lines and grooves, which stain more intensely than the surrounding tissue are associated with the shattering and holes in the tissue section and damage to the microtome knife. (H&E, ×16) (Contributed by Mr. L. E. Schellhammer)

Figure 32. *Contamination with Bone Fragments.* This is a paraffin-embedded tissue section of the brain of a rat. The gross tissue specimen was deeply impregnated with a fragment of bone by the careless technique of the prosector at the time of necropsy. The undecalcified fragment of bone, and focal areas of adjoining brain tissue were shattered by the knife during microtomy. To the right of the shattered fragment of bone, several lines are apparent in the tissue section which are due to nicks in the edge of the microtome knife which were produced by the undecalcified fragment of bone. (H&E, ×10) (Contributed by Mr. L. E. Schellhammer)

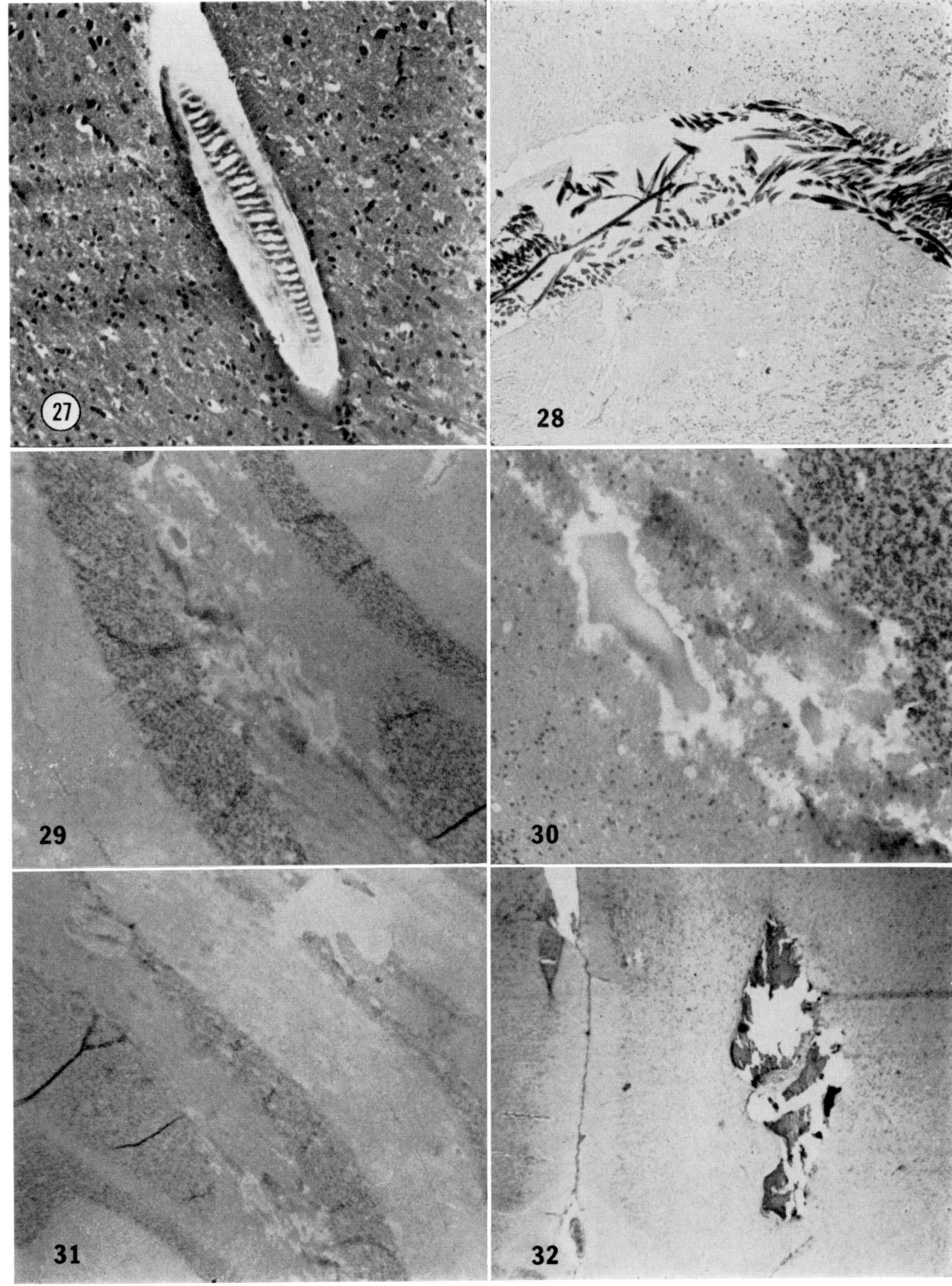

Figure 33. *Freezing Artifact*. At times, tissue specimens may be intentionally or unintentionally frozen during or prior to fixation. When frozen by conventional means the tissue becomes dehydrated owing to the extraction of moisture from the cells and large ice crystals are formed intracellularly and extracellularly. Naturally, these ice crystals melt when the specimen is finally placed in fixative leaving compressed and/or ruptured cells and disoriented interstitium as depicted in this tissue section of a specimen of the human testis which was frozen prior to fixation (see also Figures 34 through 44). (H&E, ×100) (AFIP Negative No. 72-4771)

Figure 34. *Freezing Artifact*. This tissue section was cut from a specimen of human kidney which was frozen prior to fixation (see also Figure 33). Such tissue is worthless for morphologic study and there is no satisfactory means of correcting such an artifact. (H&E, ×100) (AFIP Negative No. 72-4775)

Figure 35. *Freezing Artifact*. This is a higher magnification of a tissue section cut from the same specimen of kidney as depicted in Figure 34. The tubular epithelial cells are shrunken as a result of dehydration and although intact nuclei can be observed, cytoplasmic components of the cells are obscured. The interstitium and lumina of the tubules are dilated owing to the formation of large ice crystals. The glomerular tufts are dehydrated to the point that they are solid, hard granules of tissue which resist sectioning by the microtome knife and are pushed, rather than being cut, as the knife edge passes through the paraffin block. (H&E, ×1000) (AFIP Negative No. 72-4774)

Figure 36. *Freezing Artifact*. While tissue sections prepared from some tissues which have been frozen prior to fixation are easily identified as to the organ from which they were derived, it is difficult to identify the origin of some such specimens. This is a tissue section of the lung of a human being which was frozen prior to fixation. (H&E, ×100) (AFIP Negative No. 72-4773)

Figure 37. *Freezing Artifact*. This tissue section was cut from a specimen of human liver tissue which was frozen prior to fixation. The hepatocytes are shrunken and intensely basophilic. Although the architectural pattern of the organ is preserved, the section is unsuitable for morphologic study. (H&E, ×100) (AFIP Negative No. 72-4772)

Figure 38. *Freezing Artifact*. Dense connective tissues withstand freezing prior to fixation better than soft tissues which have a higher moisture content as seen in this section of the human aorta which was frozen prior to fixation. The vacuoles within the interstitium result from the formation of ice crystals. Such an artifact might be confused with some types of lesions since the morphology of the fibers per se has not been greatly altered. Such misinterpretation could more readily occur if other tissue specimens from the same necropsy were not frozen prior to fixation. (H&E, ×100) (AFIP Negative No. 72-5344)

Effect of fixation in absolute ethyl alcohol
Effect of fixation in Bouin's fluid
Acid hematin crystals in Bouin's-fixed tissue
Acid hematin crystals in neutral buffered 10% formalin-fixed tissue
Acid formalin hematin pigment
Effect of fixation in 10% acid formalin
Effect of fixation in neutral buffered 10% versus 10% acid formalin
Effect of refrigeration of unfixed specimens prior to fixation
Pseudocalcification due to calcium acetate
Pseudocalcification due to calcium carbonate

Figure 45. *Freezing Artifact.* Tissue specimens may be frozen subsequent to being placed in fixatives, usually by being transported in freezing weather with inadequate insulation for the fixative container and its contents. The effect is essentially the same as when the specimen is frozen prior to fixation, as seen in this specimen of human skin, except that the interstitial vacuoles and intracellular vacuoles may tend to be larger since the ice crystals formed when the freezing occurs over a longer perior of time tend to be larger than the ice crystals formed by rapid freezing (see also Chapter II). The collagen within such specimens tends to be more anisotropic than in unfrozen tissue specimens. (H&E, ×100) (AFIP Negative No. 73-4142)

Figure 46. *Freezing Artifact.* Higher magnification of a portion of Figure 45 depicting the large interstitial vacuoles within the subcutis and large intracytoplasmic vacuoles within epidermal cells resulting from the formation of large ice crystals during slow freezing of the specimen. Within many of the nonvacuolated epidermal cells there is a granular, paranuclear condensation of the cytoplasm caused by the dehydration of the cells due to freezing concomitant with the fixation of the nonaqueous cytoplasmic components. These foci of condensed cytoplasm resemble mucoid material. (H&E, ×265) (AFIP Negative No. 73-4143)

Figure 47. *Freezing Artifact.* These unidentified pieces of tissue were frozen during fixation. Intracellular and extracellular ice crystals displace the tissue components and produce vacuoles and voids. That the tissue was frozen slowly is denoted by the large clefts seen in the section. These spaces were formerly occupied by large ice crystals. If the specimen had been sharp-frozen, the crystals would have been microscopic in size and would have produced considerably less derangement of the specimen. In this instance, the ice crystal artifact was so extensive that identification of the tissue microscopically was not possible. (H&E, ×6)

Figure 48. *Saphrophytic Bacteria.* The specimen is an inadequately fixed wedge biopsy of formalin-fixed liver tissue. Fixation was delayed owing to failure to place the specimen in fixative soon enough, or the surface of the specimen adhered to the inner surface of the fixative container, or the surface of the specimen adhered to other specimens in the fixative container, or inadequate quantities of fixative were used, or the specimen was too thick at the time it was placed in the fixative. In addition, the specimen became contaminated with saphrophytic bacteria while it was being collected or handled prior to fixation. The saphrophytic bacteria within the specimen multiplied and produced autolytic changes while the fixative was attempting to penetrate the specimen from its surface. The saphrophytic bacteria stain basophlic and the liver parenchyma is autolyzed and unsuitable for morphologic study. (H&E, ×160) (AFIP Negative No. 67-2653)

Figure 49. *Autolytic Changes.* The tissue specimen is a formalin-fixed wedge biopsy of the liver. The specimen adhered to the inner surface of the fixative container and was not exposed to the fixative. In inadequately fixed tissue, even in biopsies, gas bubbles may be formed as depicted here. In such specimens, the autolytic changes may not have advanced to the point that tissue morphology is completely lost. (H&E, ×70) (AFIP Negative No. 63-3816)

Figure 50. *Autolytic Changes.* In this tissue section from an inadequately formalin-fixed wedge biopsy of the liver, the hepatocytes are disassociated. In some diseases, such as acute toxic hepatitis or Leptospirosis, such an alteration of structure might be interpreted as a lesion. However, in this instance it is an artifact produced by enzymatic digestion caused by inadequate fixation. The possible causes of inadequate fixation of this biopsy are the same as those described for Figure 48. (H&E, ×70) (AFIP Negative No. 67-2751)

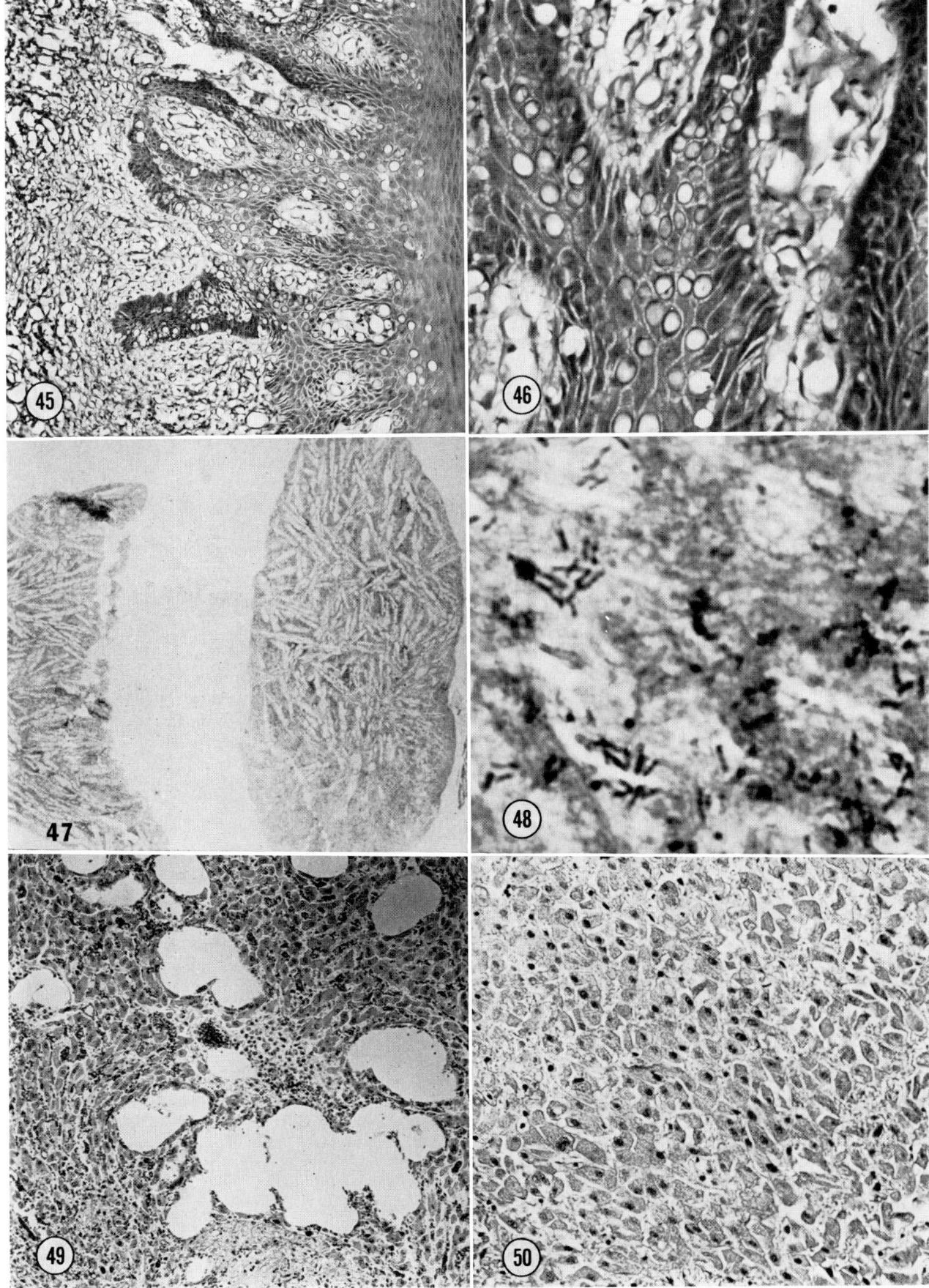

Figure 51. *Autolysis.* Focal autolysis is observed in this paraffin-embedded tissue section of a specimen of human liver which was fixed in neutral buffered 10% formalin (see also Figures 52 and 53). The autolyzed portion is the light-stained area on the left side of the photograph. The cut surface of the specimen was touching the side of the fixative container at the particular site in which autolysis was noted in the tissue section. The dissociation of the hepatocytes within the autolyzed focus resembles morphologic changes that are frequently seen in cases of Leptospirosis. (H&E, ×70) (AFIP Negative No. 72-18032)

Figure 52. *Autolysis.* Focal autolysis is observed in this paraffin-embedded tissue section of a specimen of human liver which was fixed in neutral buffered 10% formalin. The autolysed portion of the specimen was not in contact with the fixative (see also Figure 53). (H&E, ×100) (AFIP Negative No. 73-4880)

Figure 53. *Autolysis.* This is a higher magnification of the central portion of the field of view depicted in Figure 52. Note the extensive degeneration and disassociation of the hepatocytes in the focal area of autolysis. Artifacts of this type frequently occur when the tissue specimen is placed in a dry container prior to the addition of the fixative. Those surfaces of the specimen which are in contact with the dry surface of the container will not be in contact with the fixative and will undergo autolysis during fixation. (H&E, ×265) (AFIP Negative No. 73-4481)

Figure 54. *Inadequate Fixation.* The demands made upon surgical pathology services, when fresh-frozen tissue sections are not adequate for a diagnosis, frequently do not provide for adequate periods of time for exposure of tissue specimens to fixatives. Tissue which has been inadequately fixed will differ in some morphologic aspects from adequately fixed tissue as depicted in this illustration. The specimen of liver tissue at the left is shown with a peripheral light-colored zone and inner scattered perivascular zones which represent portions of the specimen which have been penetrated by the fixative during a brief period of fixation. These zones are adequately fixed. The darker zones surrounded by the peripheral, adequately fixed shell have not been penetrated by the fixative in sufficient concentration or for a sufficient period of time to provide for adequate fixation. The area of the specimen which is adequately fixed will contain cells which have crisply stained nuclear chromatin, distinct and acidophilic nucleoli, and very little cellular shrinkage as depicted by the hepatocyte at the upper right. The area of the specimen which is inadequately fixed, which is usually the center of the specimen, contains cells which are shrunken, exhibit clumping of cytoplasm, less distinct nuclear chromatin and basophilic nucleoli as depicted by the hepatocyte at the lower right.

Figure 55. *Inadequate Fixation.* As has been mentioned previously, fixation may be inadequate because the tissue specimen is too large in relation to the volume of fixative or because the time allowed for fixation was too short in duration. The fixation of this specimen of human liver in neutral buffered 10% formalin was inadequate in that the time allowed for fixation was too short in duration. The hepatocytes are shrunken and the sinusoids appear dilated. The nuclei of the hepatocytes are small and there is no distinctive chromatin staining although the volume of fixative used and the thickness of the specimen were both adequate. (H&E, ×200) (AFIP Negative No. 71-12159-7)

Figure 56. *Inadequate Fixation* (see also Figure 55). In this instance, the tissue specimen is from a human lymph node which was fixed in neutral buffered 10% formalin. Although the specimen was trimmed to an adequate thickness and the volume of fixative to tissue was also adequate, the total fixation procedure was inadequate because the specimen was not exposed to the fixative for a sufficient period of time. The net result is an artifact which is characterized by condensation of nuclear chromatin. (H&E, ×530) (AFIP Negative No. 72-3739)

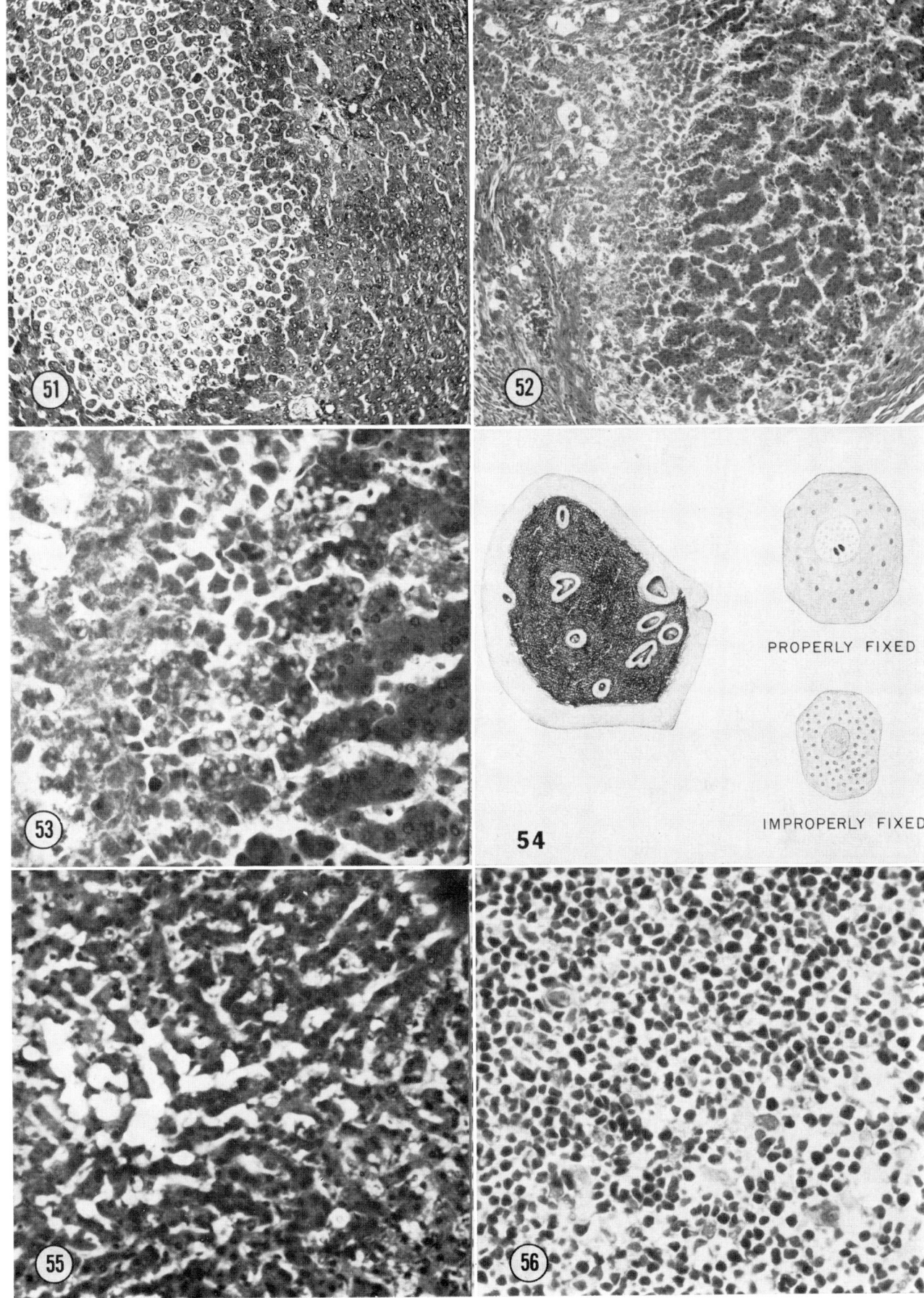

Figure 57. *Inadequate Fixation*. As mentioned previously, fixation may be inadequate because the tissue specimen is too large in relation to the volume of fixative or because the time allowed for fixation was too short in duration. This specimen of human liver tissue was fixed in formalin and fixation was inadequate because the specimen was too thick (greater than 6 mm). Only the periphery of the specimen is fixed, forming a shell of firm tissue surrounding a central mass of autolyzed tissue (see Color Plate 1, Figure 1).

Figure 58. *Inadequate Fixation* (see also Figures 55, 56, and 59). In this instance, the tissue specimen is from a human kidney which was fixed in 10% neutral buffered formalin. Fixation is inadequate, even though the thickness of the specimen and the volume of fixative used were adequate, because the specimen was not exposed to the fixative for a sufficient period of time. The usual practice is to fix tissues for a period of twenty-four hours and then change the tissues to 20 volumes of fresh fixative (per volume of tissue) for an additional twenty-four-hour period. Fixation is usually complete at the end of the forty-eight-hour period and the tissues are ready for processing. If the tissue specimens are slightly thicker than 6 mm or they are unusually dense, longer periods of fixation may be required. The tissue section shown here was prepared from a portion of the gross specimen which was removed from the fixative after the first twenty-four hours of fixation. It appears to be shrunken, particularly the glomeruli, and there is a lack of staining of the nuclear chromatin. (H&E, ×50) (AFIP Negative No. 72-6169)

Figure 59. *Inadequate Fixation*. This tissue section was prepared from a portion of the same gross specimen as used for the section depicted in Figure 58. In this instance, the fixative solution (20 volumes per volume of tissue) was changed after the first twenty-four hours and the portion was left in the fixative for an additional twenty-four hours (total of 48 hours). The section does not present the shrunken appearance noted in Figure 58 and the staining of all cellular components is crisper and more definitive. (H&E, ×50) (AFIP Negative No. 72-6168)

Figure 60. *Inadequate Fixation*. Artifacts may result from inadequate fixation. Fixation may be inadequate because the tissue specimen is too large in relation to the volume of fixative or because the time allowed for fixation was too short in duration. This specimen of human kidney was fixed in formalin. Fixation was inadequate because the specimen was too thick. Only the periphery of the specimen was fixed, forming a shell of firm, fixed, cortical tissue (see Figure 61) surrounding an autolyzed mass of medullary tissue as depicted here. Note that the erythrocytes have been completely autolyzed and tubular walls have shrunken and become indistinct. Also, notice that the nuclear elements have been altered. (H&E, ×145) (AFIP Negative No. 72-6165)

Figure 61. *Inadequate Fixation*. This is a section of the same kidney depicted in Figure 60. This portion of the kidney was well fixed (compare with Figure 60). Notice that erythrocytes and the morphologic detail of other tissue components have been preserved. The fixative could not penetrate the thick specimen rapidly enough to prevent autolysis in the deeper portions of the specimen. The maximum thickness of a specimen should not exceed 6 mm and for each volume of tissue 20 volumes of fixative should be used. (H&E, ×145) (AFIP Negative No. 72-6166)

Figure 62. *Barium Contaminants*. An anisotropic crystalline contaminant is noted in this tissue section of a human lung which had been fixed in 10% formalin. This artifact resulted from contamination of the gross specimen with barium salts of the type used in barium solutions employed in radiology. The tissue specimen had been fixed in a container which had originally been used for barium meal. Supposedly, the container had been thoroughly washed before being used as a tissue specimen jar. It will be noted that there is no tissue reaction to the presence of these crystals. (H&E, partial polariscopy, ×80)

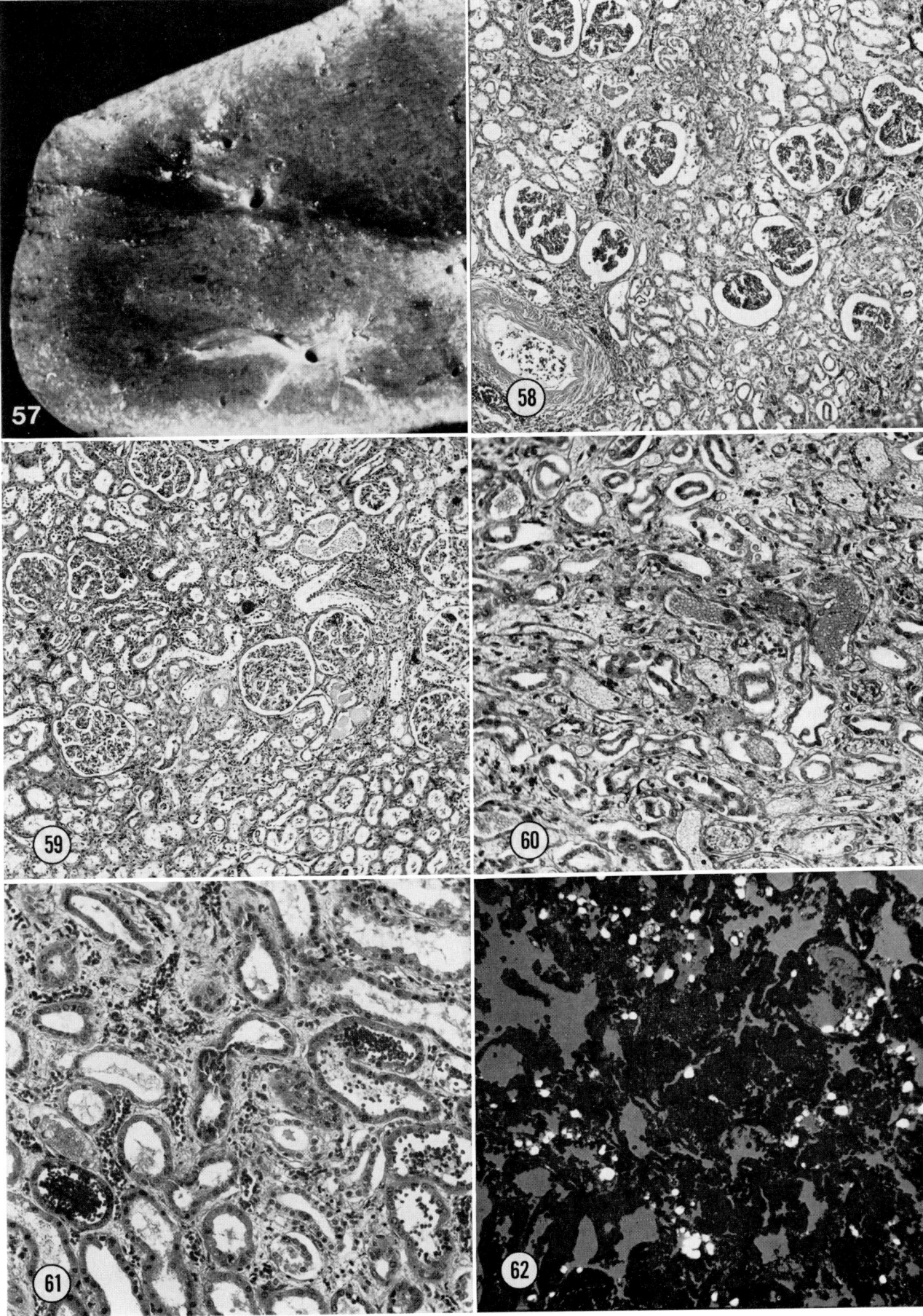

Figure 63. *Oxidation Contaminants.* If the gasket of the fixative container is loose, or the metal cap is not securely affixed to the container, or the metal cap is rusty initially, or the specimen is held in the fixative for prolonged periods of time, fixatives such as formalin undergo oxidation and cause the metal cap to rust as shown in this picture. Rust will flake from the inner surface of such a metal cap (seen at left) and contaminate the fixative within the container (seen at the right). The grayish haze seen on the internal wall of the container is a positive Prussian blue reaction denoting the presence of iron as a contaminate within the fixative (see Color Plate 1, Figure 2).

Figure 64. *Oxidation Contaminants.* The gross specimen of the human eye shown here was fixed in the container shown in Figure 63. The external surface of the specimen was covered with a fine reddish-brown precipitate of rust which was derived from the rusty metal cap of the container. The surface of such a specimen will yield a positive Prussian blue reaction for iron (see Color Plate 1, Figure 3). (AFIP Negative No. 62-6179)

Figure 65. *Oxidation Contaminants.* This tissue section was prepared from a portion of the human eye depicted in Figure 64. Brownish-colored granular precipitates were observed upon the external surface of the cornea and within the interstitium of the peripheral portion of the cornea. This precipitate resembled hemosiderin and yielded a positive Prussian blue reaction for iron. The artifact was the result of contamination of the gross specimen with rust during fixation (see Color Plate 1, Figure 4). (Prussian blue reaction for iron, ×40)

Figure 66. *Foreign Material Contaminants.* This specimen of liver tissue from a rat was contaminated with animal hair during fixation. Such forms of surface contamination of tissue specimens can also occur during necropsy procedures (see Figures 25 and 26). However, in this instance, the contamination occurred due to the fact that pieces of skin and attached hair were placed in the same container of fixative as the specimen of liver tissue. Specimens of skin and attached hair (fur) should be fixed in separate containers. Such surface contaminants frequently are not removed by washing the tissue specimens subsequent to fixation and should be removed at the time the specimen is macrosectioned prior to processing and infiltration (see Figure 26). As described in the legend for Figure 26, such surface contaminants, depending upon their orientation to the cutting face of the tissue block, can cause considerable damage to tissue sections during microtomy. (H&E, ×40) (Contributed by Mr. L. E. Schellhammer)

Figure 67. *Foreign Material Contaminant.* This paraffin-embedded tissue section of a specimen of the kidney of a rat was fixed in neutral buffered 10% formalin. Tissue specimens from twenty-two organs and tissues of the same rat were placed in the same fixative container including a portion of a femur which had been detached from the leg with bone cutters. Splinters of bone adhered to the capsule of the kidney. This was not removed during the postfixation washing of the specimen or trimming of the specimen prior to processing. In addition, metallic particles from unfiltered washwater adhered to the same specimen and were not removed during trimming prior to processing. These contaminants caused the tissue section to split as it was being cut on the microtome because they are harder than the surrounding paraffin-infiltrated tissue. The microtome knife pushed the contaminants through the tissue section. (H&E, ×40) (Contributed by Dr. W. L. Wooding)

Figure 68. *Foreign Material Contaminants.* This is a higher magnification of a portion of the tissue section depicted in Figure 67. The surface of tissue specimens should be examined for such contaminants during macrosectioning and removed from the specimen prior to processing and embedding. If such surface contaminants are embedded with the tissue specimen they may appear in the paraffin of the tissue block as small dark or chalk specks. If located near the surface of the block they can be more readily detected with a hand lens or dissecting microscope. Such contaminants may nick the edge of the knife during sectioning and cause the sections to split or the specimen to crumble and drop out of the wax as they are cut. If located on or near the surface of the block they may be dissected out with a teasing needle. If they cannot be removed in this fashion the blocks should be melted down and the specimen washed, infiltrated, and embedded in fresh paraffin. (H&E, ×140) (Contributed by Dr. W. L. Wooding)

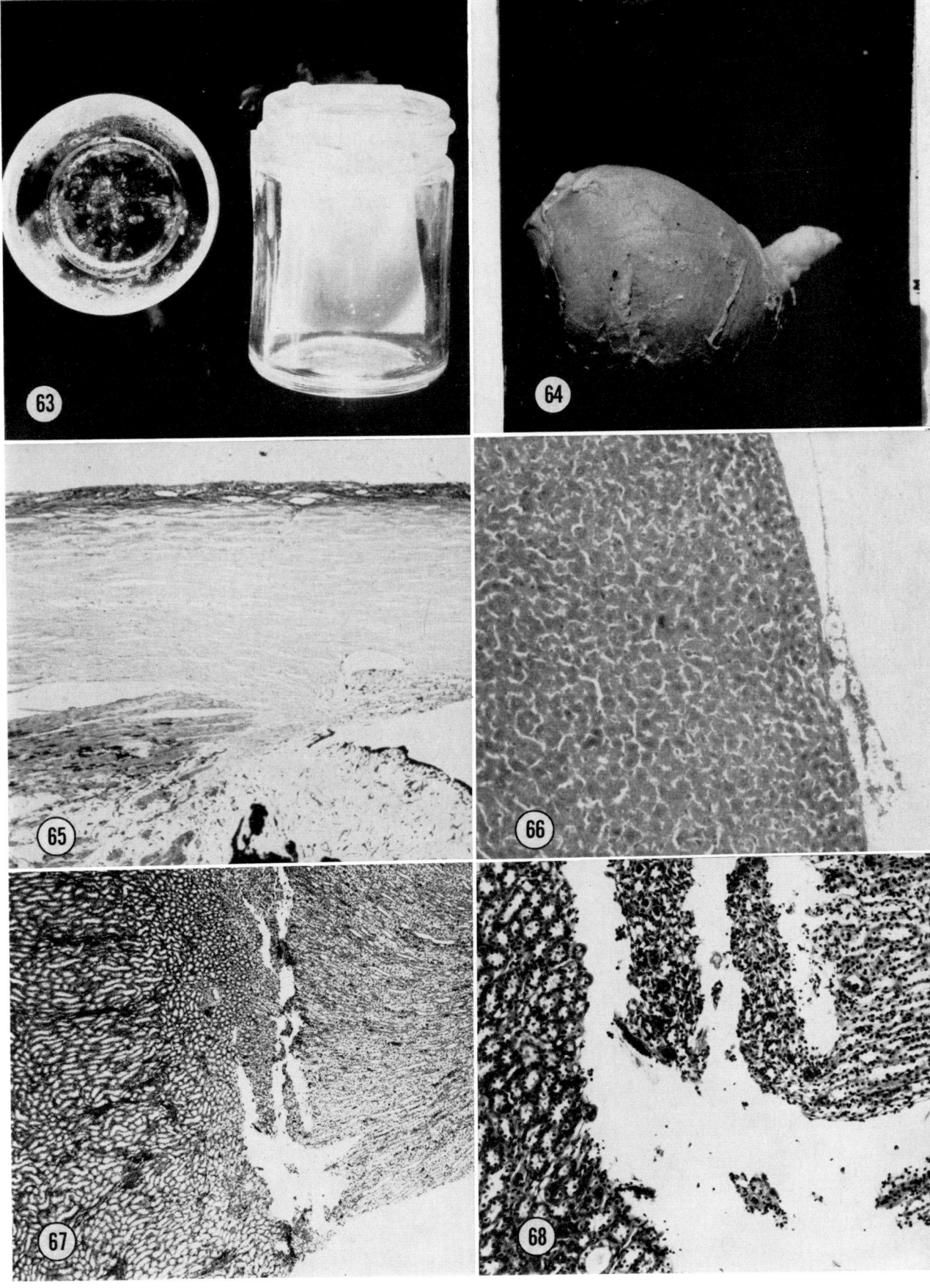

Figure 69. *Comparative Effects on Nuclear Morphology.* This is a paraffin-embedded tissue section prepared from a tissue specimen of human skin which was fixed for twenty-four hours in 10% unbuffered formalin, pH 4.4. This tissue section was stained with thionine. No counterstain was employed. This and the following eight photographs are presented to depict the effect of various fixatives upon tissue morphology. Compare with the nuclear staining effects achieved with other fixatives as depicted in Figures 70 through 76. (Thionine, ×750) (AFIP Negative No. 68-1235)

Figure 70. *Comparative Effects on Nuclear Morphology.* This tissue specimen of the skin of the same human being (same site) as depicted in Figure 69 was fixed for twenty-four hours in 10% buffered formalin, pH 6.7. The fixative was prepared with formaldehyde which did not contain the 10% methyl alcohol which is usually added to stock formaldehyde to prevent polymerization. Embedding and staining procedures were the same as described for Figure 69. Compared with the nuclear staining achieved with other fixatives as depicted in Figure 69 and Figures 71 through 76. (Thionine, ×750) (AFIP Negative No. 68-1239)

Figure 71. *Comparative Effects on Nuclear Morphology.* This tissue specimen of the skin of the same human being (same site) as depicted in Figures 69 and 70 was fixed for twenty-four hours in 10% formol-saline (not isotonic), pH 3.8. Embedding and staining procedures were the same as described for Figure 69. Note the nuclear shrinkage and condensation of chromatin. Compare with the nuclear staining achieved with other fixatives as depicted in Figures 69 and 70 and Figures 72 through 76. (Thionine, ×750) (AFIP Negative No. 68-1237)

Figure 72. *Comparative Effects on Nuclear Morphology.* This tissue specimen of the skin of the same human being (same site) as depicted in Figures 69 through 71 was fixed for twenty-four hours in 10% formol-calcium, pH 3.0. Embedding and staining procedures were the same as described for Figure 69. Compare with the nuclear staining achieved with other fixatives as depicted in Figures 69 through 71 and Figures 73 through 76. (Thionine, ×750) (AFIP Negative No. 68-1236)

Figure 73. *Comparative Effects on Nuclear Morphology.* This tissue specimen of the skin of the same human being (same site) as depicted in Figures 69 through 72 was fixed for twenty-four hours in absolute ethyl alcohol. Embedding and staining procedures were the same as described for Figure 69. Notice the extensive nuclear shrinkage and condensation of chromatin. Compare with the nuclear staining achieved with other fixatives as depicted in Figures 69 through 72 and Figures 74 through 76. (Thionine, ×750) (AFIP Negative No. 68-1242)

Figure 74. *Comparative Effects on Nuclear Morphology.* This tissue specimen of the skin of the same human being (same site) as depicted in Figures 69 through 73 was fixed for twenty-four hours in Bouin's fluid, pH 1.4. Embedding and staining procedures were the same as described for Figure 69. Compare with the nuclear staining achieved with other fixatives as depicted in Figures 69 through 73, 75, and 76. (Thionine, ×750) (AFIP Negative No. 68-1243)

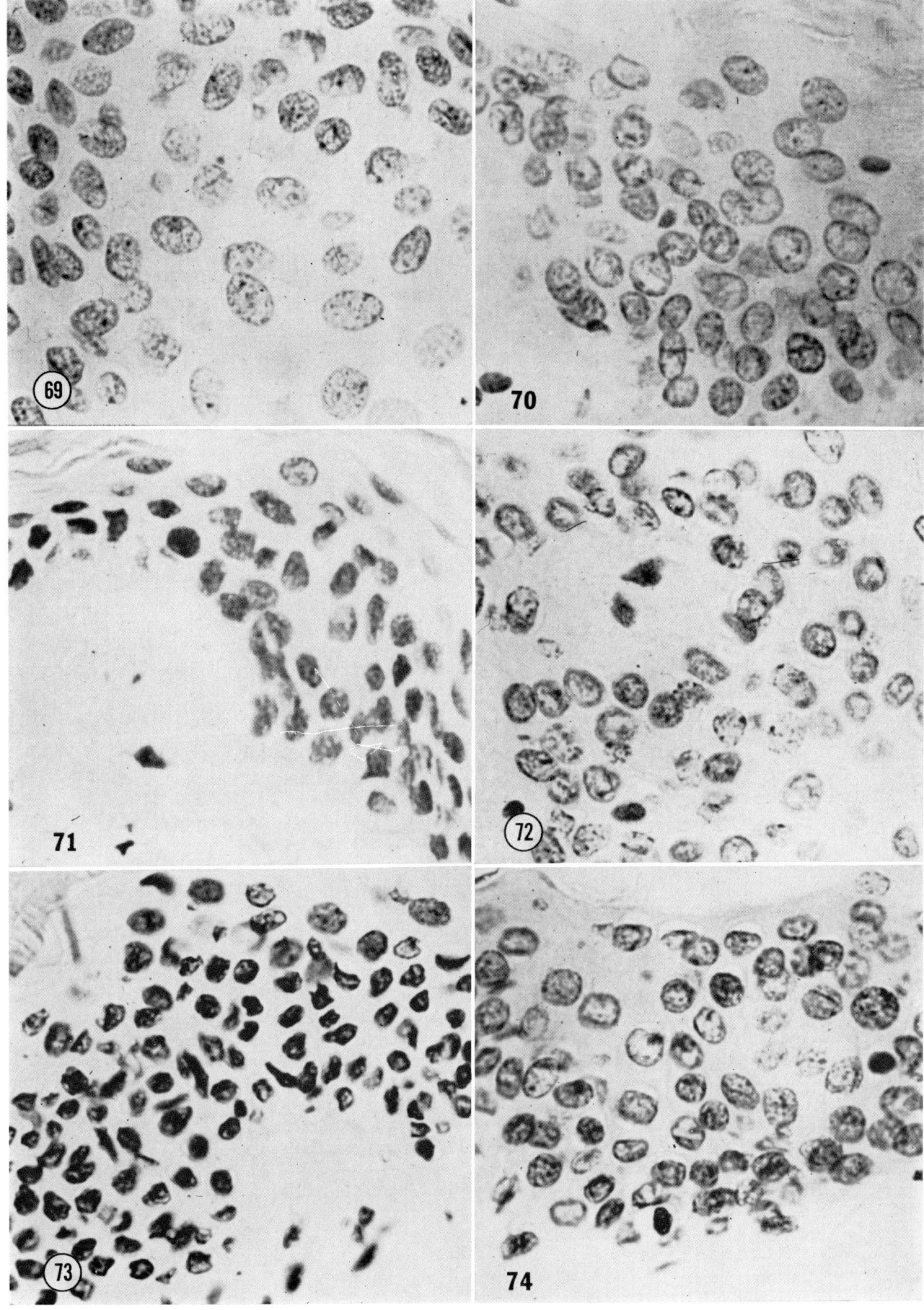

Figure 75. *Comparative Effects on Nuclear Morphology.* This tissue specimen of the skin of the same human being (same site) as depicted in Figures 69 through 74 was fixed for twenty-four hours in glutaraldehyde, pH 7.5. Embedding and staining procedures were the same as described for Figure 69. Notice the nuclear shrinkage and condensation of chromatin. Compare with the nuclear staining achieved with other fixatives as depicted in Figures 69 through 74 and 76. (Thionine, ×750) (AFIP Negative No. 68-1240)

Figure 76. *Comparative Effects on Nuclear Morphology.* This tissue specimen of the skin of the same human being (same site) as depicted in Figures 69 through 75 was fixed for twenty-four hours in paraformaldehyde, pH 7.4. Embedding and staining procedures were the same as described for Figure 69. Notice the distortion of nuclear morphology and inadequate demonstration of chromatin. Compare with the nuclear staining achieved with other fixatives as depicted in Figures 69 through 75. (Thionine, ×750) (AFIP Negative No. 68-1241)

Figure 77. *Comparative Effects of Various Fixatives.* It is well established that the morphology of a tissue specimen may be altered by the use of different fixatives. This tissue section of a specimen of human skin illustrates the excellent morphologic detail which can be expected by fixation in neutral buffered 10% formalin. Compare this photograph with Figures 78 through 82 to ascertain the effect produced by different fixatives on duplicate tissue specimens taken from the skin of the hypogastric region. (H&E, ×575) (AFIP Negative No. 68-2668)

Figure 78. *Comparative Effects of Various Fixatives.* This tissue section was prepared from a specimen of human skin which was fixed in neutral buffered 10% formalin which had been prepared with methanol-free formaldehyde. Compare with Figure 77 and note the swelling of the tissue components which has been produced by methanol-free formaldehyde. The swelling is similar to the effect produced by fixation with Bouin's fluid (see Figure 80). Methanol-free formaldehyde should not be used as a fixative unless one is familiar with the changes in morphology which it may produce. (H&E, ×575) (AFIP Negative No. 68-2673)

Figure 79. *Comparative Effects of Various Fixatives.* This tissue section of a specimen of human skin demonstrates the effect of fixation with formalin-saline solution which contains the same concentration of formaldehyde as 10% formalin but is not buffered and in addition contains 0.9% sodium chloride. Notice the extensive shrinking and homogeneity of the nuclear chromatin compared to the specimens fixed in neutral buffered 10% formalin (Figure 77), or Zenker's fluid (Figure 82), or Carnoy's fluid (Figure 81), or Bouin's fluid (Figure 80). (H&E, ×575) (AFIP Negative No. 68-2670)

Figure 80. *Comparative Effects of Various Fixatives.* This tissue section of a specimen of human skin demonstrates the effect of fixation with Bouin's fluid. This fluid is composed of formaldehyde, saturated picric acid, and acetic acid. Formaldehyde tends to harden tissue excessively which is supposedly offset by the picric acid. The acetic acid component tends to offset the tissue shrinkage associated with picric acid and produced moderate swelling of the tissue similar to the effect produced in Carnoy's fixed tissue (Figure 81). Bouin's-fixed tissue compares more favorably with neutral buffered 10% formalin-fixed tissue (Figure 77) than Zenker's-fixed tissue (Figure 82) insofar as shrinkage is concerned. Deoxyribonucleic acid may be removed from tissue fixed in Bouin's fluid resulting in considerable variability in the intensity of nuclear staining and a dramatic difference in morphology of Bouin's-fixed versus the neutral buffered 10% formalin-fixed (Figure 77) specimens. (H&E, ×575) (AFIP Negative No. 68-2672)

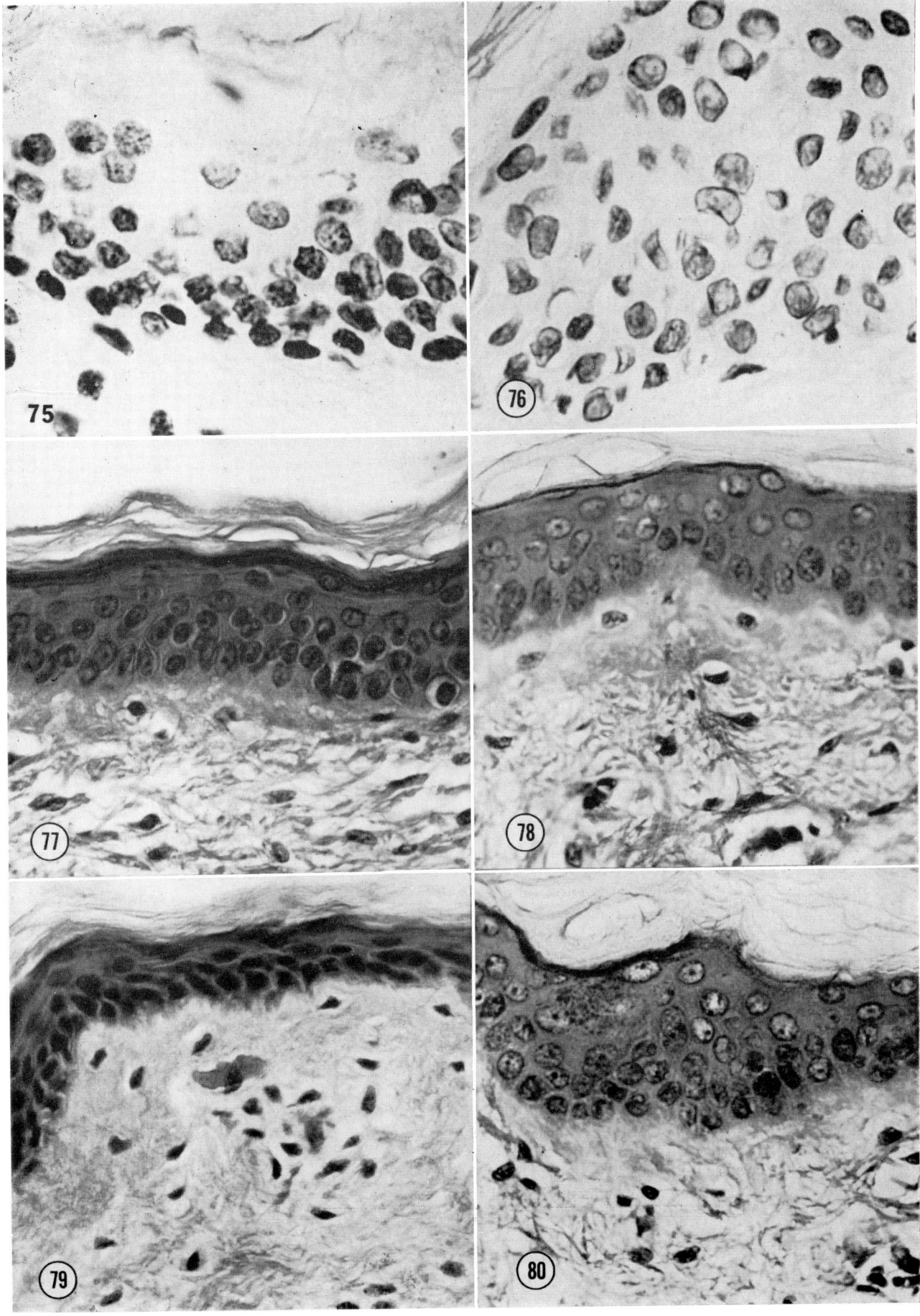

Figure 81. *Comparative Effects of Various Fixatives.* This tissue section of a specimen of human skin demonstrates the effect of fixation with Carnoy's fluid. This fluid is composed of alcohol, glacial acetic acid, and chloroform. The chloroform acts as an adjuvant to increase the rate of alcohol penetration. Alcohol tends to dehydrate and cause increased shrinkage of the tissue which is supposedly offset by the swelling effect produced by acetic acid. The Carnoy's-fixed specimen compares more favorably with the 10% neutral buffered formalin-fixed specimen (Figure 77) than the Zenker's-fixed specimen (Figure 82) insofar as shrinkage is concerned. However, there is still a dramatic difference in the morphology of the Carnoy's-fixed specimen versus the 10% neutral buffered formalin-fixed (Figure 77) specimens. (H&E, ×575) (AFIP Negative No. 68-2669)

Figure 82. *Comparative Effects of Various Fixatives.* This tissue section of a specimen of human skin demonstrates the shrinking effect that takes place during the first phase of fixation in Zenker's fluid. By comparison with Figure 77 it is evident that this specimen is inadequately fixed. There is a dramatic difference in the morphology of the Zenker's-fixed versus 10% neutral buffered formalin-fixed specimens. See Figure 83 for a hypothesis of the three stages of Zenker's fixation. (H&E, ×575) (AFIP Negative No. 68-2671)

Figure 83. *Effect of Fixation in Zenker's Fluid.* These three drawings of a cell illustrate a hypothesis developed by L.G.L. for the changes a cell undergoes during the process of fixation in Zenker's fluid. During the initial one to four hours of exposure to Zenker's fluid (upper left), a great deal of shrinkage of the nucleus occurs and a separation between the nucleus and the cytoplasm is produced (see Figure 82). During this period the nuclear chromatin granules cannot be discerned. During the ensuing four to seven hours (upper right), swelling of the nucleus occurs and the initial separation of the nucleus and cytoplasm disappears. At this stage, the nuclear chromatin is distinct and the nucleolus is prominent. It is at this point that optimal fixation has been accomplished. If fixation is prolonged for several hours beyond optimal fixation (lower center), "Over-Zenkerization" occurs. Tinctorially, there is no color differentiation between the nucleus and cytoplasm in stained tissue sections. In hematoxylin and eosin-stained tissue sections, both the nucleus and cytoplasm are stained a washed-out purple color (see Figures 84 to 87). Fortunately, the effect of "Over-Zenkerization" can be corrected by exposure of decerated tissue sections to a 10% aqueous solution of sodium bicarbonate for six to eight hours followed by staining with hematoxylin and eosin.

Figure 84. *Zenker's Overfixation.* This specimen of human splenic tissue was left in Zenker's fluid for a prolonged period of time (> eight hours). Tissue sections prepared from the specimen were not pretreated with iodine and sodium thiosulfate prior to staining. Tissues which are overexposed to Zenker's fixative will not exhibit the usual hematoxylin staining characteristics. Overexposure to Zenker's fluid (eight hours or longer) produces acidophilia and a loss of basophilia (see Color Plate 1, Figure 5). Chromatin material cannot be differentiated chromatically and, in general, nuclei are not distinct. Zenker's fluid is not intended to be used for the wet storage of gross tissue specimens. Tissues should not be exposed to the fixative in excess of seven hours. In addition to mercuric chloride crystals and loss of basophilia, another type of artifact associated with Zenker's fixation is noted in this tissue section. Zenker's fluid will often crystallize erythrocytes (see Figures 88 and 89). Microscopically, the erythrocytes will exhibit a transparent or translucent appearance and anisotropism. (H&E, ×250) (AFIP Negative No. 71-12159-2)

Figure 85. *Zenker's Overfixation.* This is a duplicate tissue section prepared from the same specimen of splenic tissue depicted in Figure 84. The tissue section was decerated and treated with iodine and sodium thiosulfate and was then placed in 10% aqueous sodium bicarbonate for six to eight hours. It was subsequently placed in running tap water for ten minutes and then stained with hematoxylin and eosin (see Color Plate 1, Figure 6). This technique is usually successful in restoring the basophilia to tissues which have been overexposed to Zenker's fluid. *Note:* The extent of the improved chromatic results obtained by this treatment is not depicted well in black and white photographs. Microscopically, the results are quite dramatic. (H&E, ×250) (AFIP Negative No. 71-12159-4)

Figure 86. *Zenker's Overfixation.* This specimen of Zenker's-fixed tissue exhibits several artifacts related to overfixation in Zenker's fluid, as well as mercuric chloride crystals. The tissue section was not pretreated with iodine and sodium thiosulfate prior to staining. However, such pretreatment would do little to eliminate the separation of hepatocytes produced by overfixation in Zenker's fluid. Prolonged fixation in mercurial sublimate type fixatives hardens tissue excessively and results in increased eosinophilia (see Color Plate 2, Figure 7). Basophilia can be restored by pretreatment prior to staining with 10% aqueous sodium bicarbonate for six to eight hours. (H&E, ×305) (AFIP Negative No. 73-4281)

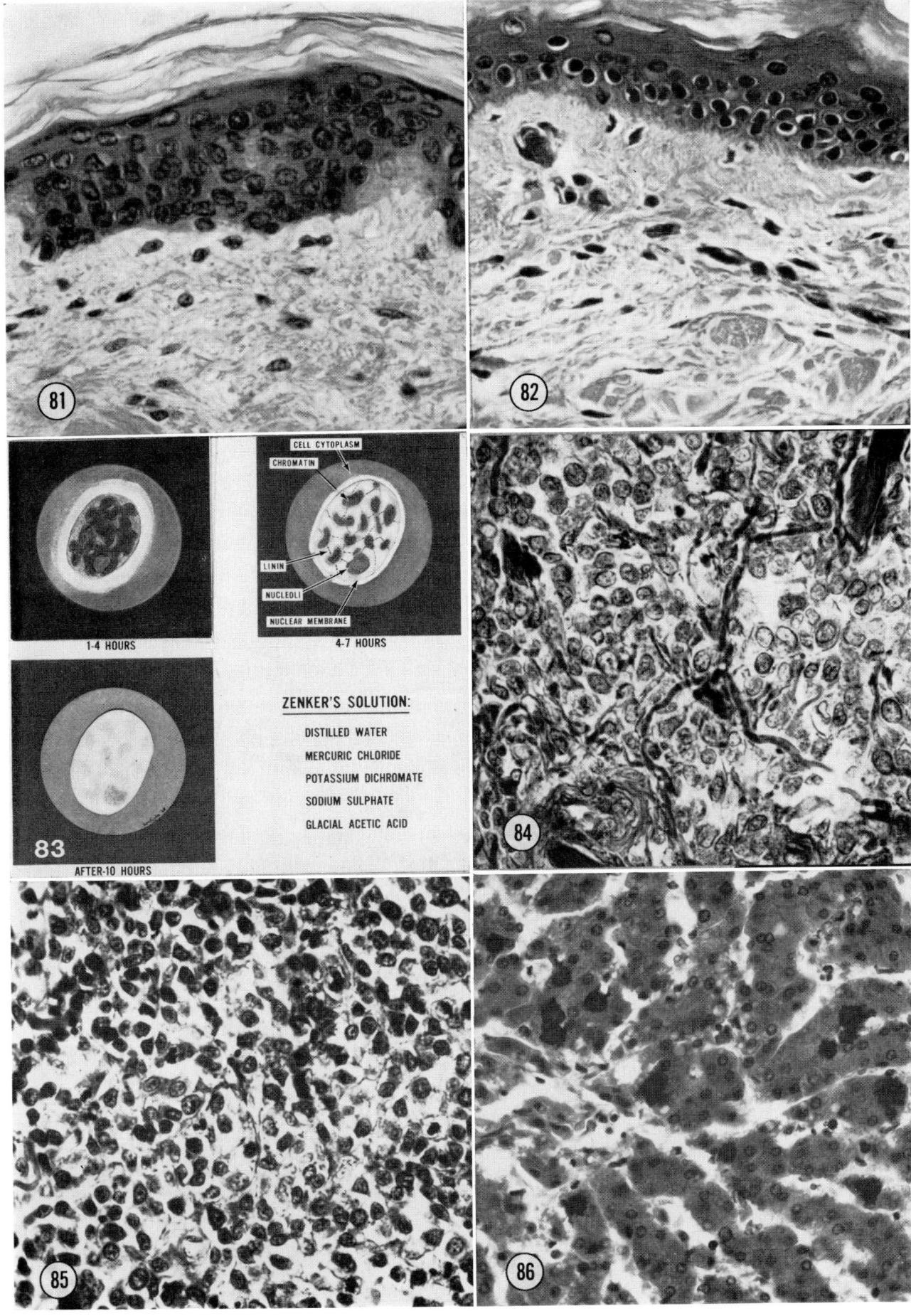

Figure 87. *Zenker's Overfixation.* The dark-stained streaks observed in the capsular stroma of this tissue section of a specimen of human spleen which was fixed in Zenker's fluid resulted from excessive dehydration from prolonged exposure (eight hours or longer) of the tissue to mercurial sublimate fixation (see also Figure 86). Chromatically, this dehydrated zone assumes a purplish tint after staining with hematoxylin and eosin and frequently simulates the staining results that may be obtained with minute foci of calcium deposition. (H&E, ×165) (AFIP Negative No. 73-4913)

Figure 88. *Zenker's Overfixation.* One of the least commonly observed effects of Zenker's fluid on animal tissues is the crystallization of erythrocytes as observed in this paraffin-embedded tissue section of a specimen of liver tissue from a human being which has been fixed in Zenker's fluid. The erythrocytes can be seen throughout the photomicrograph as clear, haloed structures. (H&E, ×530) (AFIP Negative No. 72-13666)

Figure 89. *Zenker's Overfixation.* This is the same tissue section and field of view as depicted in Figure 88 as seen with partial polariscopy. The crystallized erythrocytes which have resulted from Zenker's fixation are anisotropic. (H&E, ×530) (AFIP Negative No. 72-13665)

Figure 90. *Mercurial Sublimate Crystals.* When tissue specimens are fixed with mercurial sublimate fixatives, such as Zenker's fluids, anisotropic crystals of mercuric chloride are deposited in the tissue specimen. The recommended procedure is to fix the specimens for six hours followed by washing the specimen in running tap water for fourteen to sixteen hours. However, unless the tissue sections prepared from such specimens are treated to remove the mercuric chloride crystals, prior to staining, they remain as artifacts in the finished tissue section. Such artifacts are depicted in this tissue section of the spleen of a human being which had been fixed in Zenker's acetic fluid. In the classic form, these crystals are spheroid with an irregular periphery. Numerous other forms of the crystals have also been observed including needle shaped and polymorphic configurations (see Figures 91 through 103). (H&E, ×40) (Contributed by Mr. L. E. Schellhammer)

Figure 91. *Mercurial Sublimate Crystals.* This is the same tissue section as depicted in Figure 86, in the discussion of Zenker's overfixation, as viewed by means of partial polariscopy to demonstrate the anisotropism of mercurial sublimate crystals in tissue sections. (H&E, ×42) (AFIP Negative No. 71-11700)

Figure 92. *Mercurial Sublimate Crystals.* By treating tissue sections prepared from Zenker's-fixed tissue with a solution of iodine in 60% ethyl alcohol for ten to fifteen minutes, followed by treatment with 5% sodium thiosulfate for five minutes, it is possible to remove mercuric chloride crystals prior to staining. This is a tissue section of the same splenic tissue shown in Figure 90. It was treated with iodine and sodium thiosulfate prior to being stained. It is apparent that the crystals of mercuric chloride have been adequately removed from the tissue section. Such pretreatment of the tissue section prior to staining should be carried out routinely with tissues which are freshly fixed in Zenker's fluids. (H&E, ×40) (Contributed by Mr. L. E. Schellhammer)

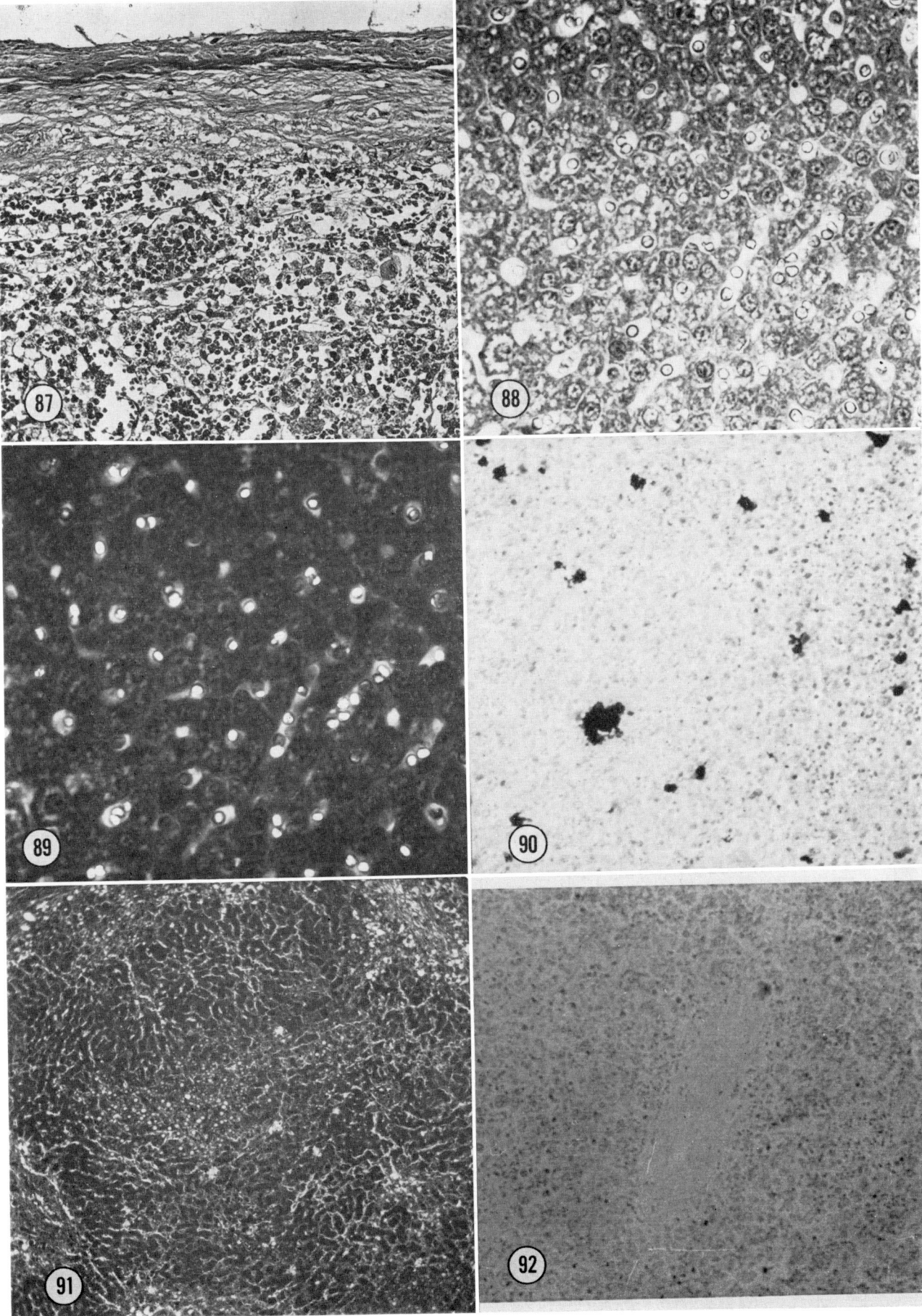

Figure 93. *Mercurial Sublimate Crystals.* Mercuric chloride crystals are deposited in Zenker's-fixed tissue in many sizes, shapes and forms. The following five photomicrographs (Figures 94 through 98) were made of paraffin-embedded tissue sections from a specimen of human liver tissue which was fixed in Zenker's fluid and which contained multiple mercuric chloride crystals. The tissue section was decerated and mounted without staining. Close observation of the photomicrograph reveals a wide variety of crystals of diverse sizes, shapes, and forms, including the large black mercuric chloride crystals which are most commonly seen in Zenker's-fixed tissue. The small clear mercuric chloride crystals are not commonly seen in hematoxylin and eosin-stained tissue sections of Zenker's-fixed specimens because of their refractive index. However, the latter type of crystals can be demonstrated by Luna's technique (see Figure 100). (Unstained, ×220) (AFIP Negative No. 73-4283)

Figure 94. *Mercurial Sublimate Crystals.* This section is similar to the one depicted in Figure 93. The unstained tissue section was photographed during partial polariscopy to better illustrate the variety of sizes, shapes, and forms of anisotropic mercuric chloride crystals which can be observed in Zenker's-fixed tissue specimens. (Unstained, ×220) (AFIP Negative No. 73-4285)

Figure 95. *Mercurial Sublimate Crystals.* This is a higher magnification of the central portion of the unstained tissue section depicted in Figure 93. The variety of sizes, shapes, and forms of mercuric chloride crystals which may be observed in unfixed tissue sections of Zenker's-fixed tissue specimens is more readily discernable at this magnification. (Unstained, ×485) (AFIP Negative No. 73-4282)

Figure 96. *Mercurial Sublimate Crystals.* This is the same tissue section and field of view depicted in Figure 95 as observed under partial polariscopy. All of the various sizes, shapes, and forms of mercuric chloride crystals observed in Figure 95 are strongly anisotropic. (Unstained, ×485) (AFIP Negative No. 73-4284)

Figure 97. *Mercurial Sublimate Crystals.* Unusual crystalline deposits can be seen scattered throughout this tissue section of a specimen of human cardiac muscle which had been fixed in Zenker's fluid. The form of these mercurial sublimate crystals is slightly different from the numerous other forms depicted in this chapter since the crystals blend with the general architecture of the cardiac muscle bundles. Several pathologists who examined this specimen failed to identify these forms as mercurial sublimate crystals since they were moderately clear and did not react tinctorially in the same fashion as crystals observed in hematoxylin and eosin-stained tissue sections from the same specimen. In the latter preparations, the mercurial sublimate crystals were a characteristic dark brown color. It should never be assumed that mercurial sublimate crystals are easily identified since they can occur in many forms and colors. (Luna-Parker Stain, ×305) (AFIP Negative No. 73-5171)

Figure 98. *Mercurial Sublimate Crystals.* This is the same microscopic field as depicted in Figure 97 as viewed by polariscopy. The irregularly shaped aggregates of anisotropic mercurial sublimate crystals are readily detected between and on cardiac muscle bundles. (Luna-Parker Stain, ×305) (AFIP Negative No. 73-5169)

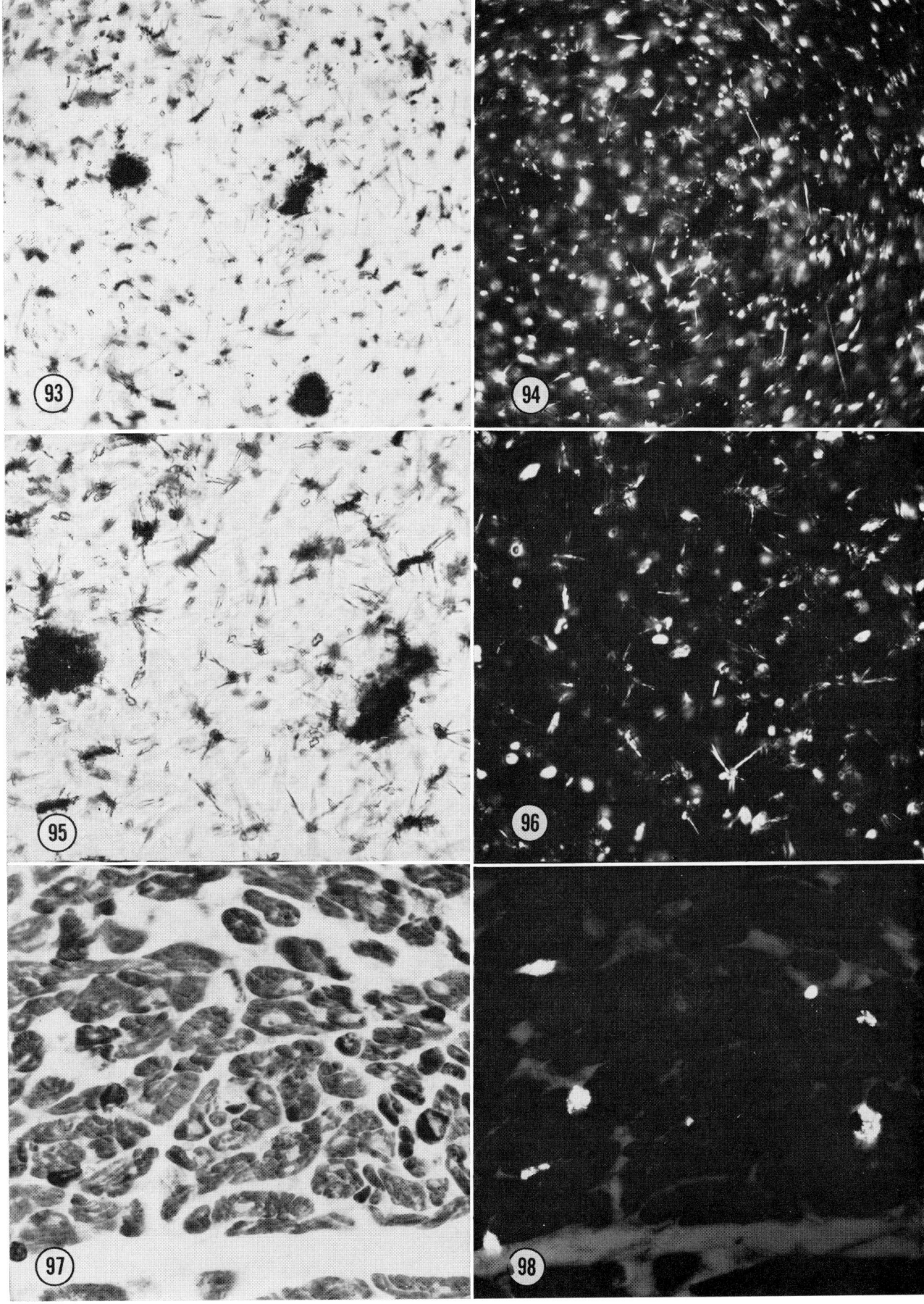

Figure 99. *Mercurial Sublimate Crystals.* This Zenker's-fixed tissue section from a specimen of human brain tissue was not pretreated with iodine and sodium thiosulfate prior to staining. The numerous forms which the aggregates of mercuric chloride crystals can assume are well demonstrated. (H&E, ×100) (AFIP Negative No. 69-6524)

Figure 100. *Mercurial Sublimate Crystals.* This is a duplicate tissue section of the specimen depicted in Figure 99. Because mercuric chloride crystals may be deposited in Zenker's-fixed tissues in other than characteristic forms, they may be confused with other crystalline material. This tissue section has been treated by Luna's technique for the demonstration of mercuric chloride as follows: (1) decerate and hydrate the tissue section in distilled water; (2) immerse in a 20% aqueous solution of ammonium hydroxide (28%) for thirty seconds; (3) rinse in distilled water (5 dips); (4) counterstain in a 0.2% aqueous solution of light green SF yellowish for thirty seconds; (5) dehydrate in two changes of 95% ethyl alcohol, absolute ethyl alcohol, and clear in xylene; (6) coverslip. The mercuric chloride crystals will appear black against a light green background. The color reaction of the crystals will fade after several weeks. Sections *cannot* be retreated with ammonium hydroxide solution if the original color reaction is light. (Luna-Parker Stain, ×100) (AFIP Negative No. 69-6523)

Figure 101. *Mercurial Sublimate Crystals.* In this tissue section of a specimen of Zenker's-fixed tissue from the snout of a pig, mercuric chloride crystals can be seen as large, intensely hematoxylinophilic structures which are scattered throughout the field. The unique feature in this example of the mercurial sublimate crystal artifact is that the crystals stained heavily with hematoxylin although the section had been exposed to iodine and sodium thiosulfate prior to staining. However, the crystals were not removed by this pretreatment because the exposure to iodine was less than the required ten to fifteen minutes. (H&E, ×325) (AFIP Negative No. 74-5207)

Figure 102. *Mercurial Sublimate Crystals.* In this specimen of human liver tissue which had been fixed in Zenker's fluid, and in which the tissue section had not been pretreated with iodine and sodium thiosulfate prior to staining, the deposits of mercuric chloride crystals are round and quite small and closely approximate to the size of the hepatocyte nucleus. (H&E, ×115) (AFIP Negative No. 71-11426)

Figure 103. *Mercurial Sublimate Crystals.* This tissue section was prepared from the same block of embedded tissue as depicted in Figure 102. It is stained by Gomori's methenamine silver nitrate stain for the demonstration of argyrophilic tissue components. The mercuric chloride crystals yield a positive reaction either because of the availability of aldehydes at the sites of deposition of the crystals (see Figure 106) or because the crystals themselves are capable of acting as reducing substances and reduce the silver of the methenamine-silver complex. This staining method is widely used for the demonstration of certain fungi in tissue sections. It is not inconceivable that such minute deposits of mercuric chloride in Zenker's-fixed tissue might at times be mistaken for protozoan parasites or fungi in tissue sections that are not pretreated with iodine and sodium thiosulfate prior to staining. (Gomori's methenamine silver stain, ×115) (AFIP Negative No. 71-11427)

Figure 104. *Mercurial Sublimate Burns.* The recommended practice is to prepare tissue sections of paraffin-embedded specimens which have been fixed in Zenker's fluid as soon as possible after they have been embedded. In tissue sections which have been prepared from Zenker's-fixed specimens several weeks to months after being embedded, the mercuric chloride crystals within the tissue section will yield an apparently positive periodic acid-Schiff reaction which is resistant to prior diastase digestion of the tissue section. In such instances, the crystals will yield a positive periodic acid-Schiff reaction as seen in this tissue section of a Zenker's-fixed specimen of human liver which was not treated with iodine and sodium thiosulfate prior to staining. (Periodic acid-Schiff reaction preceded by diastase digestion, ×100) (AFIP Negative No. 71-10670)

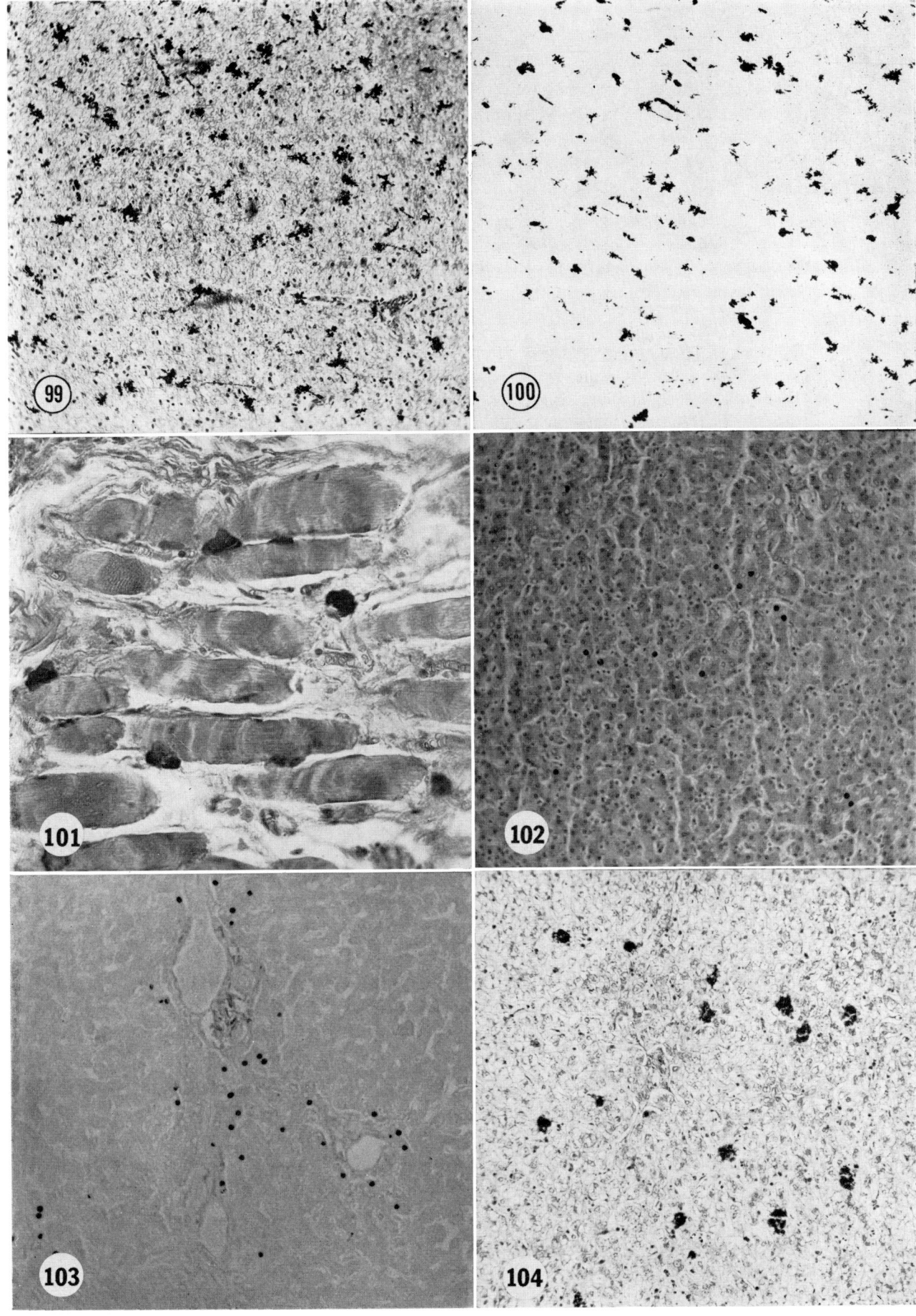

Figure 105. *Mercurial Sublimate Burns*. This is a high magnification of a portion of the tissue section depicted in Figure 104. The aggregates of "old" deposits of mercuric chloride crystals yield a positive periodic acid-Schiff reaction. (Periodic acid-Schiff reaction subsequent to diastase digestion, ×250) (AFIP Negative No. 71-10672)

Figure 106. *Mercurial Sublimate Burns*. This tissue section was prepared from the same block of embedded tissue as depicted in Figure 104. Prior to being stained, the tissue section was treated with alcoholic iodine and sodium thiosulfate to remove the mercuric chloride crystals. Although the crystals per se are no longer present in this tissue section, the former sites of deposition of the crystals are discolored (burned). However, when either Gram's iodine (iodine-1 gm, potassium iodide-2 gm and distilled water-300 ml) or Lugol's iodine solution (same formula as Gram's iodine except that only 100 ml of water is used) is used in place of alcoholic iodine in the iodine and sodium thiosulfate treatment, such discolored areas do not remain in the tissue after the mercuric chloride crystals have been removed. (H&E, ×100) (AFIP Negative No. 71-10675)

Figure 107. *Mercurial Sublimate Burns*. This is a higher magnification of a portion of the tissue section depicted in Figure 106 to show the finer detail of the burned areas that are left in the tissue after the removal of "old" mercuric chloride crystals with alcoholic iodine and sodium thiosulfate. These burned areas stain light purple with hematoxylin and eosin; dark pink with nuclear fast red; green with Giemsa stain; salmon with the colloidal iron stain; and they also yield a diastase resistant, positive periodic acid-Schiff reaction. That the crystals (see Figures 104 and 105) and/or the burned areas which remain after their removal with alcoholic iodine and sodium thiosulfate yield a positive periodic acid-Schiff reaction is not unexpected in view of the fact that mercuric chloride in Zenker's fluid can hydrolyze plasmalogen in such a way that plasmal is available for the plasmal reaction of Feulgen, for the demonstration of acetylphosphatides, without the need of further hydrolysis of the tissue specimen provided the fixation is greater than six hours. Mercuric chloride crystals in embedded tissue continue to act as oxidizing agents and will split not only the acetylphosphatides to form aldehydes, but will also oxidize unsaturated fatty acids to form aldehydes which will react with Schiff's reagent. In addition to its effect on acetylphosphatides and unsaturated fatty acids, the mercuric chloride in Zenker's fluid has an adverse effect on hyaluronic acid which cannot be demonstrated with colloidal iron techniques following Zenker's fixation. It is not known if other mucosubstances are similarly affected by Zenker's fixation. (H&E, ×250) (AFIP Negative No. 71-10674)

Figure 108. *Urea Polymers*. Urea is sometimes added to Zenker's fluid to prevent the hemolysis of erythrocytes. If tissues which are initially fixed in Zenker's urea are subsequently stored as gross tissue in 10% formalin, urea polymers will form within the tissue specimen. The section depicted here was prepared from a specimen of human heart tissue which was initially fixed in Zenker's fluid which contained urea instead of sodium sulphate and was subsequently stored in formalin. When urea and formalin react, a plastic polymer is produced in the form of round, clear-to-gray, crystalline, anisotropic deposits within hematoxylin and eosin-stained tissue sections. This heretofore undescribed artifact is difficult to see by means of bright-field microscopy (arrow). It can be differentiated from mercuric chloride crystals since it does not react (turn black) when treated with ammonium hydroxide (see Figures 114 through 116) and yields a positive reaction to the Degalantha stain for the demonstration of urates and uric acid. It is best seen by means of polariscopy. (H&E, ×180) (AFIP Negative No. 73-4906)

Figure 109. *Urea Polymers*. This is the same tissue section as depicted in Figure 108 as observed by polariscopy. The urea polymer crystals seen along the epicardium are strongly anisotropic both before and after treatment with ammonium hydroxide whereas mercuric chloride crystals do not polarize after treatment with ammonium hydroxide (see Figures 114 through 116). In addition, mercuric chloride crystals appear to be slightly above the tissue surface while the urea crystalline polymer is embedded in the tissue. (H&E, ×180) (AFIP Negative No. 73-4902)

Figure 110. *Urea Polymers*. In hematoxylin and eosin-stained tissue sections the urea polymer stains darker at its periphery as depicted in this tissue section of a specimen of the myocardium of a human being. (H&E, ×130) (AFIP Negative No. 73-6276)

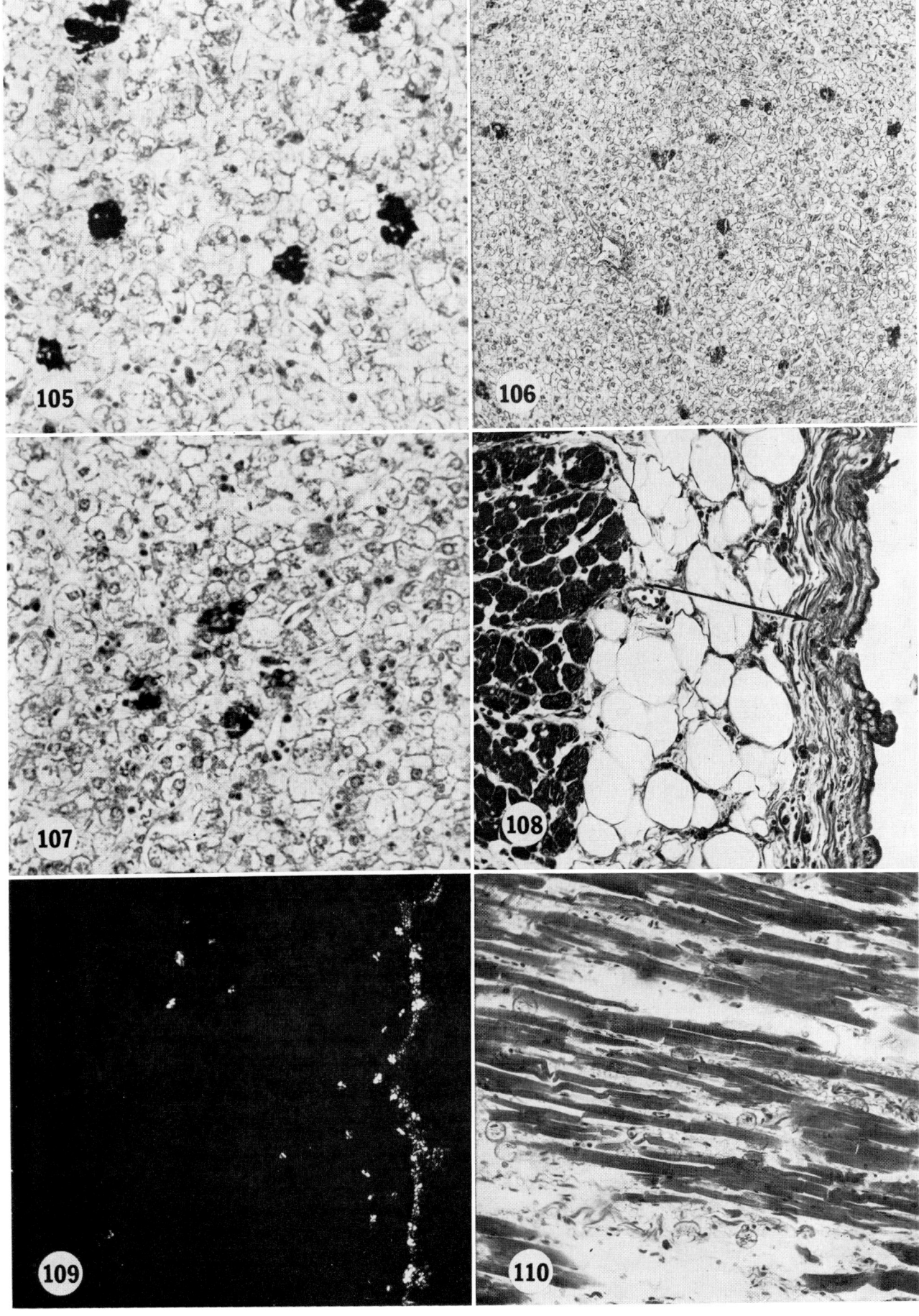

Figure 111. *Urea Polymers*. This is the same field of view depicted in Figure 110 as viewed by means of partial polariscopy. Urea polymer deposits are anisotropic and are readily detected by means of polariscopy. Urea polymer artifacts are not seen in Zenker's urea fixed tissues that have not been exposed to formalin. (H&E, ×130) (AFIP Negative No. 73-6275)

Figure 112. *Urea Polymers*. The effects produced by urea polymers (arrows) are well illustrated in this photomicrograph of a tissue section prepared from a specimen of a human heart which was initially fixed in Zenker's urea and subsequently stored in formalin (see also Figures 108 and 109). Microscopically, the rounded crystals appear to be a morphologic change in the structure of the tissue. Urea polymer crystalline artifacts are decidedly different from other types of crystalline artifacts. (H&E, ×130) (AFIP Negative No. 73-4921)

Figure 113. *Urea Polymers*. This is the same tissue section as depicted in Figure 112 as observed by partial polariscopy. Partial polariscopy demonstrates the morphology of the typical urea polymer crystals. (H&E, ×130) (AFIP Negative No. 73-4896)

Figure 114. *Mercurial Sublimate and Urea Polymer Crystals*. This photomicrograph depicts mercuric chloride and urea polymer crystals in a tissue section prepared from a specimen of human heart which was initially fixed in Zenker's fluid to which urea had been added and was subsequently stored in 10% neutral buffered formalin. The tissue section was treated by Luna's procedure for the demonstration of mercuric chloride crystals as described in the legend for Figure 100. The black-colored polymorphic crystals seen in the photomicrograph are mercuric chloride crystals which have turned black after being treated by Luna's procedure. The urea polymer crystals (arrows) remain uncolored after exposure to Luna's procedure. (Luna's reaction for mercuric chloride, ×50) (AFIP Negative No. 73-4900)

Figure 115. *Mercurial Sublimate and Urea Polymer Crystals*. This is a higher magnification of the central portion of the tissue section depicted in Figure 114. The fine detail of the mercuric chloride (black) and urea polymer (arrows) crystals is more readily discernable than with low power objectives. (Luna's reaction for mercuric chloride, ×305) (AFIP Negative No. 73-4898)

Figure 116. *Mercurial Sublimate and Urea Polymer Crystals*. This is a view of the central portion of the field of view depicted in Figure 115 as observed by polariscopy. Following treatment of the tissue section by Luna's procedure, mercuric chloride crystals are isotropic, whereas urea polymer crystals retain their anisotropism. (Luna's reaction for mercuric chloride, ×305) (AFIP Negative No. 73-4920)

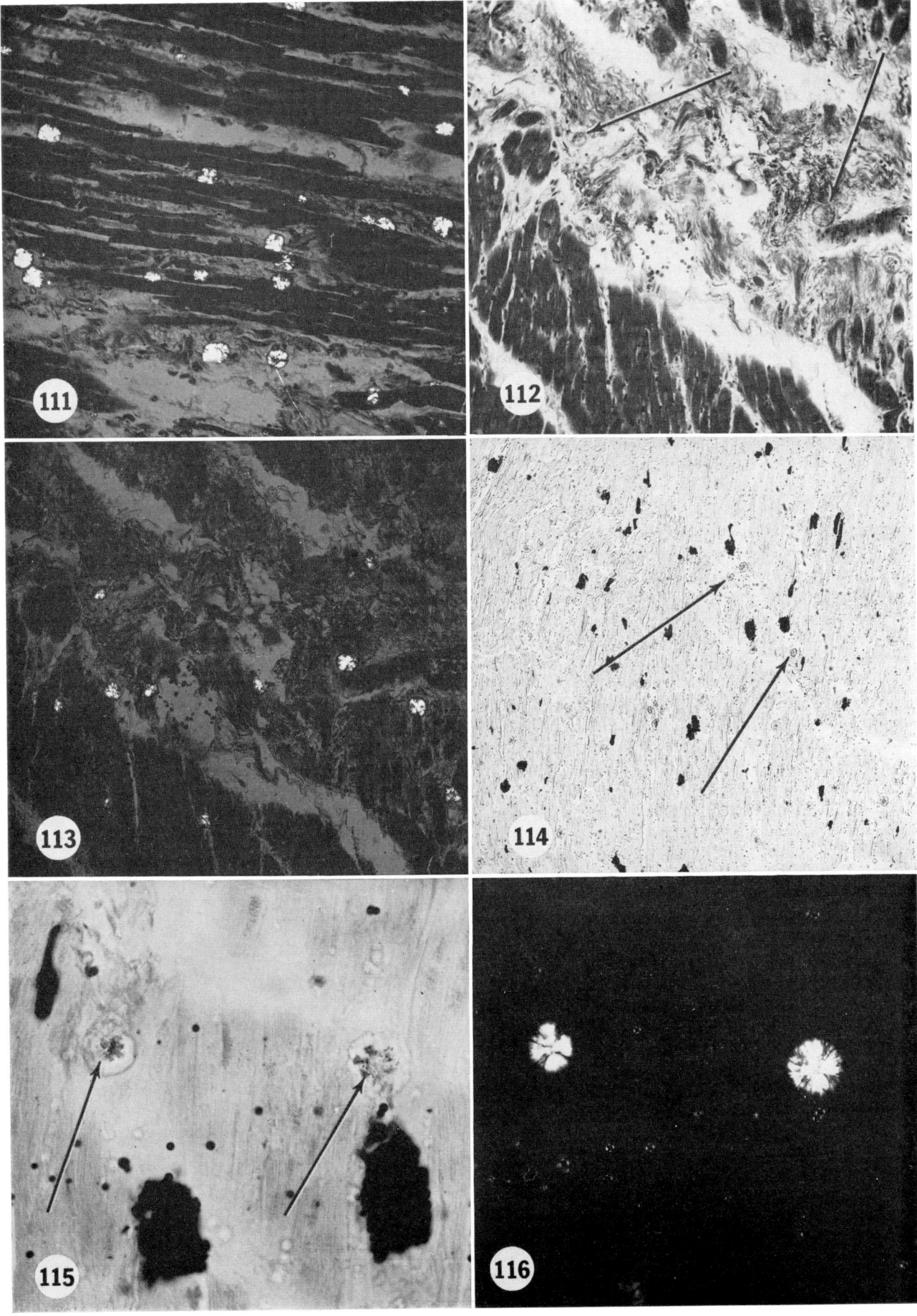

Figure 117. *Effect of Neutral Buffered 10% Formalin on Glycogen.* Glycogen exists as an intracytoplasmic colloid and is precipitated in a granular form when fixatives are used. As seen in this photograph of a paraffin-embedded section of a specimen of human liver, fixed in neutral buffered 10% formalin, conventional means of fixation generally cause glycogen to migrate to one side of the cell. Such artifacts are not observed in tissues prepared by freezing-substitution or freezing-drying techniques. The latter method is considered to be one of the most efficient for the preservation of soluble tissue glycogen. Numerous fluid fixatives have been recommended for the preservation of tissue glycogen. Anhydrous fixatives are frequently used because of the known solubility of glycogen in water or trichloroacetic acid. Glycogen is demonstrable in tissues fixed in formalin, even after prolonged washing in water subsequent to fixation. However, alcoholic-formalin fixatives give better and more consistent preservation of glycogen. Either neutral buffered 10% formalin or alcoholic-formalin is preferable to alcohol, Bouin's fluid, or Zenker's fluid for the preservation of tissue glycogen. (Periodic acid-Schiff reaction, ×205) (AFIP Negative No. 71-11707)

Figure 118. *Absolute Ethyl Alcohol.* Alcohol is frequently used as an anhydrous fixative for the preservation of water soluble components of tissue. This specimen of human liver tissue was fixed in absolute ethyl alcohol. The usual procedure is to fix specimens no thicker than 2 to 3 mm in 20 volumes of absolute ethyl alcohol for four hours and then change the tissues to 70% ethyl alcohol (20 volumes per volume of tissue) until fixation is complete but not for longer than seventy-two hours. Alcohol penetrates tissues rather quickly and it has the ability to denature protein by coagulation and rapid dehydration. In this respect, its action is similar to the effect of heat upon tissues. However, it is not intended to be a general purpose fixative since the dehydration is naturally associated with extensive shrinking of the tissues and morphological alterations of many of its components. In alcohol-fixed tissues, erythrocytes are lysed, leukocytes shrunken and distorted, hemosiderin pigment is slightly altered in staining qualities, and peripheral cells are completely dehydrated and collapsed as seen in this photomicrograph. (Periodic acid-Schiff reaction subsequent to diastase digestion, ×210) (AFIP Negative No. 72-7020)

Figure 119. *Bouin's Fluid.* It is generally believed that, once a tissue specimen has been embedded in paraffin, it makes little difference in the quality of the slides which will be obtained if one cuts the tissue sections immediately or later after a considerable time lapse. This may be the case with formalin-fixed tissue, but it is not the case with all types of fixatives. The paraffin-embedded tissue section depicted in this photograph was prepared from a specimen of human liver fixed in Bouin's fluid. The section was cut and stained within twenty-four hours after the specimen was embedded in paraffin. The result is an excellent tissue section. (H&E, ×220)

Figure 120. *Bouin's Fluid.* The tissue section depicted in this photograph was cut from the same block of paraffin-embedded, Bouin's-fixed, tissue as depicted in Figure 119. All things are identical to the procedures used with the previous tissue section with the exception that the section was cut twelve weeks after the specimen had been embedded in paraffin. The stains are diffused, some cellular boundaries are indistinct, and the cytoplasm of some of the hepatocytes has a hyalin appearance. The picric acid within Bouin's fluid is rarely completely removed during the processing of gross specimens. Some picric acid remains in the embedded tissue to be finally removed from the exceedingly thin tissue section during the actual staining procedure. This picric acid continues to act upon tissue components, adjacent to its site of deposition, even in the embedded tissue specimen. The longer one waits to cut and stain the tissue section, the greater is the influence exerted by the picric acid residues in the embedded tissue specimen. (H&E, ×220)

Figure 121. *Acid Hematin in Bouin's-Fixed Tissue.* A dark brown, anisotropic, microcrystalline, iron-negative pigment which is quite similar to acid formalin hematin may be formed in the spleen and other blood-rich tissues which have been fixed in Bouin's fluid, as observed in this tissue section of the luminal contents of a blood vessel of the skin of a human being. Bouin's fluid contains saturated aqueous picric acid, formaldehyde, and glacial acetic acid. Although acid formalin hematin is not formed in tissues which have been fixed in Bouin's fluid that contain at least 1.1% acetic acid and 1% picric acid, it may be formed in tissues fixed in Bouin's fluid which contain increased proportions of formaldehyde and decreased proportions of picric acid and/or acetic acid. Such artifacts result from faulty formulation of the Bouin's fluid in which decreased quantities of acetic acid in relation to the concentration of picric acid and formaldehyde occur in the fixative. Such errors may occur readily since the acetic acid component of the fluid is added to a stock solution of picric acid and formaldehyde immediately before the fixative is to be used. (H&E, ×250) (AFIP Negative No. 72-6138)

Figure 122. *Preformed Acid Hematin in Neutral Buffered 10% Formalin-fixed Tissue.* This tissue section was prepared from a specimen of canine kidney which was fixed in neutral buffered formalin. Strongly anisotropic pigment seen within the cytoplasm of the renal tubular epithelial cells is preformed acid hematin in that it did not result from the simultaneous action of acid and formaldehyde on hemoglobin. The pigment is thought to result from the action of acid on hemoglobin prior to fixation. Such pigments may be the pigment which is formed in autolyzed stomachs and spleens when fixed in neutral formalin rather than acid formalin hematin. The pigment may be removed from tissue sections prior to staining by means of the same techniques which are used for the removal of acid formalin hematin (see Figure 133). (H&E, partial polariscopy, ×300)

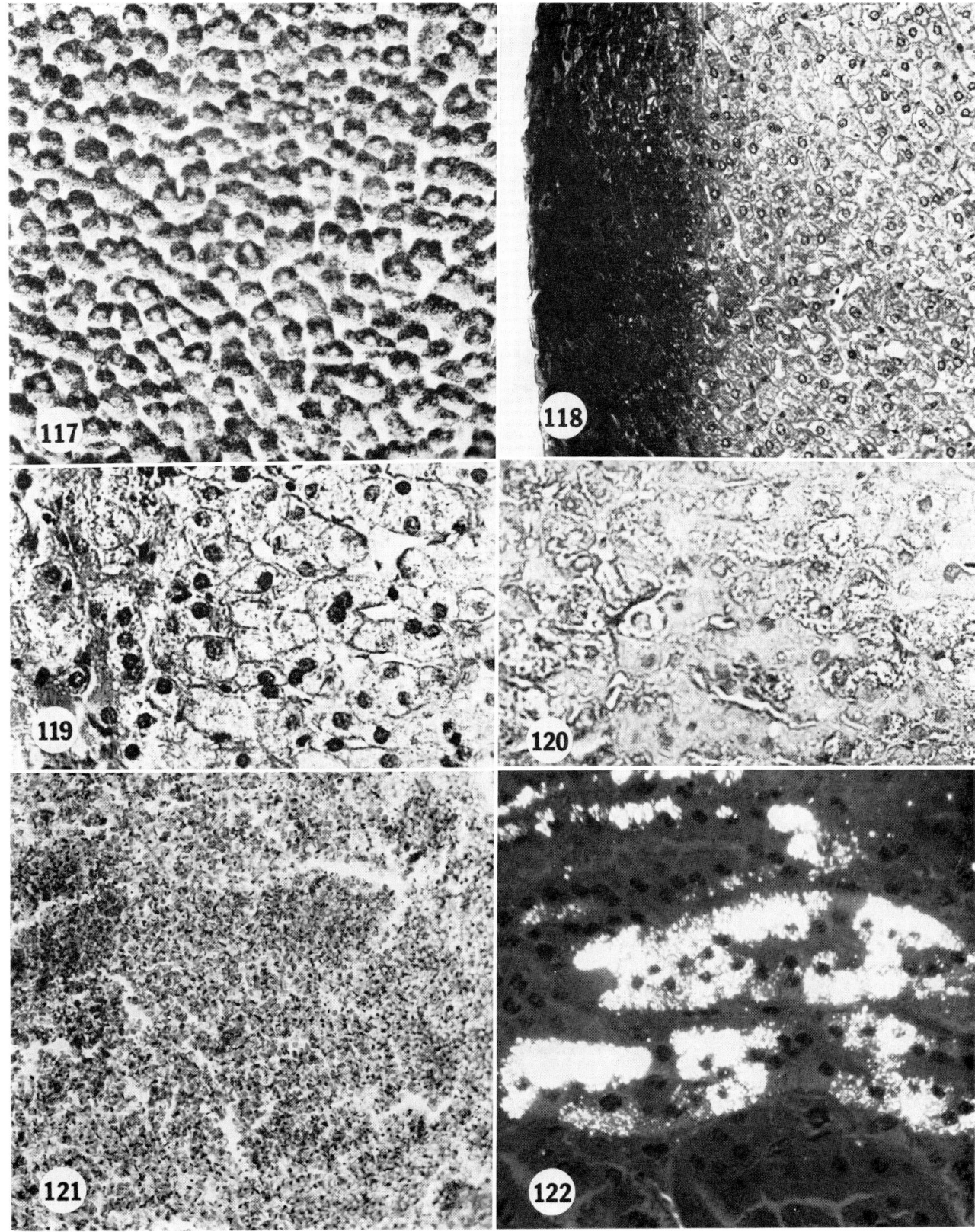

Figure 123. *Acid Formalin Hematin Pigment.* As previously mentioned, acid formalin hematin pigment is produced by the reaction of formic acid of unbuffered formalin with the heme of hemoglobin. Therefore, one may erroneously assume that the pigment will only be seen in, on, or around erythrocytes within tissue sections. However, this is not always the case and the pigment may be encountered in a wide variety of sites of deposition within tissue specimens since these sites may contain heme (the iron-containing portion of hemoglobin). In this photograph of a portion of a paraffin-embedded tissue section of a specimen of human kidney, acid formalin hematin has been deposited in an orderly pattern within a glomerulus rather than the rather disorganized pattern of deposition which is more frequently encountered. (H&E, ×275) (AFIP Negative No. 74-7448)

Figure 124. *Acid Formalin Hematin Pigment.* This is a lower power view of the same field depicted in Figure 123 as seen via partial polariscopy. Notice that the anisotropic acid formalin hematin pigment is predominantly deposited in the glomerular tuft. (H&E, ×180) (AFIP Negative No. 74-5742)

Figure 125. *Acid Formalin Hematin Pigment.* This photograph is from a different portion of the same tissue section depicted in Figure 123 in which a small focal hemorrhage was observed within the renal cortex. Notice that a dark-colored (acid formalin hematin) pigment has been deposited upon the intima of segments of an interlobular vein. (H&E, ×145) (AFIP Negative No. 74-5739)

Figure 126. *Acid Formalin Hematin Pigment.* This is the same field of view as depicted in Figure 125 as viewed by partial polariscopy. Notice that the anisotropic acid formalin hematin pigment is predominantly deposited on the intima of the segments of the interlobular vein. Comparatively little pigment is deposited on the erythrocytes within the lumen of the vein and in the focal hemorrhage surrounding the vein or in the glomeruli (compare with Figure 124). (H&E, ×145) (AFIP Negative No. 74-5744)

Figure 127. *Acid Formalin Hematin Pigment.* This is a higher magnification of a portion of the field depicted in Figure 125 to better illustrate the acid formalin hematin pigment which is deposited on the intima of a segment of the interlobular vein which is surrounded by focal hemorrhage. Note the paucity of pigment on erythrocytes within the lumen of the vessel or the focus of hemorrhage. (H&E, ×400) (AFIP Negative No. 74-7447)

Figure 128. *Acid Formalin Hematin Pigment.* This is a photograph from another portion of the same tissue section depicted in Figures 123 through 127. Numerous segments of an interlobular vein, surrounded by focal hemorrhage, are present within the field. Very little acid formalin hematin pigment is deposited within the glomeruli (compare with Figures 123 and 125) or on the intima (compare with Figures 125 and 127) of the vein seen within this field. (H&E, ×145) (AFIP Negative No. 74-5740)

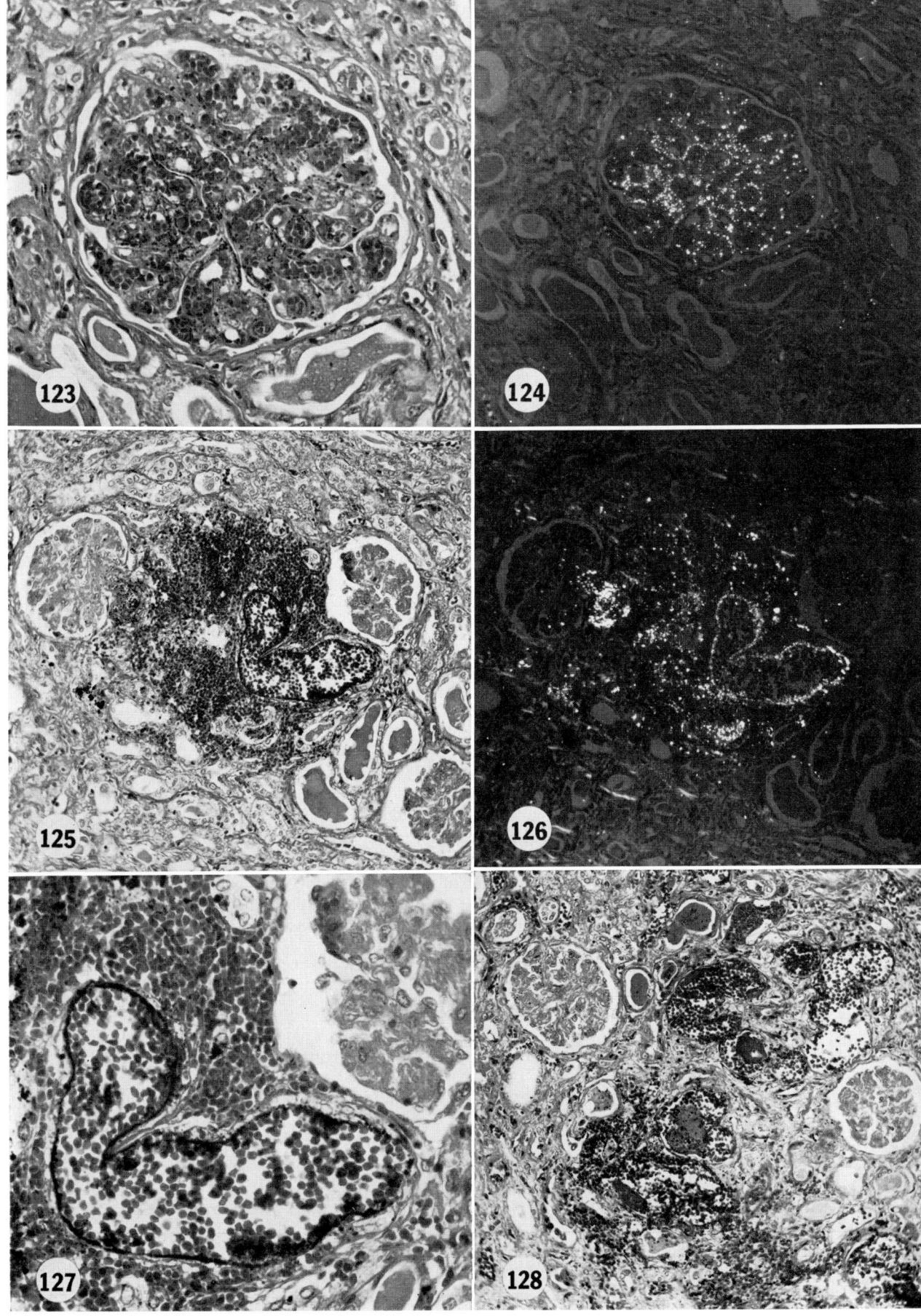

Figure 129. *Acid Formalin Hematin Pigment*. This is the same field depicted in Figure 128 as viewed by means of partial polariscopy. Note the paucity of anisotropic acid formalin hematin pigment within the glomeruli and its absence from the intima of the segments of the interlobular vein. In this field, the pigment is deposited upon erythrocytes within the lumens of the segments of the vein and in the foci of paravascular hemorrhage. In addition, deposits of the pigment are seen within tubular casts, renal tubular epithelial cells, and cortical interstitium. (H&E, ×145) (AFIP Negative No. 74-5743)

Figure 130. *Acid Formalin Hematin Pigment*. Clusters of acid formalin hematin pigment are observed in this tissue section of a specimen of human kidney which was fixed in acid (unbuffered) formalin. They are observed within the lumina of renal tubules and branches of the arcuate artery. The pigment has no pathologic significance but its presence in tissue sections is a nuisance when one is conducting various types of histochemical studies or polariscopy. (H&E, ×165) (AFIP Negative No. 72-3738)

Figure 131. *Acid Formalin Hematin Pigment*. This tissue section was prepared from a portion of the same specimen of the kidney as depicted in Figure 130. The pigment is deposited upon the walls of tubules (arrow) (see Color Plate 2, Figure 8) and on erythrocytes within the lumina of blood vessels. (H&E, ×130) (AFIP Negative No. 72-4768)

Figure 132. *Acid Formalin Hematin Pigment*. In addition to deposits of acid formalin hematin pigment in the lumina of blood vessels in this tissue section of a human kidney which was fixed in acid (unbuffered) formalin, minute deposits are seemingly present within the cytoplasm of renal tubular epithelial cells. (H&E, ×300) (AFIP Negative No. 73-4288-10)

Figure 133. *Acid Formalin Hematin Pigment*. This tissue section was prepared from the same specimen of kidney as depicted in Figures 130, 131, and 135. It has been treated prior to staining to remove the acid formalin hematin pigment. The pigment can frequently be removed by treating the tissue section with a variety of organic and inorganic agents. One should ascertain that other pigments in the tissue section, which are of interest, will not be simultaneously removed from the section or otherwise adversely affected (see Thompson, pp. 1110-1271). The most frequently used methods for the removal of acid formalin hematin pigment from tissue sections are: decerate and hydrate to water, rinse well in distilled water and (1) place in saturated alcoholic (absolute ethyl) picric acid solution for three hours and then wash well in running tap water; or (2) place in 100 ml of 70% ethyl alcohol plus 2 ml of 28% ammonium hydroxide for three hours, rinse in tap water followed by rinsing in a 1% aqueous glacial acetic acid solution, wash well in distilled water; or (3) place in a solution composed of 50 ml of acetone plus 50 ml of 3% hydrogen peroxide plus 1.0 ml of 28% ammonium hydroxide for one hour or more, wash well in running tap water followed by distilled water; or (4) place in a solution composed of 50 ml of 95% ethyl alcohol plus 15 ml of 28% ammonium hydroxide for one hour, wash well in running tap water. (H&E, ×575) (AFIP Negative No. 73-4288-11)

Figure 134. *Acid Formalin Hematin Pigment*. The anisotropism of acid formalin hematin pigment is demonstrated in this tissue section of the lesions of *Pneumocystis corinii* in the lung of a human being. At the left the pigment is observed as it is seen by means of conventional bright-field microscopy and at the right the pigment is seen as it is observed by means of polariscopy. Acid formalin hematin reduces silver which results in a positive reaction with all silver staining procedures. The pigment should be removed from tissue sections (see Figure 133) prior to exposure of the sections to a silver staining procedure. This will eliminate any possible confusion of acid formalin hematin with other argyrophilic tissue components. (Grocott's methenamine silver stain for fungi, ×575) (AFIP Negative No. 71-10681)

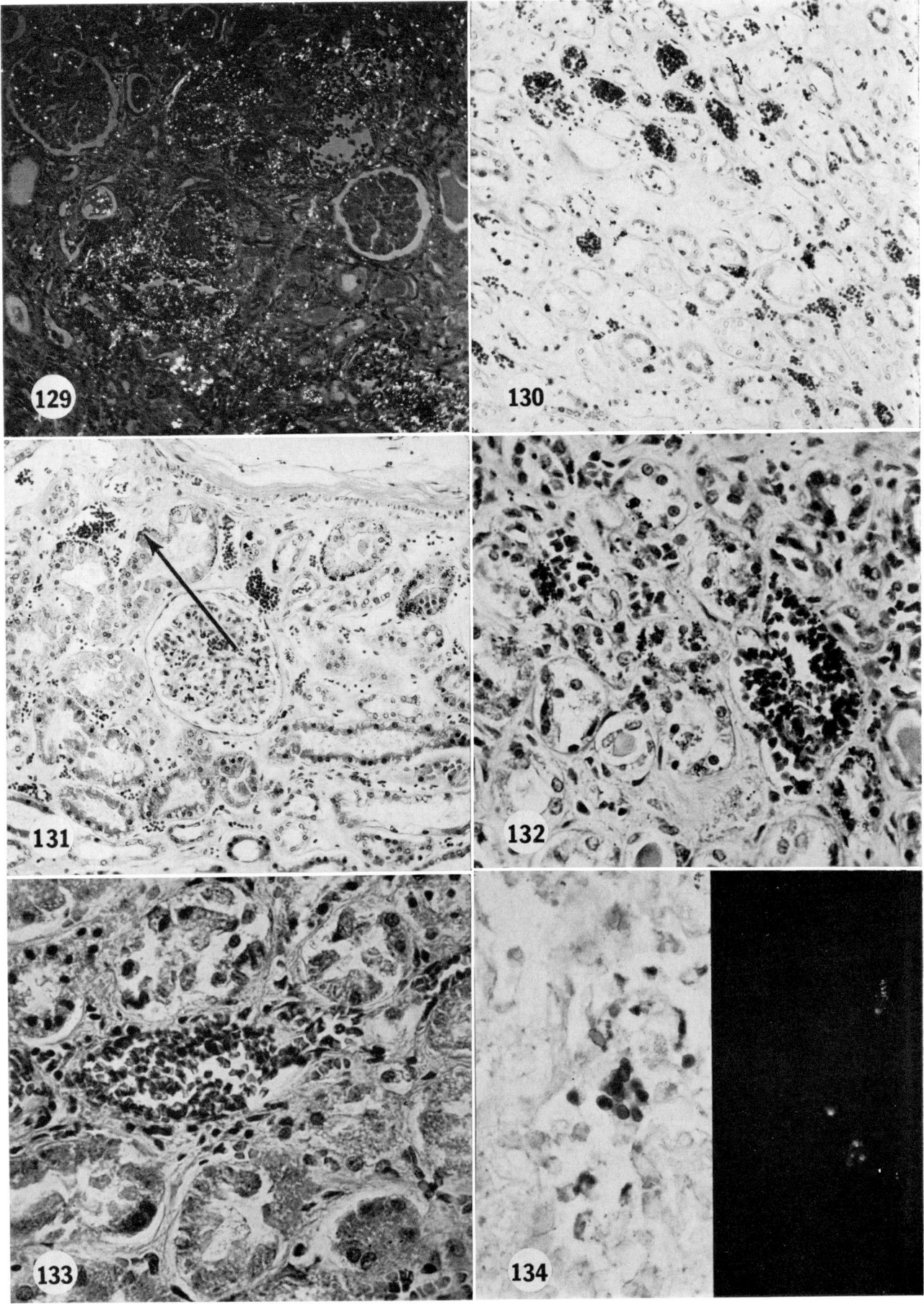

Figure 135. *Acid Formalin Hematin Pigment.* This is a higher magnification of a tissue section prepared from a portion of the same specimen of kidney as depicted in Figures 130 and 131. In addition to the deposition of the pigment upon erythrocytes, note the presence of the pigment within the cytoplasm of renal tubular epithelial cells at the basal aspect of the cells. (H&E, ×575) (AFIP Negative No. 72-4768)

Figure 136. *Acid Formalin Hematin Pigment.* As observed in this tissue section (arrows) of a specimen which was fixed in unbuffered formalin, acid formalin hematin (acid formaldehyde hematin, formalin pigment) is a dark brown, anisotropic, microcrystalline, iron-negative pigment. It occurs in blood-rich organs which have been fixed in acid aqueous or alcoholic formalin which has a pH lower than 6.0 owing to the simultaneous action of acid and formaldehyde on hemoglobin. (H&E, ×210) (AFIP Negative No. 71-11049)

Figure 137. *Acid Formalin Hematin Pigment.* A duplicate photograph of Figure 136, taken with partial polariscopy, is shown here to depict the anisotropism of the pigment. A somewhat similar pigment is produced by fixation in solutions of acetic and formic acid in alcohols or acetone (see Figure 121). However, these latter pigments are considered to be acid hematins, rather than acid formalin hematin. (H&E, ×210) (AFIP Negative No. 11051)

Figure 138. *Acid Formalin Hematin Pigment.* Within the vacuoles of fat cells in this tissue section of a specimen of human bone marrow, acid formalin hematin pigment appears black chromatically. The pigment is evident in the vacuoles left within fat cells by dehydrating and clearing agents. It is important to realize that this pigment is not always deposited in or near hemoglobin. Acid formalin hematin pigment may be deposited in many crystalline forms of varied colors and in a variety of sites within a tissue specimen including the cytoplasm of cells. The pigment is not deposited in tissues fixed in neutral, buffered formalin and this fact should be sufficient cause to discontinue the use of unbuffered formalin as a fixative. (Hematoxylin-phloxine-saffron, ×80) (AFIP Negative No. 73-6305)

Figure 139. *Acid Formalin Hematin Pigment.* This is the same field as seen in Figure 138 as observed by means of partial polariscopy. It is not uncommon to find anisotropic acid formalin hematin pigment in the vacuoles remaining from fat cells after the fat has been dissolved by dehydrating and clearing agents in the processing of tissue fixed in unbuffered formalin (see Color Plate 2, Figure 9). (Hematoxylin-phloxine-saffron, ×80) (AFIP Negative No. 73-6304)

Figure 140. *Acid Formalin.* These tissue sections were prepared from blocks of human liver tissue which were fixed in 10% unbuffered formalin. The specimen at the left was fixed for a period of less than twenty-four hours. The specimen at the right was fixed for a period of three months. The patient was afflicted with Wilson's disease and both tissue sections were stained by the rubeanic acid method for the demonstration of copper. Deposits are present throughout the tissue section at the left (< twenty-four hours fixation) but are absent from the tissue section at the right (three months fixation). This example illustrates that routine unbuffered formalin fixation will alter or remove some pathologic tissue components such as copper, iron, and calcium. (Rubeanic acid, ×575) (AFIP Negative No. 70-7684)

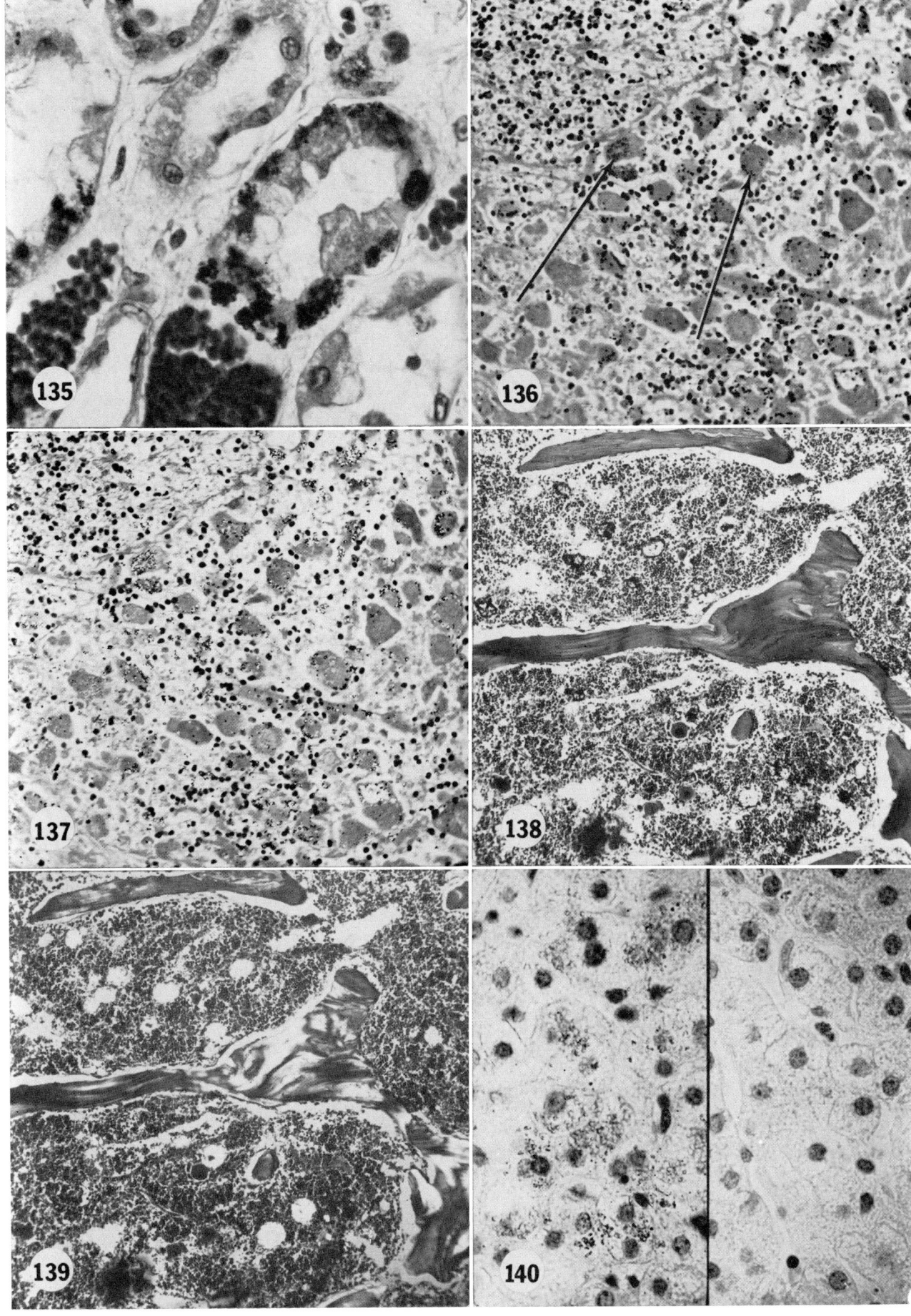

Figure 141. *Acid Formalin.* The use of acid formalin (nonbuffered) for the fixation of tissue should be discontinued due to its deleterious effect on many normal tissue components and/or pathologic entities. An example of this problem is well illustrated in this photomicrograph of a paraffin-embedded tissue section of a specimen of human skin which was fixed and stored in acid formalin for four months prior to processing. Paget cells in the epidermis yield a negative aldehyde fuchsin reaction (arrow) (compare with Figure 142). (Gomori's aldehyde-fuchsin stain, ×90) (AFIP Negative No. 73-3923)

Figure 142. *Acid Formalin.* This section was prepared from a duplicate specimen of the same piece of human skin as depicted in Figure 141. However, this specimen was only fixed in acid formalin for approximately ten hours before it was processed and embedded. The tissue section was cut and stained within twenty-four hours after removal from the host. The Paget cells within the epidermis yield an intensely positive aldehyde fuchsin reaction (compare with Figure 141). (Gomori's aldehyde fuchsin reaction, ×90) (AFIP Negative No. 73-3922)

Figure 143. *Neutral Buffered 10% Versus Acid Formalin.* In this tissue section of a paraffin-embedded specimen of human kidney, which was fixed for three months in neutral buffered 10% formalin, calcium salts are present beneath the tubular basement membrane and within glomeruli. These deposits are pathologic and were not adversely affected by fixation. (H&E, ×150) (AFIP Negative No. 73-2482)

Figure 144. *Neutral Buffered 10% Versus Acid Formalin.* This tissue section was prepared from a specimen of the same kidney depicted in Figure 143. However, this specimen was fixed in acid formalin for three weeks. The pathologic deposits of calcium salts are no longer present within the specimen, indicating that decalcification was achieved by the use of unbuffered formalin. The loss of the pathologic deposits of calcium salts was an undesirable effect of fixation. Many pigments and minerals, both pathologic and normal, are removed from tissue specimens by fixation in unbuffered formalin. (H&E, ×150) (AFIP Negative No. 73-2488)

Figure 145. *Refrigeration of Unfixed Specimens.* A practice which is not quite as disastrous as the freezing of gross specimens prior to fixation is to hold the gross specimen in a refrigerator for varied periods of time prior to fixation. This specimen of the lymph node of a domestic animal was divided into two parts at the time of necropsy. One half was fixed in formalin at the time of necropsy. The other half was held in a refrigerator at 4°C for sixteen hours before it was placed in formalin. The two specimens were subsequently processed in an identical fashion. At the left is the tissue section from the specimen that was placed in fixative at the time of necropsy. At the right is the tissue section from the specimen which was held at 4°C for sixteen hours prior to being placed in fixative. The cells in the tissue section at the right display artifactitious crenation. (H&E, ×500) (AFIP Negative No. 73-4288-5)

Figure 146. *Refrigeration of Unfixed Specimens.* These tissue sections are from two halves of a lymph node from the same animal and handled in the same fashion as described in Figure 145. In this case Bouin's fluid was the fixative employed. At the left is a tissue section which was prepared from the half of the specimen which was placed in fixative at the time of necropsy. The tissue section at the right is from the half of the lymph node which was held in a refrigerator for sixteen hours (overnight) prior to being placed in the fixative. The cells in the tissue section at the right display artifactitious crenation. (H&E, ×500) (AFIP Negative No. 73-4288-7)

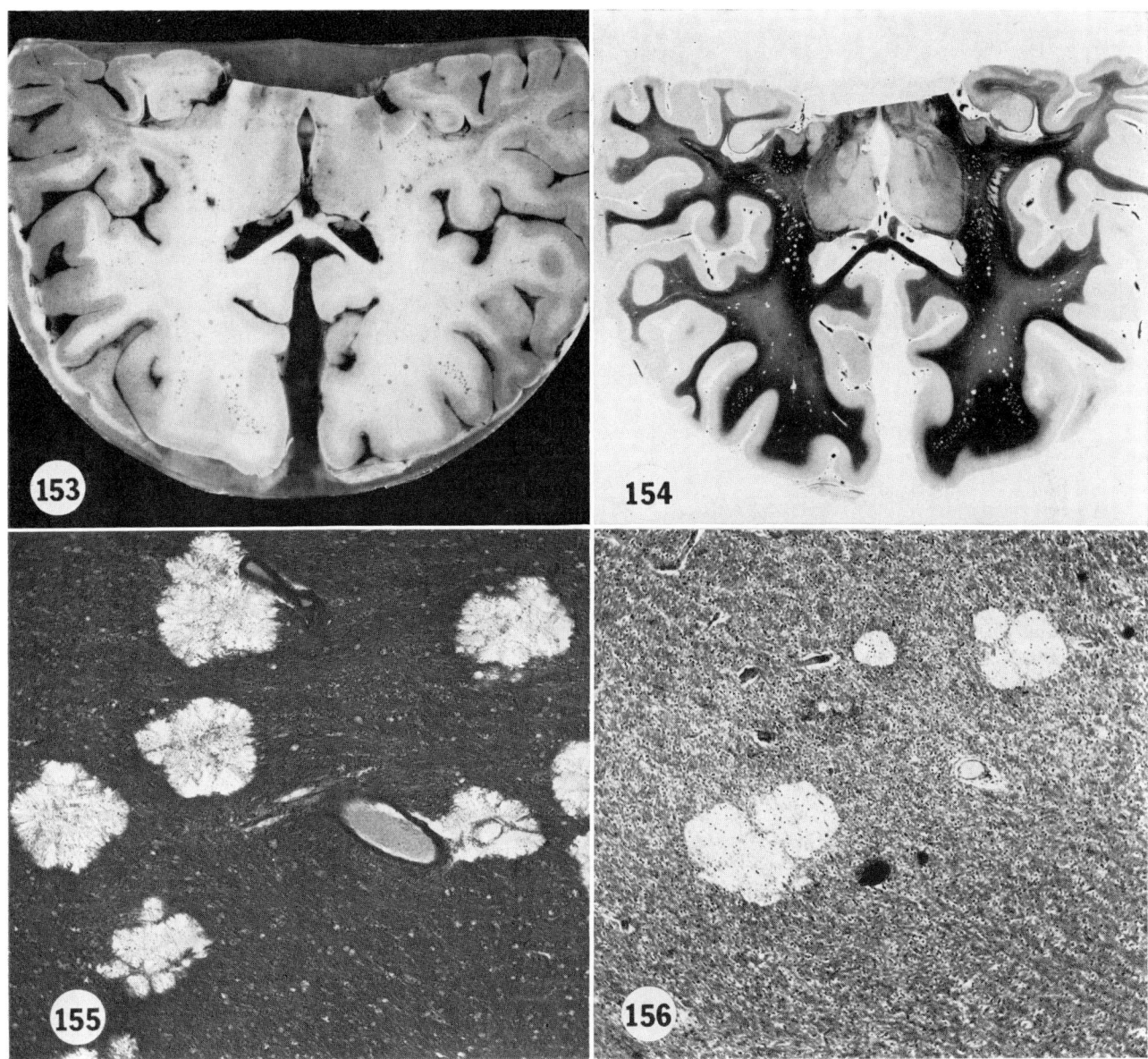

IV

Artifacts Resulting from Processing Procedures

INTRODUCTION

MANY OF THE ARTIFACTS which may be observed in microscopic tissue sections that are the result of processing procedures are the fault of the prosector in that tissue specimens were too thick to allow for adequate fixation or the time allowed for fixation of specimens of adequate thickness was too short. However, the fault for numerous artifacts resides with the individuals who grossed the fixed specimens prior to processing or selected inappropriate schedules for the processing of the tissues. In addition, some of the artifacts resulting from processing procedures are caused by malfunction of automatic tissue processors. Examples of such processing artifacts included in this chapter are:

- Inadequate period of fixation and its effect on clearing
- Denaturization due to inadequate fixation
- Transfer of mercurial sublimate crystals to formalin-fixed tissue
- Contamination of tissue during postfixation washing
- Contamination of tissue with talcum powder during trimming
- Contamination of bone by macrosawing
- Contamination of trimmed specimen with tissue debris
- Contamination of trimmed specimen with marking media for surface identification
- Dehydration during processing
- Residues of clearing fluids
- Inadequate dehydration
- Inadequate infiltration with paraffin
- Dehydration during paraffin infiltration
- Shrinkage of bone marrow during processing and paraffin infiltration

Figure 157. *Effect of Inadequate Fixation on Clearing.* This tissue section was prepared from a specimen of human skin which was exposed to neutral buffered 10% formalin for an inadequate period of time and was subsequently cleared in chloroform during processing. The net effect of poor fixation and clearing in chloroform is excessive shrinkage of the tissue components. (H&E, ×350) (AFIP Negative No. 72-13668)

Figure 158. *Effect of Inadequate Fixation on Clearing.* This tissue section was prepared from a specimen of human skin which was exposed to neutral buffered 10% formalin for an inadequate period of time and was subsequently cleared in xylene. The shrinkage of tissue components produced by xylene is considerably greater than the shrinkage produced by chloroform (compared with Figure 157). The shrinkage produced by clearing in xylene is proportional to the adequacy of fixation. The less adequate the fixation the greater the shrinkage induced by xylene. Very little shrinkage is expected upon clearing in either chloroform or xylene if the tissue has been adequately fixed. (H&E, ×575) (AFIP Negative No. 72-13667)

Figure 159. *Denaturization.* This paraffin-embedded tissue section of a curetted specimen from a human being depicts indistinct staining with hematoxylin and eosin which is due to denaturization as a result of improper fixation. The denatured portion of the section appears grayish-white in the photograph (see also Figures 160 and 161). (H&E, ×115) (AFIP Negative No. 73-11820)

Figure 160. *Denaturization.* This is a higher magnification of a portion of the tissue section depicted in Figure 159. Denaturizaton generally takes place in the clearing agents and/or during the process of infiltration with paraffin. Denatured tissue can be identified by uneven staining of the tissue section which is seen as grayish-white areas in the photograph. (H&E, ×305) (AFIP Negative No. 73-11821)

Figure 161. *Denaturization.* This is a higher magnification of a portion of the tissue section depicted in Figure 159 taken from an area which was not denaturized. Compare with Figure 160. (H&E, ×305) (AFIP Negative No. 73-11182)

Figure 162. *Mercurial Sublimate Crystals.* This is a paraffin-embedded tissue section of a specimen of the myocardium of a dog which was fixed in neutral buffered 10% formalin. It was processed in alcohols, clearing agents and infiltrated with paraffin which had previously been used for the processing of Zenker's-fixed tissue specimens (see also Chapter VIII). Anisotropic, brown to black, mercurial sublimate crystals, which had previously contaminated the processing solutions and wax, are scattered throughout the section. (H&E, partial polariscopy, ×120) (Contributed by Dr. W. L. Wooding)

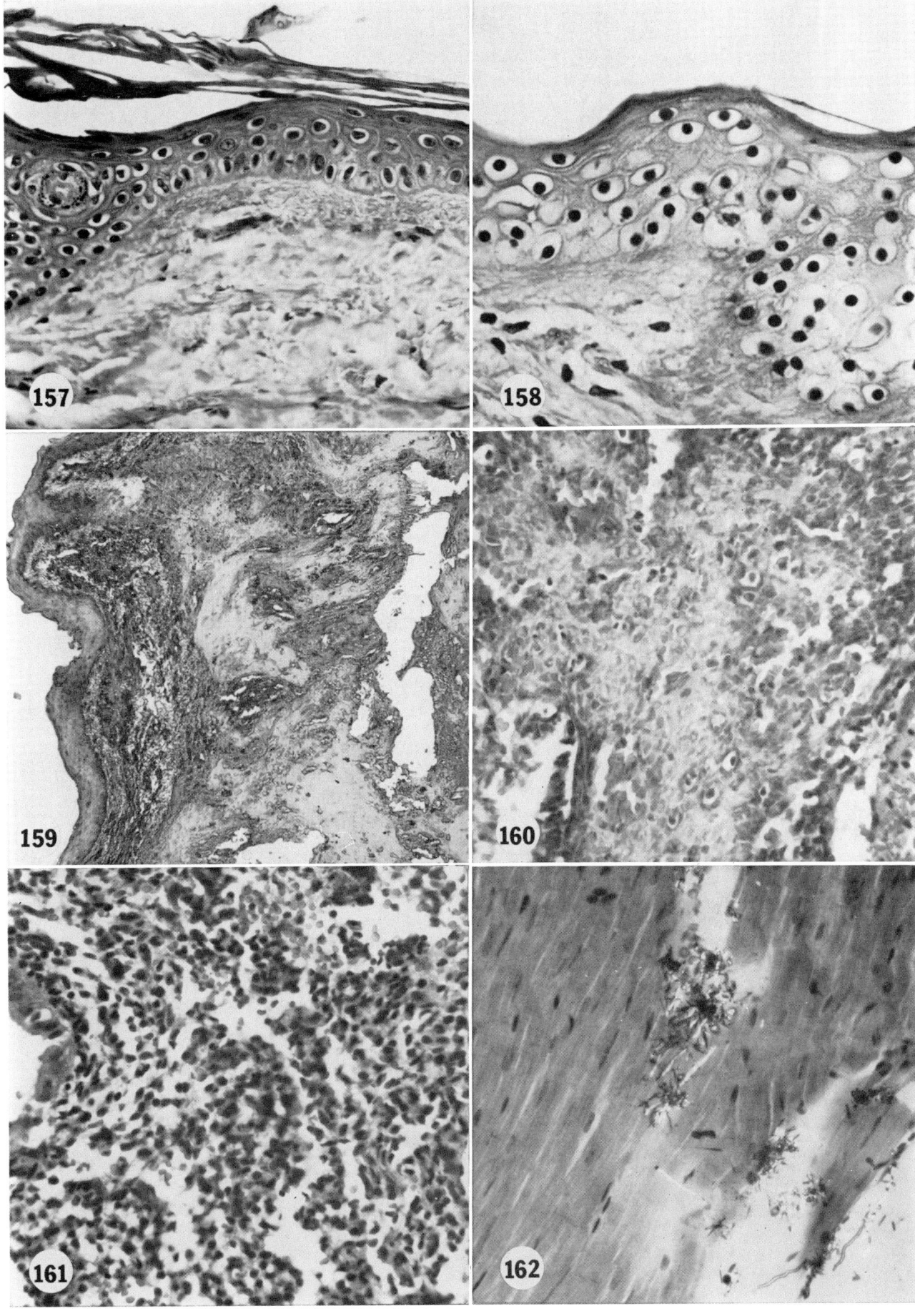

Figure 163. *Mercurial Sublimate Crystals.* In this formalin-fixed, paraffin-embedded tissue section of the liver of a rat numerous black particles are observed. Some are in the same focal plane as the cells within the field and appear to be extracellular. Other particles are not in the focal plane and appear to be out of focus and in some instances they appear to be intracellular. The tissue was processed in a vacuum tissue processor. Although the tissue was formalin-fixed, other specimens which were being processed, either prior to the processing of this specimen or concomitantly, in the same processor were fixed in a mercurial sublimate fixative. The particulate material seen in this tissue section is mercurial sublimate which impregnated the tissue under vacuum from contaminated tissue processing fluids. To correct such artifacts it is necessary to empty all fluid containers on the processor, thoroughly clean each such container and refill with fresh uncontaminated fluids. To prevent such artifacts one should refrain from using the same processor for processing formalin-fixed tissue and mercurial, sublimate-fixed tissue. (H&E, ×160) (Contributed by Mr. L. E. Schellhammer)

Figure 164. *Washing of Gross Specimens.* At times the water source used for the washing of tissue specimens has a high mineral content, particularly of iron. In such instances it is necessary to install a filter between the water source and the exit flow of water which is used for washing the tissue specimens. Such a filter is shown in this photograph.

Figure 165. *Washing of Gross Specimens.* Here a new filter cone from the device depicted in Figure 164 may be observed alongside a cone that has been used for forty-eight continuous hours. The used cone is darkened by the entrapment of impurities that were in the water which had been filtered through it. If this filter is placed in acidified ferrocyanide it will yield a positive Prussian blue reaction for iron. *Note:* Water with a high iron content may produce a positive Prussian blue reaction. The presence of iron in the water can be tested for by the following procedure: (1) fill a small glass container with the water to be tested; (2) discard the water and allow the container to dry; (3) pour 10 ml of acidified ferrocyanide (Gomori's iron reaction working solution) into the glass container and swirl solution in the container. A high iron content in the water will result in a positive Prussian blue reaction on the inside wall of the glass container.

Figure 166. *Washing of Gross Specimens.* After fixation and prior to further processing of tissue specimens, they are usually washed in running tap water to remove the excess of fixative fluids. The device shown here consists of a cold water pipe fitted with multiple faucets. Rubber tubing is fitted to the faucets, which is a common practice in many laboratories.

Figure 167. *Contamination of Specimens During Postfixation Washing.* At the left, artifacts can be noted within a tissue section of a specimen of skeletal muscle which was washed after fixation using a device similar to that which is depicted in Figure 166. The foreign material consists of slime (basophilic) from the rubber tubing which was fitted to the faucets of the washing device. At the right, there are similar fragments of slime which were isolated from the exit flow of water from the rubber tubing shown in Figure 166. This problem can be reduced considerably by the use of plastic tubing. (H&E, ×65) (AFIP Negative No. 73-4288-12)

Figure 168. *Contamination of Specimens During Postfixation Washing.* This tissue section was prepared from a specimen of human kidney which was washed after fixation using a device similar to that which is depicted in Figure 166. The foreign material consists of fragments of basophilic slime from the rubber tubing which was fitted to the faucets of the washing device. The distribution of the slime particles simulates the pattern of distribution of acid formalin hematin pigment (see Chapter III); however, slime particles are isotropic and basophilic. (H&E, ×100) (AFIP Negative No. 72-6170)

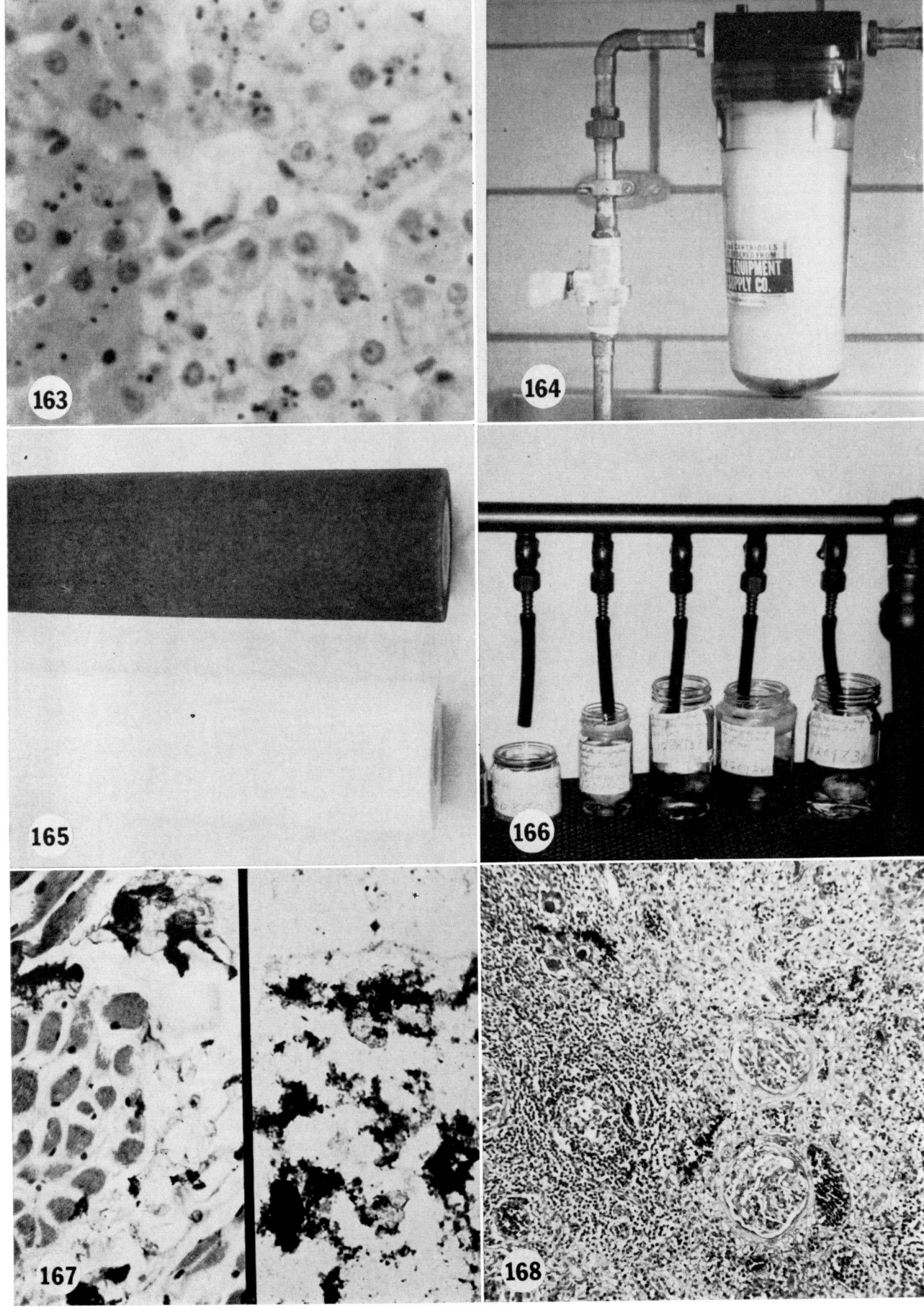

Figure 169. *Contamination of Specimens During Postfixation Washing.* This tissue section is from a specimen of canine kidney which was washed for twenty-four hours in unfiltered running tap water. It is stained by the Prussian blue reaction for iron. The water had a high mineral content and the specimen was contaminated with iron particulate matter, not only on its surface but also within its interstitial and vascular spaces which were penetrated by the running tap water. In conventionally stained tissue sections, this iron contaminate will appear as moderate to dark brown, extracellular, granular pigment. It will frequently be seen in the same focal plane as the cellular components of the microscopic field. It will resemble hemosiderin pigment, which can also occur extracellularly, and will yield a positive Prussian blue reaction for iron as depicted by the pigment within the glomerular tuft shown in this photograph. (Prussian blue reaction with a nuclear fast red counterstain, ×66) (Contributed by Mr. L. E. Schellhammer)

Figure 170. *Contamination of Specimens During Postfixation Washing.* This specimen of a rat's brain was washed in unfiltered tap water subsequent to formalin fixation and prior to processing (see Figures 164 and 165). The dark-colored, irregularly shaped, granular material seen at the center of the field is iron particulate matter which contaminated the specimen during the washing procedure. In this paraffin-embedded tissue section the artifact is not seen at the same focal plane as the tissue section (see Figure 169) since it was dislodged by the microtome knife during the cutting procedure. For this reason the artifact is observed above the focal plane of the tissue section per se, adjacent to its former site of deposition in a Virchow-Robin space. The artifact yields a positive Prussian blue reaction for iron (see also Figures 169, 171, and 172). (H&E, ×35) (Contributed by Dr. W. L. Wooding)

Figure 171. *Contamination of Specimens During Postfixation Washing.* This specimen of the pituitary gland of a rat was washed in unfiltered tap water subsequent to formalin fixation and prior to processing (see Figures 164 and 165). The dark-colored, irregularly shaped, granular material seen within the lumina or adjacent to sinusoids scattered throughout this paraffin-embedded tissue section is iron particulate matter which contaminated the specimen during the washing procedure. These artifacts yield a positive Prussian blue reaction for iron (see also Figures 169, 170, and 172) (H&E, ×35) (Contributed by Dr. W. L. Wooding)

Figure 172. *Contamination of Specimens During Postfixation Washing.* This is a higher magnification of the central portion of the tissue section depicted in Figure 171. The iron particulate matter is observed to be within the lumina of numerous vascular structures and in these locations it is in the same focal plane as the tissue section. However, numerous particles can also be seen which are above the focal plane of the tissue section per se, having been dislodged by the microtome knife during microtomy (see also Figure 170). All of the particulate matter yields a positive Prussian blue reaction for iron (see also Figures 169, 170, and 171). (H&E, ×175) (Contributed by Dr. W. L. Wooding)

Figure 173. *Talcum Powder.* In this tissue section of a specimen of perirenal adipose tissue from a rat, particles of talcum powder (starch and hydrous magnesium silicate) are present (see also Chapters I and II). This common artifact resulted from contamination of the fixed tissue specimen with dusting powder used in surgical gloves worn by the prosector during the trimming of the fixed gross specimen prior to processing and paraffin infiltration. As seen within tissue sections, the classic appearance is a hexagonal crystal. The crystal stains gray with hematoxylin and eosin as seen within this photomicrograph. It is periodic acid-Schiff-positive and stains green with Giemsa-type preparations. (H&E, ×70) (Contributed by Dr. W. L. Wooding)

Figure 174. *Talcum Powder.* This is the same tissue section as depicted in Figure 173 as seen by partial polariscopy. By polariscopy the crystal of talcum powder appears as a Maltese cross. These crystals pose no particular problem but are objectionable if seen in large numbers. This is especially true if the slide is to be photographed or if polariscopy is required for the identification of other crystalline materials. This artifact cannot be removed from tissue sections, and particular care should be taken during macrosectioning to eliminate its introduction during this procedure. (H&E, partial polariscopy, ×70) (Contributed by Dr. W. L. Wooding)

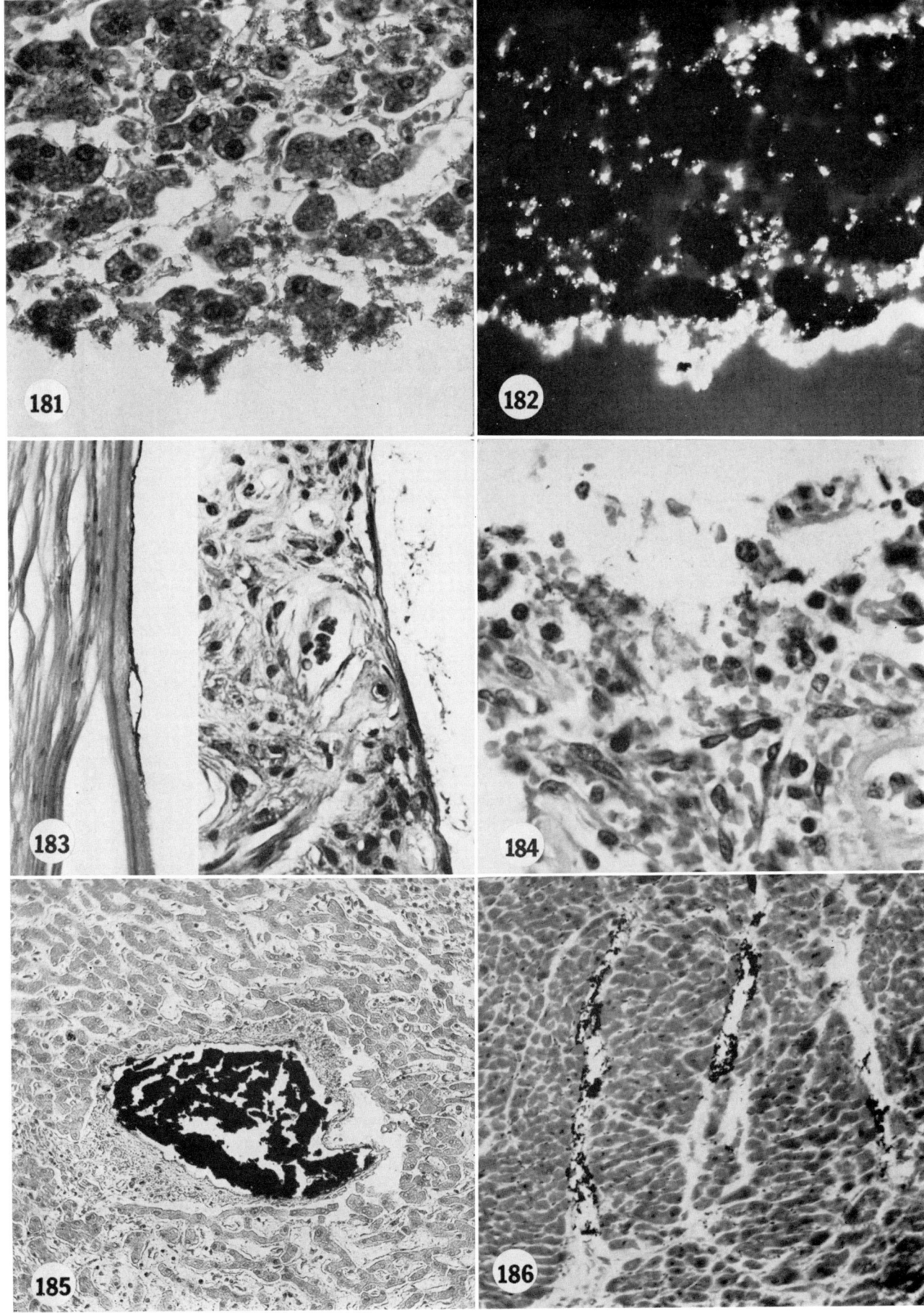

Figure 187. *Marking of Gross Specimens.* In the embedding of tissue specimens, it is a common practice to mark the specimen surface which is to be embedded, facing up, with India ink. If the marked surface of the specimen is porous or if an excess quantity of India ink is used, the ink may penetrate the tissue specimen. In this tissue section of a specimen of canine skeletal muscle, the black material seen within intracellular spaces is not a pigment. This artifact is India ink which was applied excessively to the specimen during the macrosectioning procedure prior to processing. The section was stained by the Prussian blue reaction for the demonstration of iron and the suspected pigment (India ink) yielded a negative reaction (see Color Plate 3, Figure 14). (Prussian blue reaction with a nuclear fast red counterstain, ×66)

Figure 188. *Tissue Processors.* A rather antiquated model of an automatic tissue processor is depicted in this photograph. The basic principle of most automatic tissue processors, even later models, is the same. The chromium basket shown at the top of the processor is used to automatically carry fixed tissue specimens through the different processing fluids. The processor is operated by a clock mechanism and at specified time intervals the machine automatically raises the chromium basket up out of one fluid and transfers it to the fluid in the adjacent beaker. If the machine is improperly adjusted or a power failure occurs, the basket may remain elevated during transfer and the tissue specimens may become dehydrated by exposure to air. As shown in this photograph, the solution containers are inadequately filled which would produce similar results. Such difficulties may develop even when manual processing is employed.

Figure 189. *Dehydration.* This is a tissue section of a specimen of human lung. The artifact observed here, as depicted at the top of the figure, resulted from dehydration by exposure of the tissue to air for prolonged periods of time during the tissue processing schedule due to inadequate filling of the solution containers of the tissue processor as shown in Figure 188. In the lower portion of the figure, vacuoles can be observed within interstitial cells which also resulted from dehydration during processing for paraffin embedding. (H&E, ×500) (AFIP Negative No. 73-4288-14)

Figure 190. *Dehydration.* This photograph illustrates a low- and high-power view of a tissue section of a specimen of unknown origin, which was overly dehydrated during processing because the tissue carrier malfunctioned and remained suspended between solution containers. The result is similar in appearance to the artifact depicted in Figure 189 although the means of producing the dehydration is different. The tissue section has a dry homogeneous appearance. (H&E ×100 & 500) (AFIP Negative No. 73-4288-13)

Figure 191. *Dehydration.* This tissue section of collagen was prepared from a specimen of human skin which was exposed to air for an excessive period of time during processing and infiltration with paraffin (see also Figures 189 and 190). The extreme dehydration which resulted is not dissimilar to dehydration of tissue by heat (thermal knife) during biopsy procedures as discussed in Chapter I. (H&E, ×130) (AFIP Negative No. 67-2643)

Figure 192. *Dehydration.* A "venetian blind" artifact is noted at the periphery of a tissue section and scratch marks within a paraffin-embedded tissue section of a specimen of unidentified tissue. The venetian blind effect at the periphery of the section is due to the fact that the tissue in the block of paraffin is harder than the surrounding tissue owing to overprocessing which resulted in excessive dehydration of the periphery of the specimen. As the knife passes through such a specimen, the tissue moves or vibrates within the paraffin, producing an artifact that is quite similar to artifacts produced with a loose knife or tissue block (see Chapter VI). The lengthwise scratches are produced by fragments of hard tissue from the periphery of the specimen being dragged through the section by the edge of the microtome knife. Soaking the surface of the block prior to sectioning will eliminate this problem. (H&E, ×11) (AFIP Negative No. 67-2658)

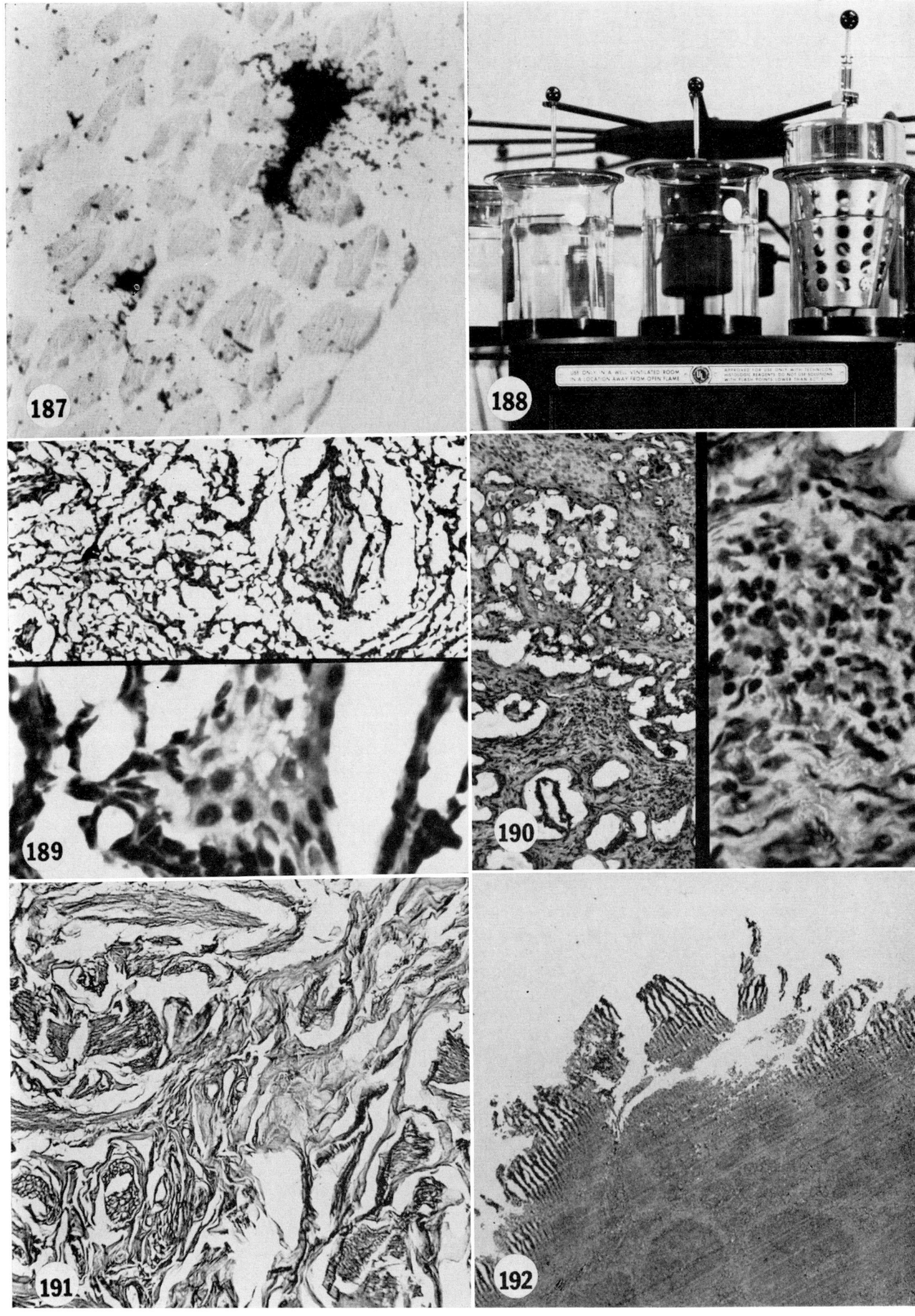

Figure 193. *Dehydration.* The moth-eaten effect observed in this tissue section of a paraffin-embedded specimen of the human liver resulted from overprocessing of the specimen prior to embedding. The specimen became excessively dehydrated during the prolonged processing. The moth-eaten effect is produced while rough-cutting (facing) the block of embedded tissue on the microtome. The dry (overly dehydrated) tissue chips out as the knife travels through the specimen. This artifact can be eliminated by soaking the block prior to cutting (see Chapter VI). (H&E, ×42) (AFIP Negative No. 72-7030)

Figure 194. *Wrinkled Tissue Sections.* Traces of processing or clearing fluids in the embedded block of tissue may result in a variety of defects in tissue sections. Even if one obtains a usable tissue section from such poorly processed tissue, the presence of such contaminants may cause difficulty in the mounting of the section on a microscope slide. Such residues may permit water to be imbibed by the tissue section thereby allowing it to swell slightly as depicted in this paraffin-embedded tissue section of the kidney of a rat. (H&E, ×40) (Contributed by Dr. W. L. Wooding)

Figure 195. *Wrinkled Tissue Sections.* This is a higher magnification of a portion of the tissue section depicted in Figure 194. Because of the residues of clearing fluids the tissue is hydrophilic. However, when placed on the tissue flotation water bath it could not expand in proportion to the amount of water it imbibed due to the fact that it was confined by strongly hydrophobic wax. The net result is that the tissue section becomes slightly wrinkled and retains such wrinkles even after being flattened on a waterbath or microscope slide. The wrinkles usually extend the width of the section and stain more intensely since the stain has access to both surfaces of the wrinkle. Such artifacts in the tissue section due to faulty processing cannot be corrected. If possible, such embedded specimens are best discarded, new tissue block should be selected from the fixed gross specimen and care should be taken that it is processed correctly. (H&E, ×170) (Contributed by Mr. L. E. Schellhammer)

Figure 196. *Inadequate Dehydration.* During tissue processing procedures, water must first be removed from the tissue specimen prior to paraffin infiltration. Water entrapped within the block of embedded tissue is usually the result of inadequate dehydration of the specimen prior to embedding. In such instances, the tissue embedded within the block of paraffin may be surrounded by a "halo." Each block of embedded tissue should be closely inspected prior to being mounted on the microtome and subsequent to "rough-cutting." If such a "halo" is noted, although tissue sections may be obtained they will look like this paraffin-embedded tissue section of a specimen of a rat kidney when they are stained. If a "halo" is noted in the block surrounding the tissue specimen, rather than waste effort in trying to obtain a satisfactory tissue section one should attempt to correct the defect prior to proceeding further in the preparation of the tissue section (see Figures 197 and 198). The most usual cause of inadequate dehydration during processing is due to failure to (1) keep the containers of processing solutions covered when not in use to prevent absorption of moisture or evaporation and/or (2) failure to change solutions frequently. The alcohols used in processing tissues lose their effectiveness as dehydrating agents as they become diluted by moisture from the atmosphere and tissues; and the clearing agents become saturated and ineffective. (H&E, ×40) (Contributed by Mr. L. E. Schellhammer)

Figure 197. *Inadequate Dehydration.* This is a higher magnification of a portion of the tissue section depicted in Figure 195 (see also Figure 198). The specimen was inadequately dehydrated during tissue processing. Since paraffin wax is strongly hydrophobic, inadequate dehydration of the specimen will prevent adequate infiltration of the specimen by wax. When such a specimen is subsequently embedded, residues of clearing agents in the inadequately dehydrated and infiltrated specimen will ooze from the specimen and contaminate the embedding paraffin adjacent to the specimen. These residues will result in large crystal size and pronounced crystallinity of the solidified paraffin adjacent to the embedded specimen producing a "halo" which can be seen macroscopically. As depicted in this photomicrograph, the irregularly stained areas were the only portions of the specimen which were dehydrated and infiltrated during processing. (H&E, ×70) (Contributed by Mr. L. E. Schellhammer)

Figure 198. *Inadequate Dehydration.* This is a higher magnification of a portion of the tissue section depicted in Figure 196. The nondescript unstained portions of the specimen were inadequately dehydrated and therefore were not infiltrated by the paraffin. The net effect seen in a stained tissue section is somewhat similar in appearance to a tissue section which has been inadequately decerated prior to staining (see Chapter VIII). However, the artifact depicted here cannot be corrected by exposing the tissue section to a fresh supply of xylene, and an improperly decerated section is not necessarily derived from a defective block of embedded tissue. If the effects of inadequate dehydration during processing are noted in the block of embedded tissue, or the finished tissue section, one can melt down the block and wash the tissue specimen in several changes of melted paraffin to remove the former paraffin. Subsequently, one may attempt to salvage the specimen by reprocessing. Such salvage procedures are more often met with failure than success but for a valuable specimen they are at least worth the attempt. (H&E, ×70) (Contributed by Mr. L. E. Schellhammer)

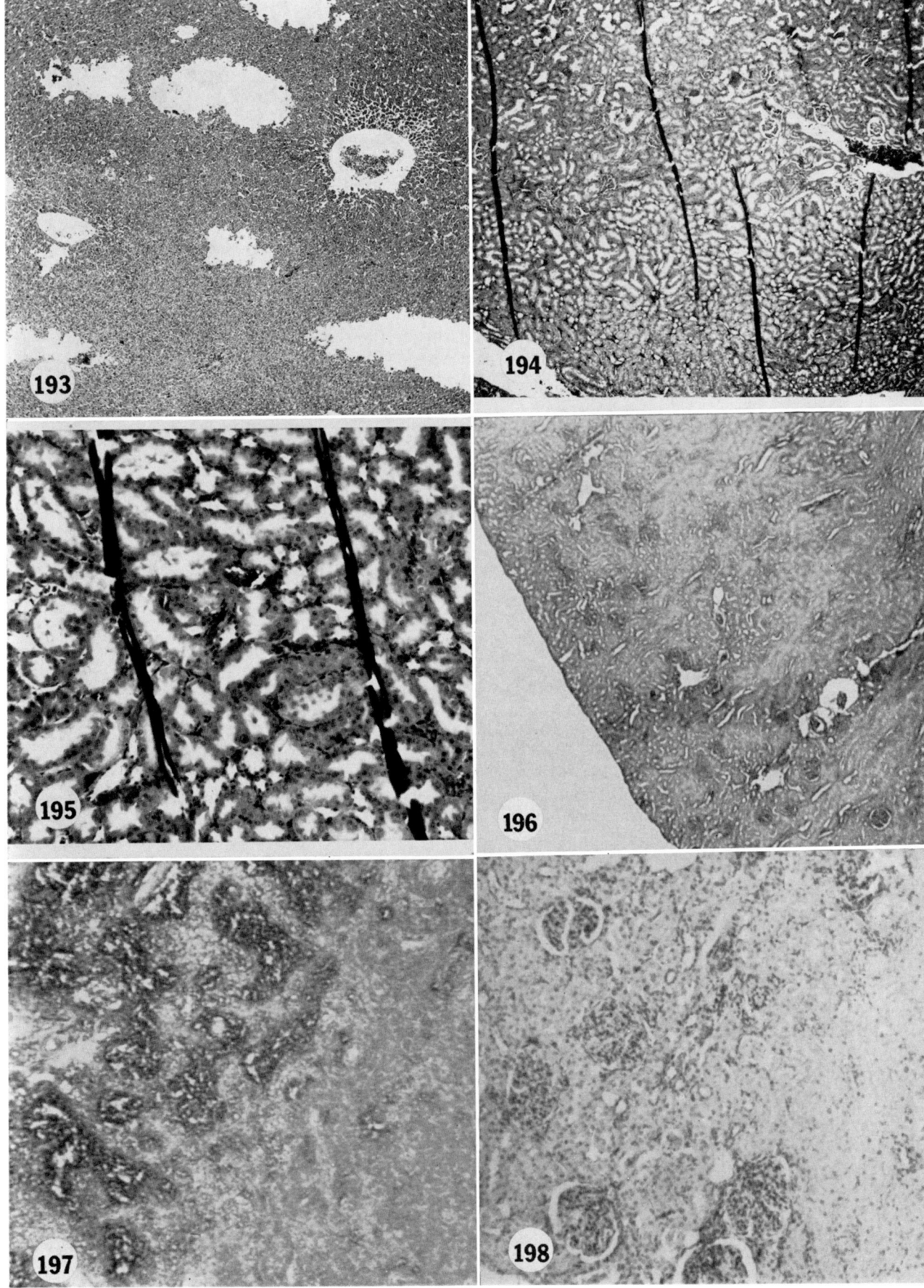

Figure 199. *Inadequate Infiltration with Paraffin.* This tissue section was prepared from a paraffin-embedded specimen of human cardiac muscle. The specimen was inadequately infiltrated with paraffin during tissue processing. When the tissue section was floated on a waterbath (see Chapter VI) it spread rapidly prior to being picked up on a glass microscope slide. A similar artifact can be produced with a properly infiltrated specimen if the water bath is too hot at the time the tissue section is floated (see Chapter VI). An improperly infiltrated paraffin-embedded tissue specimen may be identified by facing off the block (rough cut) on a microtome to expose the tissue and then applying a small, water-soaked piece of cotton to the faced surface. Tissue which has not been adequately impregnated will turn white. (H&E, ×3) (AFIP Negative No. 72-3730)

Figure 200. *Inadequate Infiltration with Paraffin.* The spreading artifact observed in this tissue section of a paraffin-embedded specimen of a human eye resulted from inadequate infiltration with paraffin during processing (see also Figure 199). There is separation of scleral structures and the cornea was similarly affected. This is a common artifact in ophthalmic pathology and its cause is the same as that described for Figure 199. (Phloxine-eosin and Mayer's hematoxylin, ×165) (AFIP Negative No. 71-12087)

Figure 201. *Inadequate Infiltration with Paraffin.* The spreading artifact observed in this tissue section of a paraffin-embedded specimen of human skin resulted from inadequate infiltration with paraffin during processing (see also Figures 199 and 200). The cause of this artifact is the same as that described for Figure 199. The artifact can be corrected by melting the paraffin block and reprocessing the specimen using an adequate processing schedule. *Note:* Inadequate infiltration of tissue may be the result of inadequate fixation, dehydration, or clearing but usually is due to insufficient time in the molten paraffin. (H&E, ×42) (AFIP Negative No. 72-5349)

Figure 202. *Inadequate Infiltration with Paraffin.* This highly distorted paraffin-embedded tissue section of a specimen of the large intestine of a human being is characteristic of what one sees if the specimen is improperly processed and/or inadequately infiltrated with paraffin at the end of the processing schedule. The tissue in the block was slightly shrunken prior to sectioning. When the surface of the embedded specimen was faced off during rough cutting on the microtome it turned white when exposed to lukewarm water (see Chapter VI) prior to fine sectioning. (H&E, ×3)

Figure 203. *Inadequate Infiltration with Paraffin.* This tissue section was made from the same specimen as depicted in Figure 202 after accomplishment of the following: The block of embedded tissue was melted and the specimen recovered; the recovered specimen was decerated in xylene and rehydrated in lukewarm water; it was then reprocessed through graded alcohols, chloroform, and infiltrated with paraffin (adequately); finally the reprocessed specimen was embedded in paraffin and subjected to microtomy. (H&E, ×3)

Figure 204. *Inadequate Infiltration with Paraffin.* Whenever wrinkles are observed running in various directions, as depicted in this photomicrograph of a paraffin-embedded tissue section of a specimen of a human kidney, it is usually indicative of inadequate infiltration of the specimen with embedding medium during processing. The most frequently encountered causes for wrinkled tissue sections are: (1) a dull knife, in which case the wrinkles tend to parallel the knife edge or (2) inadequate infiltration of the tissue with embedding medium. (H&E, ×35) (AFIP Negative No. 72-18036)

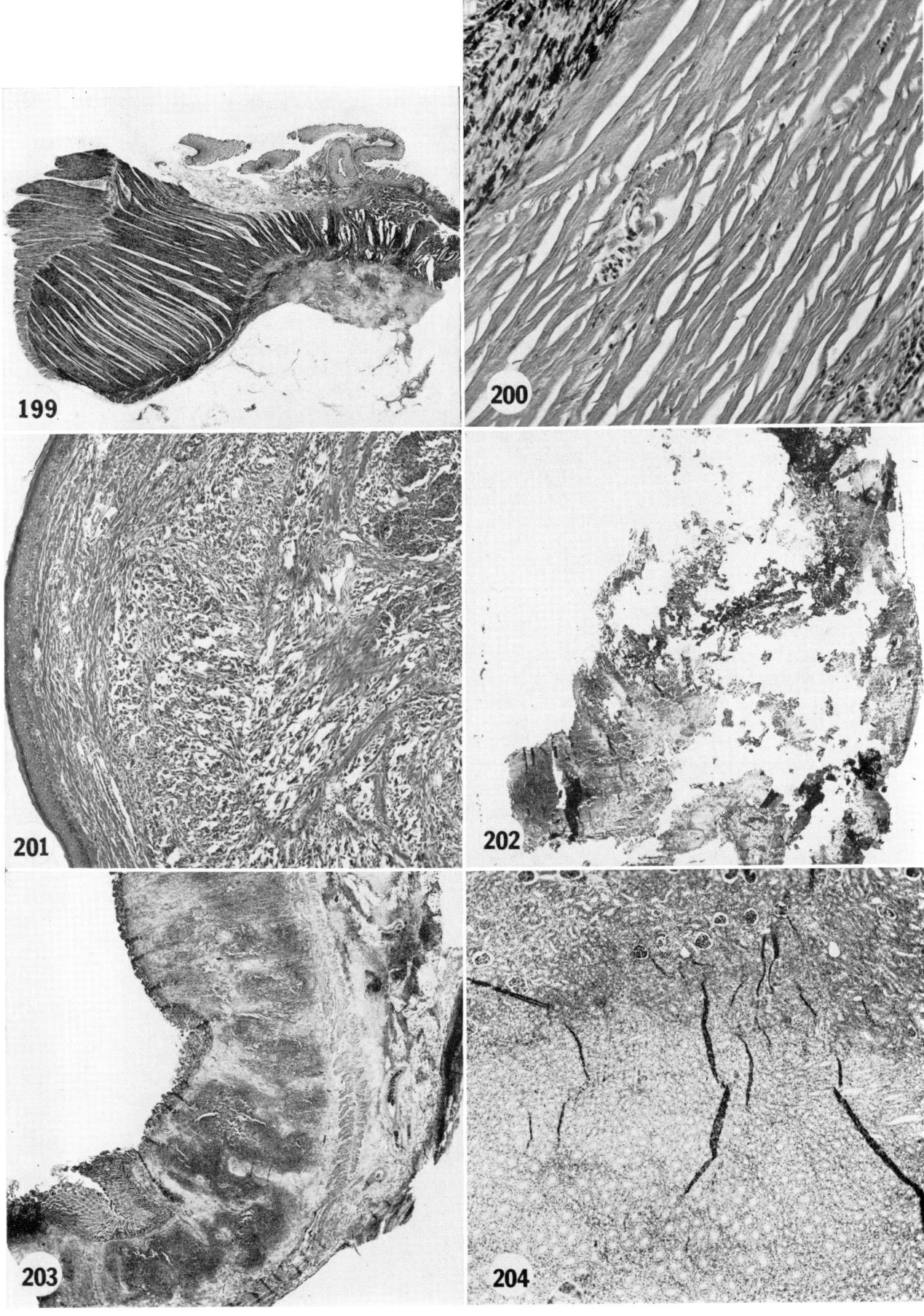

Figure 205. *Inadequate Infiltration with Paraffin.* The displaced (gouged) area seen in the dermis of this tissue section of a specimen of human skin resulted from inadequate infiltration of the specimen with paraffin during processing. Notice that only the area seen in the center of the photograph has been affected. The section cut very well which eliminated the possibility that the displaced collagen resulted from a dull microtome knife. Inadequate infiltration with paraffin can be detected by applying a piece of cotton which has been saturated with lukewarm water against the faced-off surface of the rough-cut block of embedded tissue. If the tissue is inadequately infiltrated with paraffin the faced-off surface of the embedded specimen will turn chalky white in color after fifteen to twenty seconds of exposure to the water-soaked cotton. (H&E, ×70) (AFIP Negative No. 73-3541)

Figure 206. *Inadequate Infiltration with Paraffin.* The moth-eaten effect noted in this paraffin-embedded tissue section of a specimen of splenic tissue from a human being can be produced by several faulty procedures in either tissue processing (see Figure 193) or microtomy (see Chapter VI). In addition to the causes described in the legends for the cited figure, if the specimen is incompletely infiltrated with paraffin prior to being embedded it will contain soft, spongy areas which will cause a variety of defects in the tissue sections. One of the defects that may result is that the soft, spongy areas fall or are pushed out of the tissue section as it is being cut resulting in holes in the tissue section and producing the moth-eaten effect. (H&E, ×70) (AFIP Negative No. 73-4136)

Figure 207. *Inadequate Infiltration with Paraffin.* This paraffin-embedded tissue section was prepared from a specimen of a human rib which was decalcified and processed through an automatic tissue processor in the conventional manner. The extensive distortion seen in the section is due to inadequate infiltration of the marrow spaces with paraffin. (H&E, ×8) (AFIP Negative No. 73-4274)

Figure 208. *Inadequate Infiltration with Paraffin.* This is a higher magnification of the central portion of the tissue section depicted in Figure 207. Note the radical displacement of the bone marrow and fracture of some of the trabeculae. Utilization of a vacuum oven during paraffin infiltration subsequent to processing would have obviated such an artifact. Compare with Figure 209. (H&E, ×35) (AFIP Negative No. 73-4275)

Figure 209. *Inadequate Infiltration with Paraffin.* This paraffin-embedded tissue section was prepared from a specimen of the same human rib as depicted in Figure 208. It was decalcified and processed through an automatic tissue processor and infiltrated with paraffin under vacuum. Compare with Figure 208. (H&E, ×8) (AFIP Negative No. 73-4273)

Figure 210. *Inadequate Infiltration with Paraffin.* This is a higher magnification of the central portion of the tissue section depicted in Figure 208. It illustrates the benefit of utilizing a vacuum oven during infiltration with paraffin subsequent to processing tissues which are difficult to infiltrate in the conventional manner. The small vacuoles seen in the marrow are the former sites of fat deposits. Compare with Figure 209. (H&E, ×35) (AFIP Negative No. 73-4276)

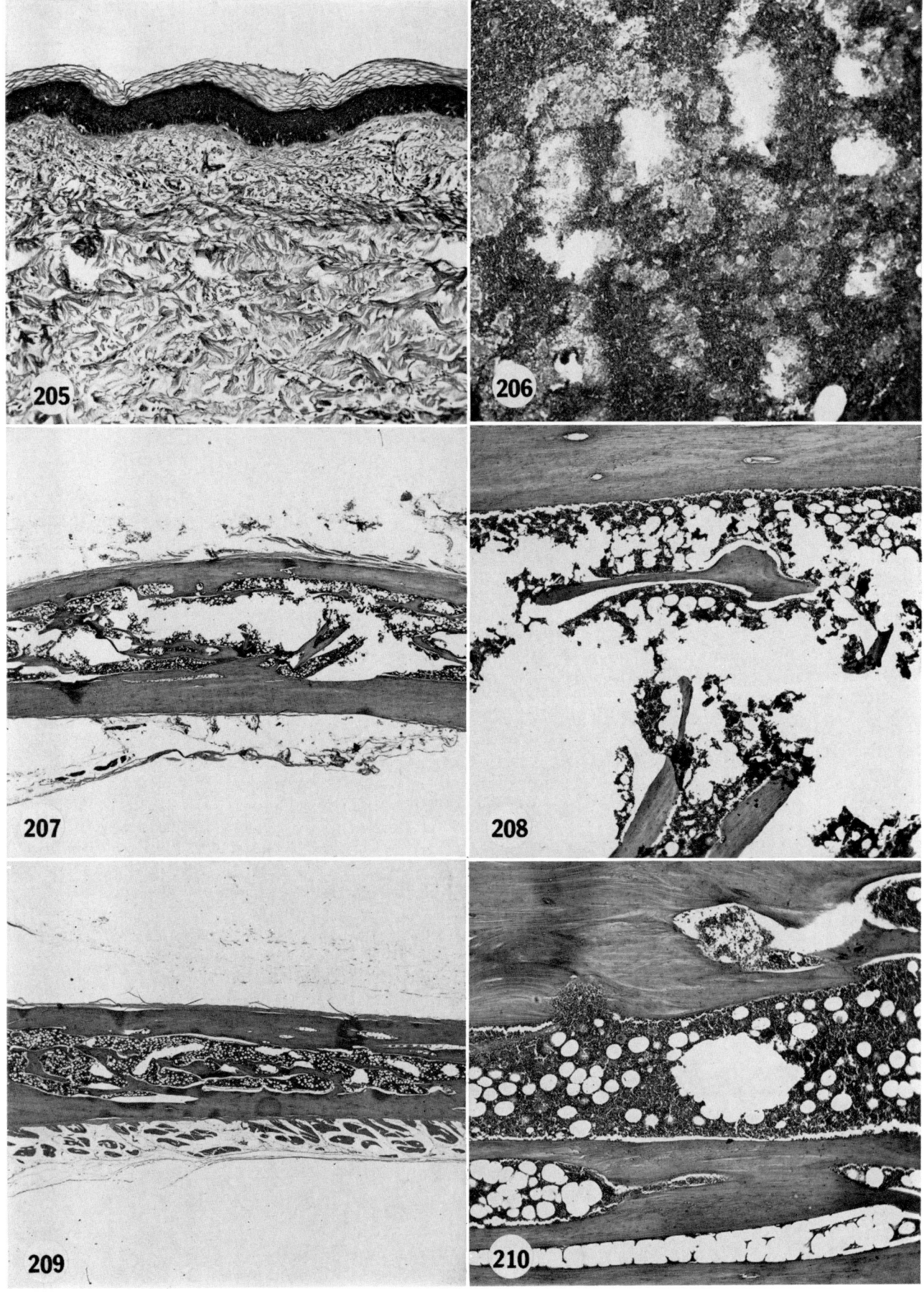

Figure 211. *Dehydration Due to Heat.* The dark-staining material at the periphery of this paraffin-embedded tissue section of a specimen of a mammary gland of a human being is a zone of burned tissue. The burn (dehydration by heat) resulted from exposure of the specimen to excessive heat during processing in an automatic tissue processor. (Modified Verhoeff's elastica stain, ×4) (AFIP Negative No. 73-4272)

Figure 212. *Dehydration Due to Heat.* This is a higher magnification of a portion of the field depicted in Figure 211. The tinctorial qualities, and the clear delineation between burned and normal tissue, which are obtainable with the modified Verhoeff's elastica stain are well illustrated. This procedure can be found in the article by Hinshaw, J. R. and Pierce, H. E. (*Surg Gyn Obstet, 103*:726-730, 1956). (Modified Verhoeff's elastica stain, ×42) (AFIP Negative No. 73-4267)

Figure 213. *Dehydration Due to Heat.* This is a higher magnification of a different portion of the field depicted in Figure 211 than shown in Figure 212. Numerous vacuoles are seen in the burned zone stained by the modified Verhoeff's elastic stain. The vacuoles are also characteristic of an artifact which can result from the freezing of tissue specimens (see Chapters II and III). If extensive work is contemplated in the staining of burned tissue, one should consult the article cited in the legend for Figure 212 since other methods are presented which may prove to be more desirable for a particular problem than the one depicted in Figures 211 and 212. (Modified Verhoeff's elastica stain, ×42) (AFIP Negative No. 73-4268)

Figure 214. *Dehydration Due to Heat.* This is a paraffin-embedded tissue section of a specimen of a kidney of a human being. The specimen was allowed to remain in excessively hot paraffin baths during processing, which resulted in the burning of the tissue. Much of the chromatic properties and good cellular morphology of the specimen was destroyed. The large blood vessel on the right depicts the characteristics of burned tissue as seen microscopically in that the erythrocytes within its lumen appear to be homogenous and are gray to greenish-yellow in their chromatic appearance (see Color Plate 3, Figure 15). It is not unusual to see this effect throughout an entire tissue section depending on the size of the specimen and the length of time it was exposed to excessively hot paraffin. The gray to greenish-yellow coloration seen in tissue sections of specimens which have been cooked in molten paraffin is never present in sections of specimens which have been dehydrated by freezing. This variable can be used to differentiate the two artifacts. (H&E, ×100) (AFIP Negative No. 73-4277)

Figure 215. *Shrinkage of Bone Marrow.* This photograph of a paraffin-embedded tissue section of a human specimen of bone and bone marrow illustrates one of the problems which occurs with the paraffin-embedding of bone marrow due to exposure of the tissue specimen to decalcifying fluids, dehydrating, and clearing agents and molten paraffin during processing. It is impossible to prevent such shrinkage artifacts when one uses paraffin-embedding techniques (see also Figure 216). (Hematoxylin-phloxine-saffron, ×115) (AFIP Negative No. 73-6303)

Figure 216. *Shrinkage of Bone Marrow.* This is another portion of the same tissue section as depicted in Figure 215. One of the primary uses of celloidin as an embedding medium is to prevent the bone marrow from shrinking away from its supporting bone trabeculi. The shrinkage artifact observed in this paraffin-embedded specimen of bone marrow and bone can be avoided by using the time-consuming celloidin-embedding technique. (Hematoxylin-phloxine-saffron, ×115) (AFIP Negative No. 73-6309)

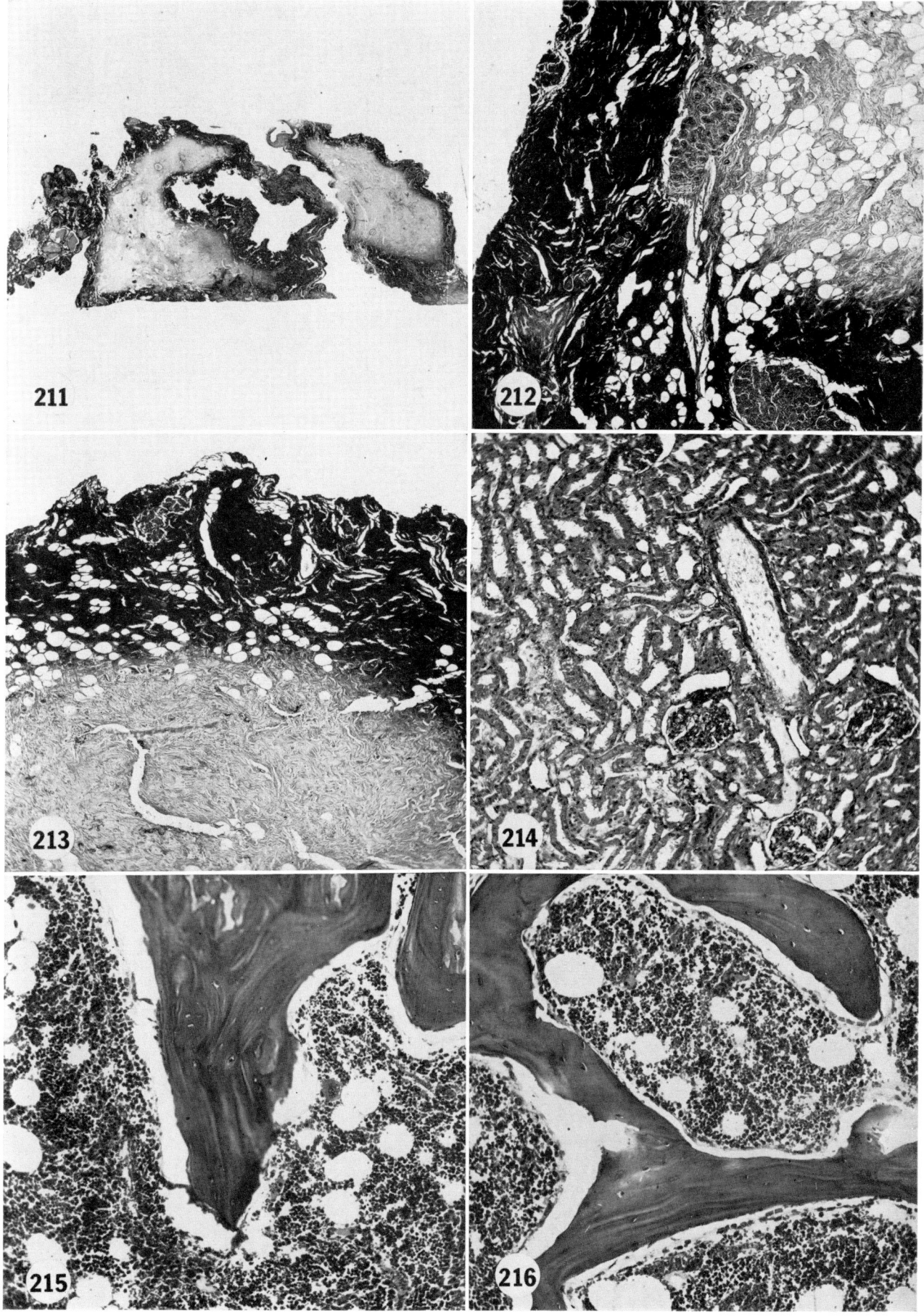

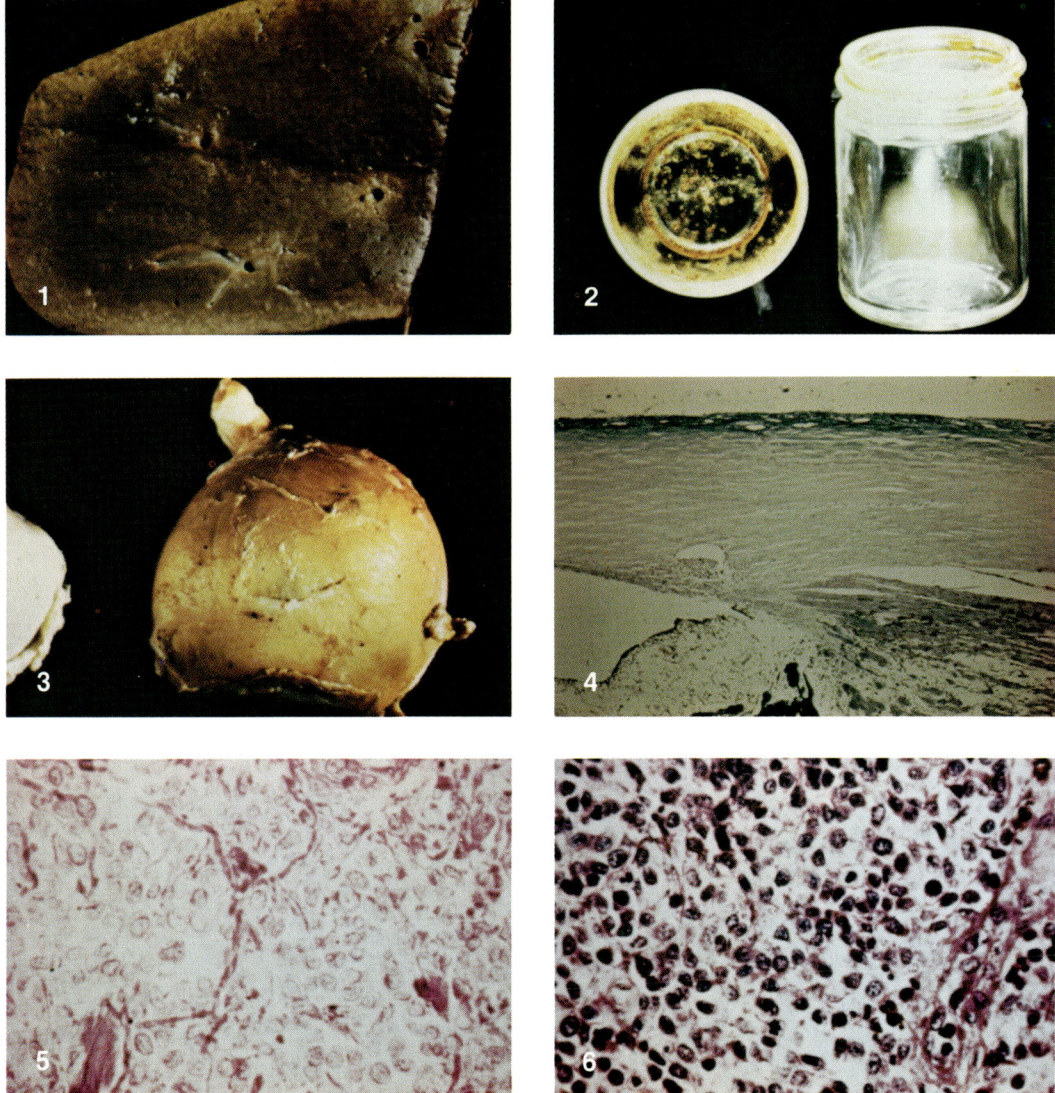

Figure 1. *Inadequate Fixation* (see Figure 57, Chapter III). This specimen of human liver tissue was fixed in formalin and fixation was inadequate because the specimen was too thick (greater than 6 mm). Only the tan-colored periphery and zones around the branches of the portal vein are fixed, forming a shell of firm tissue surrounding the central reddish-brown mass of autolyzed tissue.

Figure 2. *Oxidation Contaminants* (see Figure 63, Chapter III). Fixatives such as formalin will rust metal caps used as closures for fixative containers. The yellowish-brown material seen on the cap at the left is rust. Particles of rust contaminated the fixative within the bottle seen at the right. The bluish haze seen on the internal wall of the container is a positive Prussian blue reaction denoting the presence of iron.

Figure 3. *Oxidation Contaminants* (see Figure 64, Chapter III). The specimen of the human eye depicted here was fixed in the container shown in Figure 2. The external surface of the specimen is discolored (reddish-brown) due to the deposition of rust particles derived from the rusty metal cap of the fixative container. (AFIP Negative No. 62-6179).

Figure 4. *Oxidation Contaminants* (see Figure 65, Chapter III). The material observed on and in the corneal tissue at the top of the photograph, which is stained blue by the Prussian blue reaction, represents rust contaminants derived from the rusty metal cap of the fixative container shown in Figure 2. This tissue section is from the eye specimen shown in Figure 3. (Prussian blue reaction for iron, X40)

Figure 5. *Zenker's Overfixation* (see Figure 84, Chapter III). Overexposure to Zenker's fluid for longer than eight hours produces acidophilia and a loss of basophilia as depicted in this tissue section of a specimen of human splenic tissue. Note the lack of staining with hematoxylin. (H&E, X250) (AFIP Negative No. 71-12159-2)

Figure 6. *Zenker's Overfixation* (see Figure 85, Chapter III). The basophilia of tissue sections prepared from specimens of tissue that have been overexposed to Zenker's fluid can usually be restored. This is a duplicate tissue section of the section depicted in Figure 5. It was decerated and treated with iodine and sodium thiosulfate (see Chapter III). It was then placed in 10% aqueous sodium bicarbonate for six to eight hours and was subsequently placed in running tap water for ten minutes prior to being stained with hematoxylin and eosin. (H&E, X250) (AFIP Negative No. 71-12159-4)

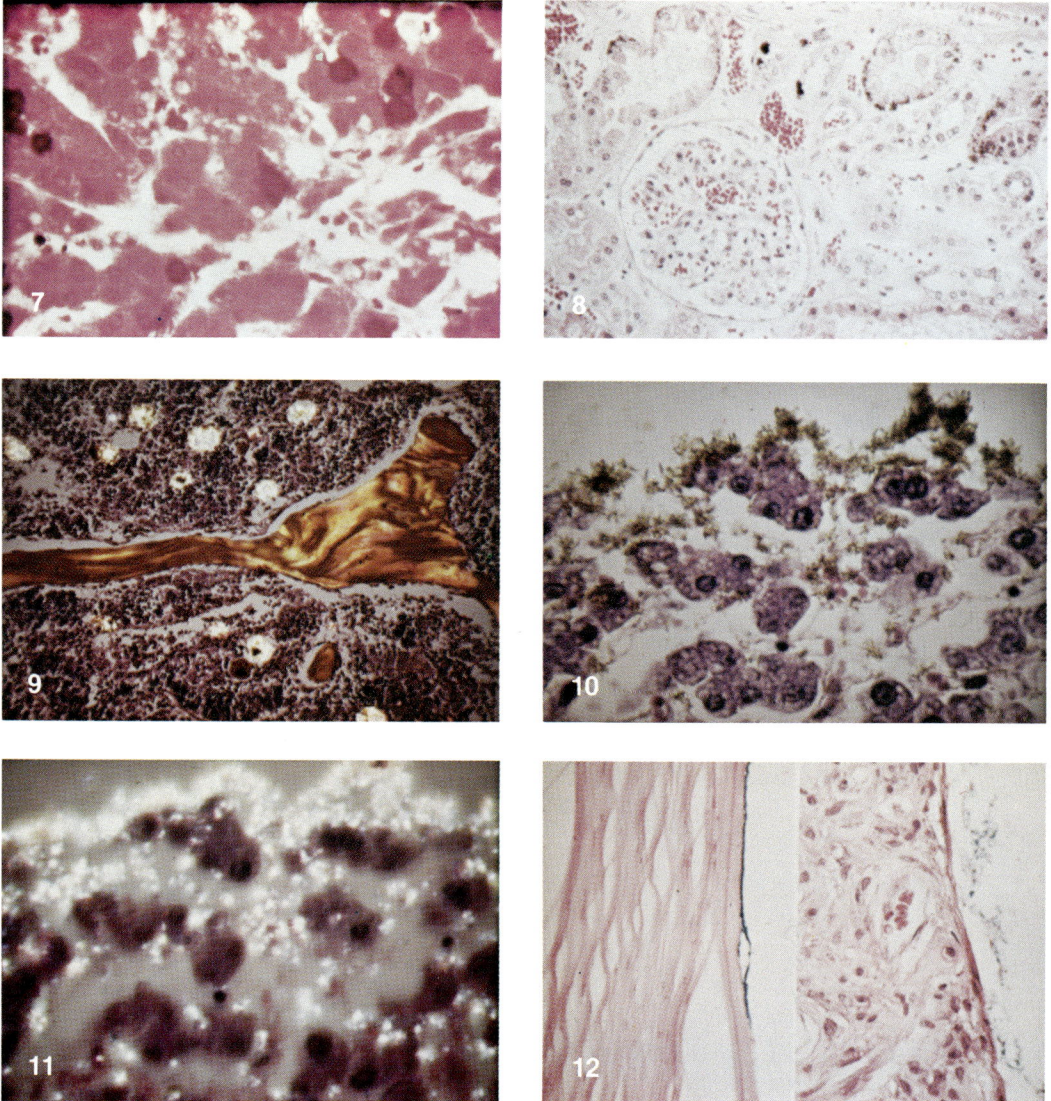

Figure 7. *Zenker's Overfixation* (see Figure 86, Chapter III). The specimen of human liver tissue from which this tissue section was derived was exposed to Zenker's fluid for longer than eight hours. The dark red blotches are caused by failure to remove mercuric chloride crystals by pretreatment of the tissue section with iodine and sodium thiosulfate (see Chapter III). The loss of basophilia can be restored by pretreatment with sodium bicarbonate and running tap water as described in the legend for Figure 6. However, prolonged exposure of tissue to Zenker's fluid also hardens tissue excessively and has resulted in the separation of the hepatocytes and this particular artifact cannot be corrected. (H&E, X305) (AFIP Negative No. 73-4281)

Figure 8. *Acid Formalin Hematin Pigment* (see Figure 131, Chapter III). Acid formalin hematin pigment is produced within fixed tissue specimens by the reaction of formic acid and the heme of hemoglobin at an acid pH. In this tissue section of a specimen of human kidney which was fixed in acid (unbuffered) formalin, the pigment is observed as brownish-black granules on the walls of tubules and on erythrocytes within the lumina of blood vessels. (H&E, X130) (AFIP Negative No. 72-4768)

Figure 9. *Acid Formalin Hematin Pigment* (see Figure 139, Chapter III). It is not uncommon to find anisotrophic acid formalin hematin pigment in the vacuoles remaining from fat cells after the fat has been dissolved by dehydrating and clearing agents in the processing of tissue fixed in acid (unbuffered) formalin. In this tissue section of human bone marrow, as viewed by partial polariscopy, the bluish white foci are clusters of anisotropic acid formalin hematin pigment. Due to the partial polariscopy a few brownish-black granules can be discerned in the center of several clusters of the pigment. Acid formalin hematin pigment is not deposited in tissues fixed in neutral buffered formalin. (Hematoxylin-phloxine-saffron, X80) (AFIP Negative No. 73-6305)

Figure 10. *Marking of Gross Specimens* (see Figure 181, Chapter IV). The yellowish-brown rhombic crystals observed on the surface and adjacent parenchyma of this paraffin-embedded tissue section of a specimen of a human liver area silver nitrate crystals. These crystals were derived from silver nitrate applicators which were used to mark the specimen surface which was to be embedded facing up. (H&E, X350) (AFIP Negative No. 72-7025)

Figure 11. *Marking of Gross Specimens* (see Figure 18182, Chapter IV). This is the same tissue section as depicted in Figure 10 as viewed by partial polariscopy to demonstrate the strong anisotropism of the rhombic silver nitrate crystals. As more dramatically shown here, if the marked surface of the specimen is porous or if an excess of silver is used, the silver nitrate may penetrate the tissue specimen. (H&E, X350) (AFIP Negative No. 72-7025)

Figure 12. *Marking of Gross Specimens* (see Figure 183, Chapter IV). In some laboratories, it is common practice to mark pathologic sites and/or specific surfaces of a specimen with a Linton-Vita® color (blue) pencil. This relatively hard pencil deposits a blue pigment on the specimen which can be identified microscopically. In these tissue sections of a human eye, the blue pigment can be seen above the tissue specimen at the right and on the corneal surface at the left. (H&E, X100) (AFIP Negative No. 73-5051-3)

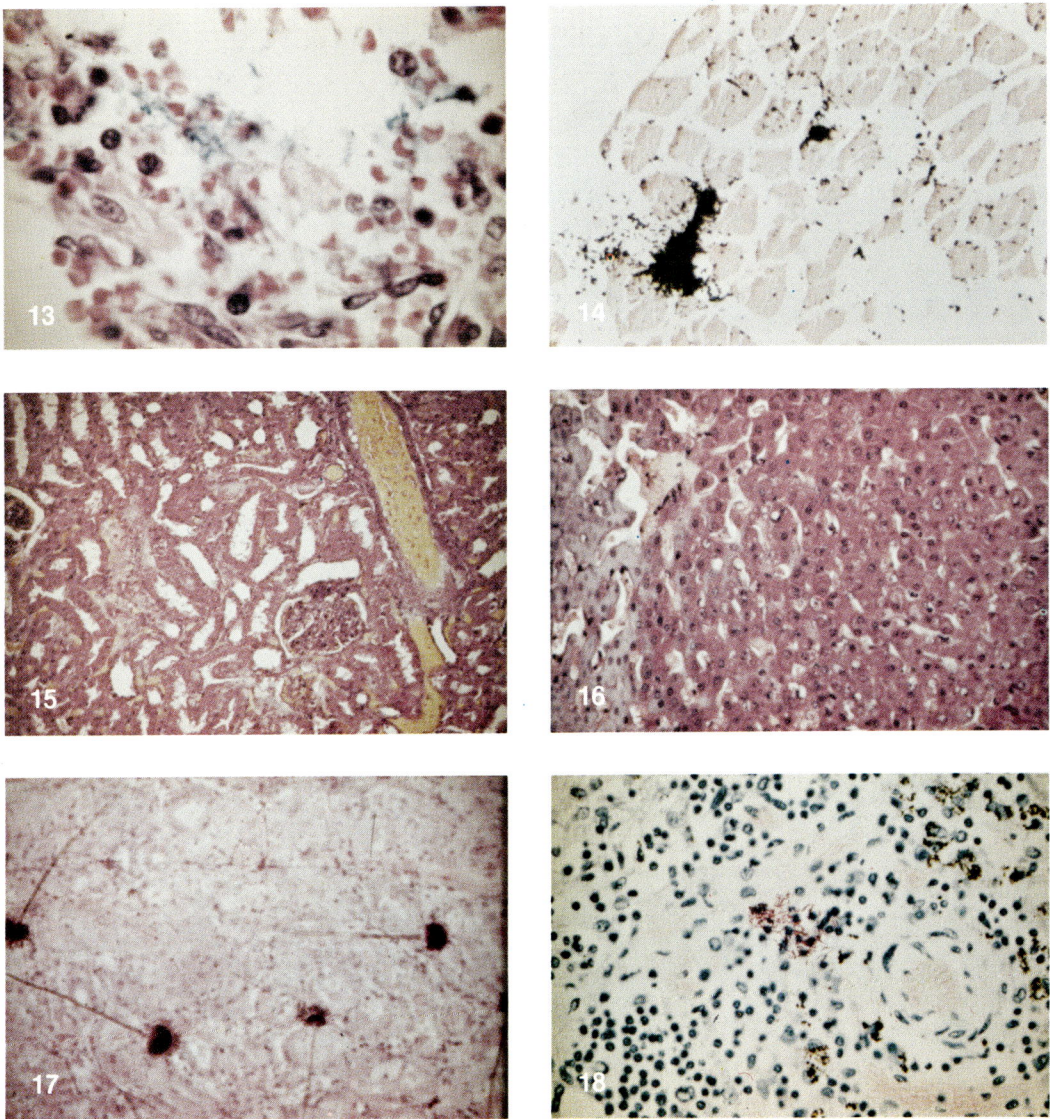

Figure 13. *Marking of Gross Specimens* (see Figure 184, Chapter IV). This is a higher magnification of the central portion of the microscopic field depicted on the right of Figure 12. Some of the blue pigment of the Linton-Vita color pencil which was used to identify the gross site of a lesion has penetrated into the interstitium of the lesion during the processing and embedding of the specimen. (H&E, X600) (AFIP Negative No. 73-3927)

Figure 14. *Marking of Gross Specimens* (see Figure 187, Chapter IV). In this tissue section of a specimen of canine skeletal muscle, the light to dark brown material seen within intracellular spaces is not a pigment. This artifact is India ink which was applied excessively to the surface of the specimen during the macrosectioning procedure, to identify the surface to be embedded facing up, prior to processing. The deposits of India ink are iron-negative. (Prussian blue reaction with a nuclear fast red counterstain, X66)

Figure 15. *Dehydration Due to Heat* (see Figure 214, Chapter IV). The specimen of a kidney of a human being from which this tissue section was prepared was allowed to remain in excessively hot paraffin baths during processing which resulted in the burning of the tissue. Much of the chromatic properties and good cellular morphology of the specimen was destroyed. The large blood vessel on the right depicts the characteristics of burned tissue as seen microscopically in that the erythrocytes within its lumen appear to be homogenous and are greenish-yellow in their chromatic appearance. (H&E, X100) AFIP Negative No. 73-4277)

Figure 16. *Dehydration* (see Figure 222, Chapter V). This tissue section was prepared from a specimen of human liver which was embedded in paraffin that was held at too high a temperature during the embedding procedure. The artifact seen at the left is a subcapsular zone of coagulated liver, produced by cooking in hot molten paraffin, which stains bluish-gray and yellow with hematoxylin and eosin. (H&E, X145) (AFIP Negative No. 72-7029)

Figure 17. *Mold Contaminants on Glass Microscope Slides* (see Figure 270, Chapter VII). This photograph depicts a paraffin-embedded tissue section of a specimen of human kidney which had been mounted on a glass microscope slide that had been obtained from a box which had mildew growing on its external surface (see Figure 267, Chapter VII). The mold had contaminated the surfaces of the glass slide. The microscope is focused on the surface of the slide beneath the tissue section to more clearly reveal the basophilic and periodic acid-Schiff-positive mold contaminants. (Periodic acid-Schiff reaction, X115) (AFIP Negative No. 72-6163)

Figure 18. *Bacterial Contaminants* (see Figure 275, Chapter VII). The acid-fast, rod-shaped structures seen in the center of this tissue section of a specimen of human splenic tissue are contaminants derived from the tissue flotation waterbath. Such waterbath contaminants simulate acid-fast bacilli in both morphology and staining characteristics. (Kinyon's acid-fast stain, X80) (AFIP Negative No. 67-8645)

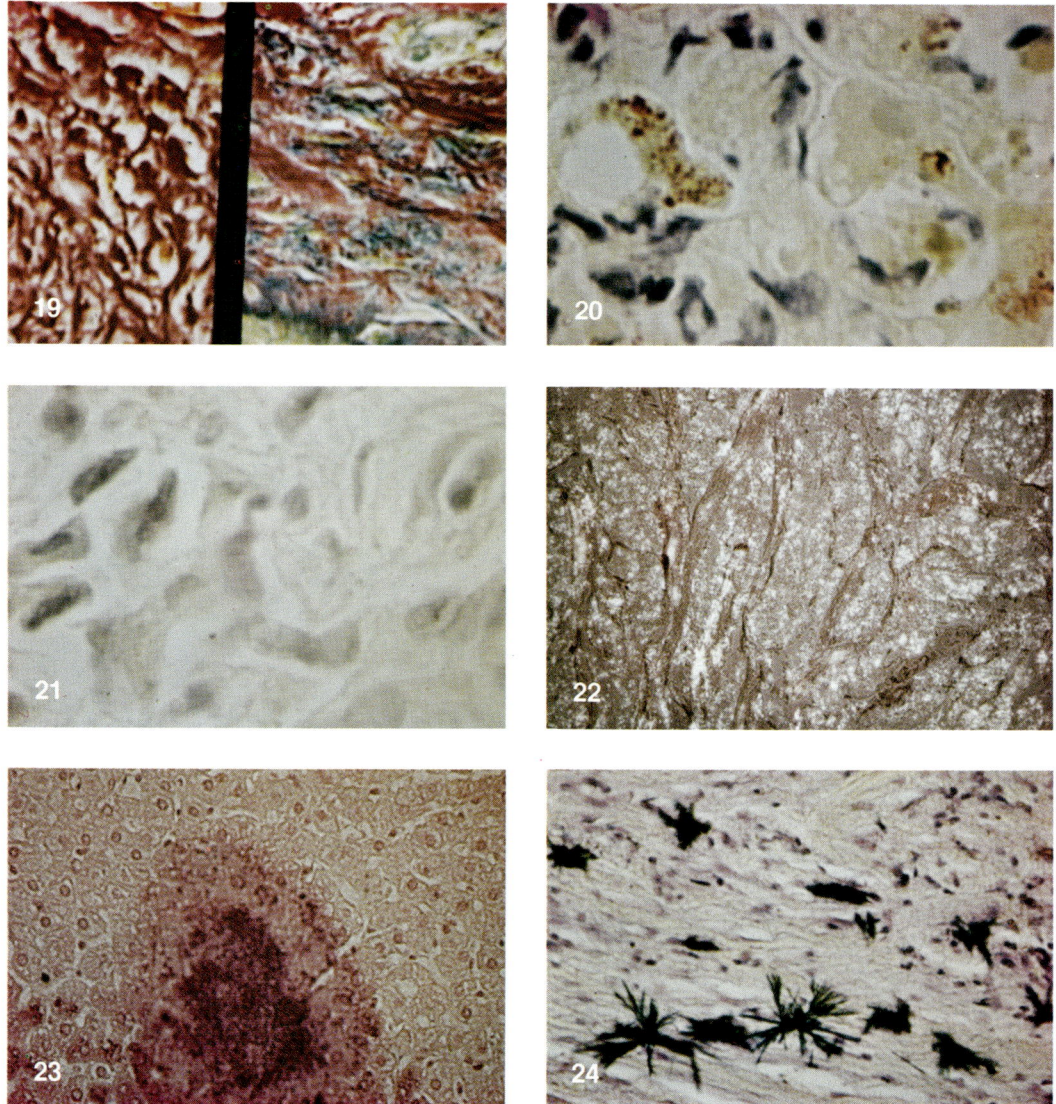

Figure 19. *Effect of Fixation on Colloidal Iron Staining* (see Figure 305, Chapter VIII). These tissue sections were prepared from duplicate specimens of human skin. The specimen on the left was fixed in Bouin's fluid and the one on the right was fixed in neutral buffered 10% formalin. A modification of Hale's colloidal iron stain, which stains acid mucopolysaccharides blue, was applied to the tissue sections prepared from each specimen. The section of formalin-fixed tissue at the right yields a positive colloidal iron staining reaction. Since acid mucopolysaccharides are not demonstrable by the colloidal iron stain in tissues fixed in Bouin's fluid, the section at the left yields a negative colloidal iron staining reaction. (Colloidal iron stain, X145) (AFIP Negative No. 71-12159-1)

Figure 20. *Effect of Fixation on the p-Dimethylaminobenzylidene Rhodanine Stain for Copper* (see Figure 307, Chapter VIII). As depicted in this paraffin-embedded tissue section of a specimen of liver, fixed in neutral buffered 10% formalin, from a human being with hepatolenticular degeneration, the granular precipitates of copper yield a red- or gold-colored reaction product. High concentrations of copper yield a red colored reaction product and low concentrations yield a gold-colored reaction product. (Rhodanine, X575) (AFIP Negative No. 72-5667)

Figure 21. *Effect of Fixation on the p-Dimethylaminebenzylidene Rhodanine Stain for Copper* (see Figure 308, Chapter VIII). This tissue section was prepared from a specimen of the same liver as depicted in Figure 20 with the exception that it was fixed in unbuffered formalin. It was stored in unbuffered formalin for six months prior to being processed and embedded. The tissue section yielded a negative reaction for copper when subjected to the p-dimethylaminebenzylidene rhodanine stain. (Rhodanine, X575) (AFIP Negative No. 72-7022)

Figure 22. *Deceration* (see Figure 319, Chapter VIII). The anisotropic bluish-white material demonstrated in and on this tissue section of a specimen of human skin, by means of polariscopy, is residual paraffin. The paraffin was not removed properly during deceration of the tissue section prior to staining. Failure to totally remove all paraffin from tissue sections prior to staining adversely affects the staining reaction. (H&E, X130) (AFIP Negative No. 73-6274)

Figure 23. *Best's Carmine Stain* (see Figure 331, Chapter VIII). Precipitated carmine dye is observed in this paraffin-embedded tissue section of a specimen of human liver which was fixed in neutral buffered 10% formalin. There is an irregular zone of diffusion of the dye into the tissue surrounding the site of deposition of the particles of precipitated dye. The tendency for tissue sections stained by this technique to develop a pink tinge within nuclei, even though counterstained with hematoxylin, is also well demonstrated. (Best's carmine with hematoxylin counterstain, X100) (AFIP Negative No. 72-5668)

Figure 24. *Cresyl Echt Violet Stain* (see Figure 336, Chapter VIII). Cresyl echt violet is routinely employed in very dilute solutions (see Chapter VIII). When solutions of the dye are improperly calculated the dye may be relatively insoluble at concentrations of 1% or higher and precipitate out of solution as needle-shaped, greenish-colored crystals which contaminate the tissue section as depicted here. (Vogt's cresyl echt violet method for nerve cell products, X145) (AFIP Negative No. 72-7798)

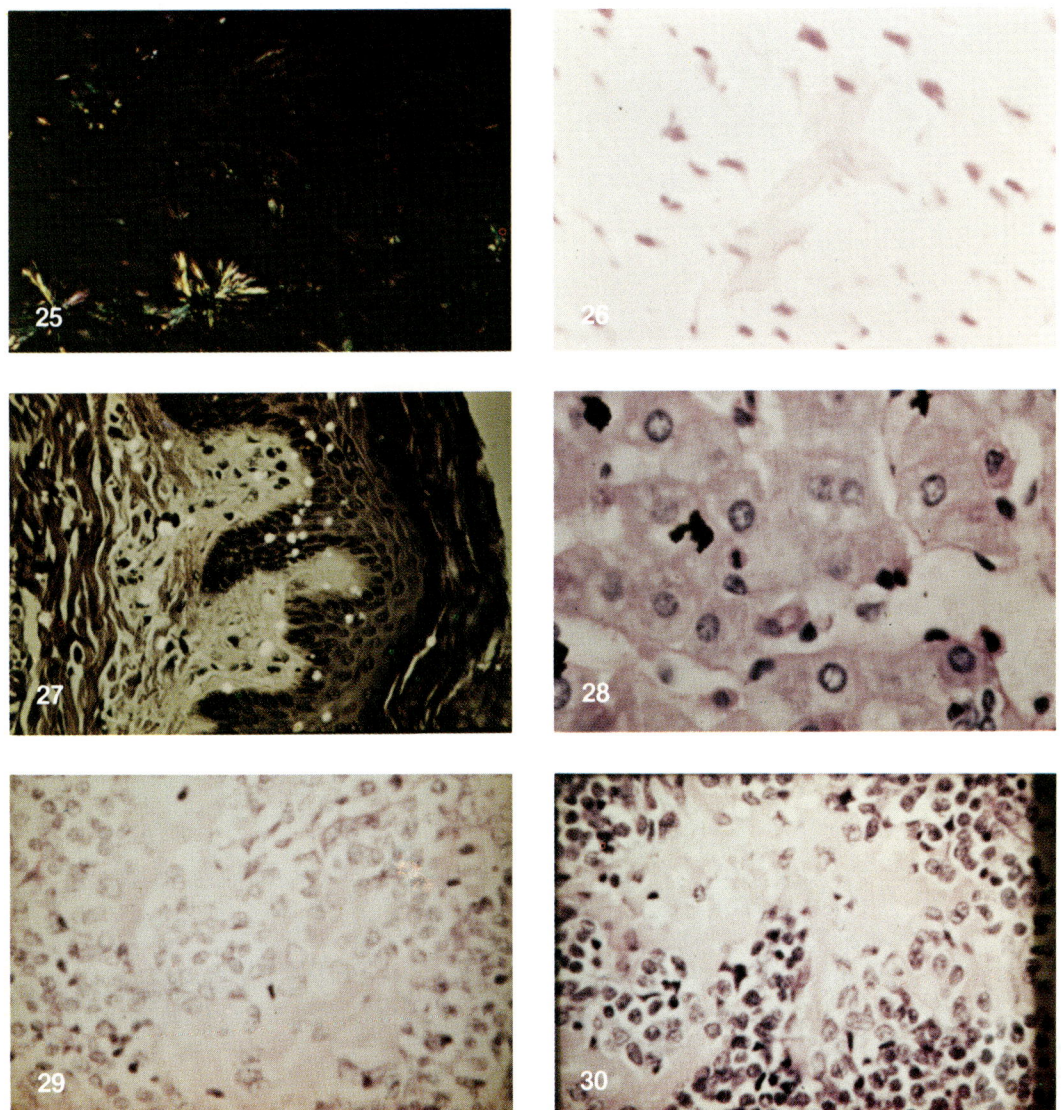

Figure 25. *Cresyl Echt Violet Stain* (see Figure 337, Chapter VIII). This photomicrograph is of the same tissue section depicted in Figure 24 taken with partially polarized light. Cresyl echt violet crystals are anisotropic. When subjected to polariscopy it is more readily apparent that the crystals are above the focal plane of the tissue section per se. (Vogt's cresyl echt method for nerve cell products, X145) (AFIP Negative No. 72-7798)

Figure 26. *Eosin* (see Figure 340, Chapter VIII). This paraffin-embedded tissue section of a specimen of the brain of a rat was stained in a working solution of eosin which had been prepared from a stock solution that had not been filtered prior to use. The irregularly shaped flake of foreign material, which resembles a hummingbird, seen above the focal plane of the tissue section is precipitated dye derived from the unfiltered stock solution. (H&E, X266) (Contributed by Mr. L. E. Schellhammer)

Figure 27. *Hematoxylin* (see Figure 345, Chapter VIII). The anisotropic bluish-white granules seen in this photomicrograph of a paraffin-embedded tissue section of a specimen of human skin, fixed in neutral buffered 10% formalin, are alum crystals from improperly prepared hematoxylin as described in the legend for Figure 344, Chapter VIII. By means of partial polariscopy, the crystals are seen to be above the focal plane of the tissue per se. When examined by bright-field microscopy the granules may simulate dark granular pigment and may appear to be within the focal plane of the tissue section. (H&E, X145) (AFIP Negative No. 64-1678)

Figure 28. *Hematoxylin* (see Figure 348, Chapter VIII). The irregularly shaped, dark-colored granules seen in this tissue section of a paraffin-embedded specimen of a human liver are hematein crystals derived from unfiltered hematoxylin solution as described in the legend for Figure 346, Chapter VIII. Within this field of view they are seen in the lumina of sinusoids where they may appear to be in the same focal plane as the cellular components of the tissue section. Where the crystals overlay hepatocytes, as seen at the left of the photograph, they are clearly observed as being above the focal plane of the tissue components. (Periodic acid-Schiff reaction with a hematoxylin counterstain, X305) (AFIP Negative No. 72-6774)

Figure 29. *Hematoxylin* (see Figure 355, Chapter VIII). This photograph of a paraffin-embedded tissue section of a specimen of soft tissue from a human being illustrates the staining effect that results with the breakdown of hematoxylin. The nuclear chromatin within individual cells is not distinctly stained. Chromatically, the tissue section appears to be very lightly stained. (H&E, X350) (AFIP Negative No. 73-6313)

Figure 30. *Hematoxylin* (see Figure 356, Chapter VIII). This tissue section was prepared from the same specimen as depicted in Figure 29. The dramatic difference in the staining resulted from using a fresh solution of hematoxylin. The nuclear chromatin within individual cells is distinctly stained. (H&E, X220) AFIP Negative No. 73-6310)

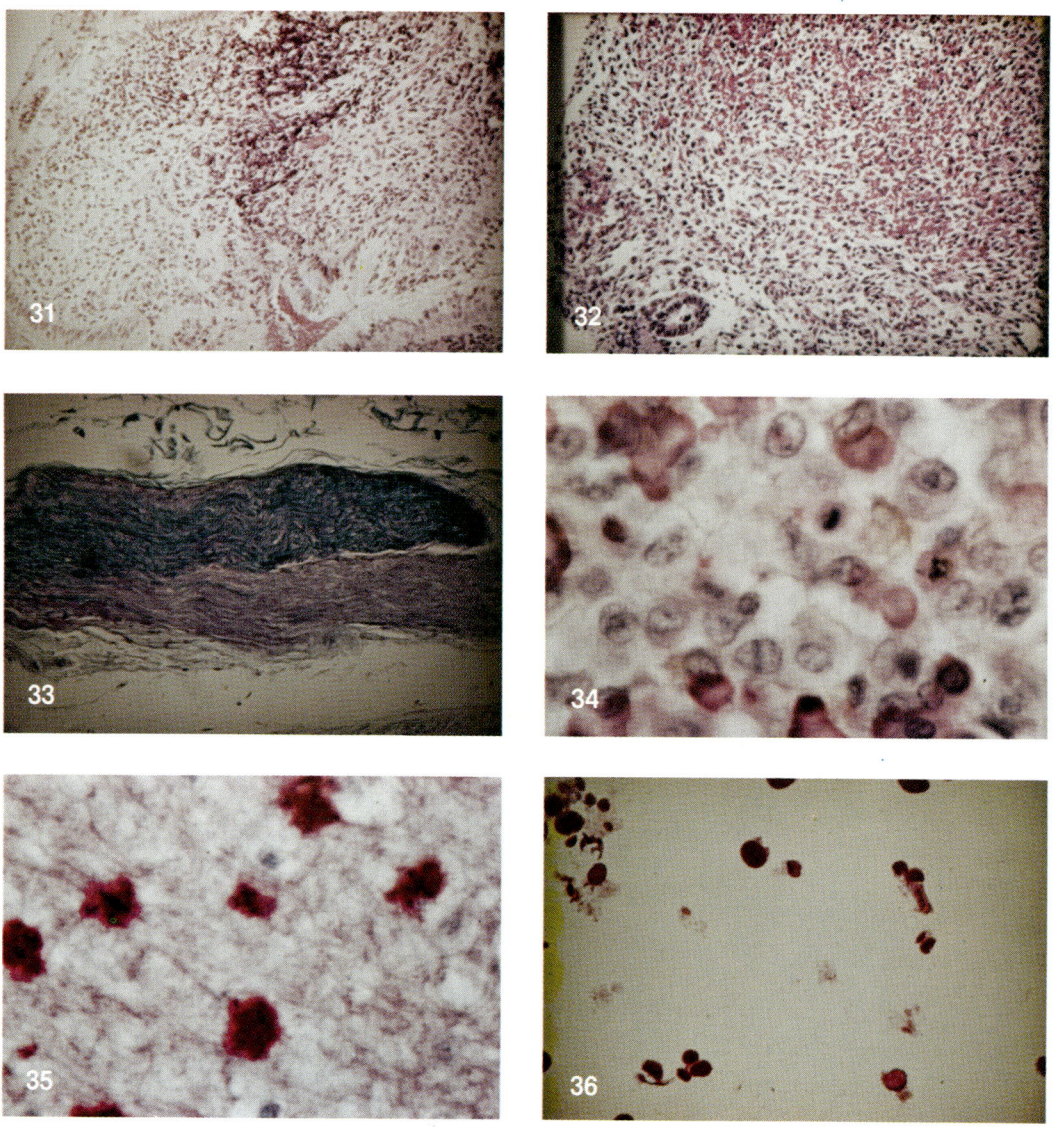

Figure 31. *Hematoxylin* (see Figure 359, Chapter VIII). Note the dark and light splotchy staining of this paraffin-embedded tissue section of an unknown specimen from a human being. The brown coloration of many of the nuclei, which gives the impresion that certain portions of the tissue section have faded, resulted from failure to expose the tissue section to a bluing procedure subsequent to staining with hematoxylin. (H&E, X115) (AFIP Negative No. 73-5614)

Figure 32. *Hematoxylin* (see Figure 360, Chapter VIII). This tissue section was prepared from the same specimen as depicted in Figure 31. Subsequent to staining with hematoxylin it exhibited the same artifact as depicted in Figure 31. However, subsequent to staining with hematoxylin it was exposed to a bluing agent which resulted in the dramatic difference noted in the quality of the staining achieved. (H&E, X115) (AFIP Negative No. 73-5618)

Figure 33. *Mallory's Iron Reaction* (see Figure 373, Chapter VIII). This paraffin-embedded tissue section was prepared from the specimen of human eye tissue depicted in Figure 3 of Color Plate 1. Oxidized iron, as a fixative contaminant, was deposited on the peripheral nerve and it subsequently yielded a positive blue reaction for iron. Unlike the microscopic deposits depicted in Figures 4 and 5 of Color Plate 1, in this instance the reaction was impossible to microscopically differentiate from true iron deposition. (Mallory's method for iron, X115) (AFIP Negative No. 72-13669)

Figure 34. *Mayer's Mucicarmine Stain* (see Figure 382, Chapter VIII). The reddish colored particulate matter seen in this paraffin-embedded tissue section of a human lymph node fixed in neutral buffered 10% formalin is undissolved fused material from the carmine stock solution. The particles, which contaminated the tissue section because of failure to filter the stock solution, resemble fungi and may be mistaken for such organisms by the inexperienced observer. (Mucicarmine, X440) (AFIP Negative No. 72-5663)

Figure 35. *Oil Red O* (see Figure 391, Chapter VIII). The red-colored precipitates seen throughout this tissue section of a specimen of human cerebrum are aggregates of crystalline oil red O which resulted from exposing the tissue section to a working solution which had too high a content of the Sudan colorant. (Oil red O, X350) (AFIP Negative No. 72-7026)

Figure 36. *Periodic Acid-Schiff Reaction* (see Figure 392, Chapter VIII). This photograph depicts granules of malt diastase which have dried on the surface of a glass microscope slide. A tissue section which was mounted on the slide had been exposed to a solution of malt diastase for the digestion and removal of glycogen prior to being subjected to the periodic acid-Schiff reaction. It is important to recognize this artifact since the malt diastase granules yield a postive periodic acid-Schiff reaction and may resemble some types of mucoid cells when they contaminate the tissue section per se. (PAS, X180) (AFIP Negative No. 73-4278)

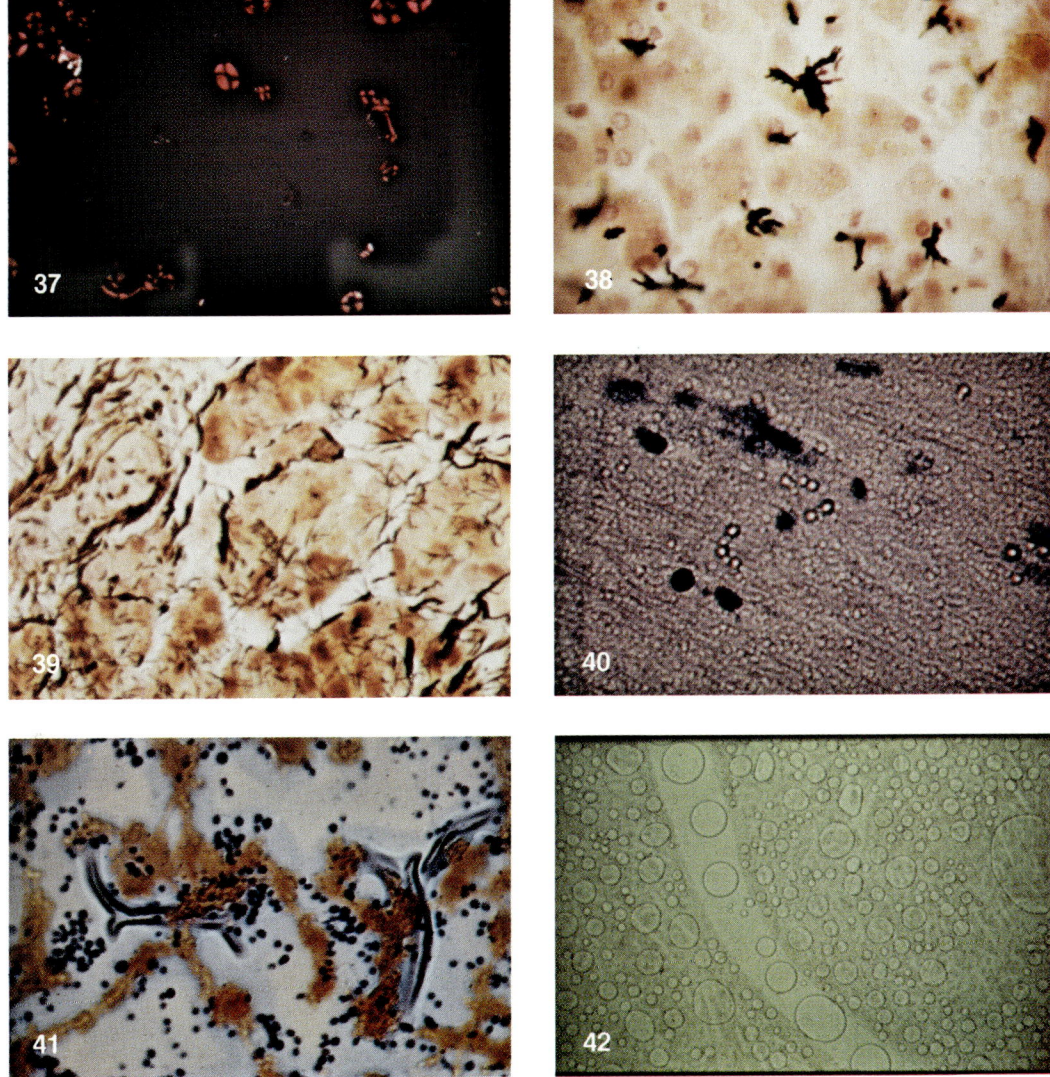

Figure 37. *Periodic Acid-Schiff Reaction* (see Figure 392, Chapter VIII). This photomicrograph is of the same field of view depicted in Figure 36 of Color Plate 6 as seen with polarized light. The periodic acid-Schiff positive granules of malt diastase which have dried on the surface of the glass microscope slide are anisotropic and are seen as reddish-white particles. They bear the Maltese cross which is the typical configureation of starch crystals when observed microscopically by means of polarized light. (PAS, X180) (AFIP Negative No. 73-4278)

Figure 38. *Rubeanic Acid* (see Figure 394, Chapter VIII). Uzman's rubeanic acid technique is frequently used for the demonstration of copper within tissue sections. The technique was employed with this paraffin-embedded tissue section of a specimen of human liver which had been fixed in Zenker's fluid. Although copper cannot be demonstrated in Zenker's fixed tissue, the mercuric chloride crystals which result from such fixative procedures are turned black by some unknown chemical reaction with rubeanic acid. (Rubeanic acid, X350) (AFIP Negative No. 73-4886)

Figure 39. *Sevier-Munger Silver Method for Neural Tissues* (see Figure 395, Chapter VIII). Brown-to-black granular precipitates of silver are observed in this paraffin-embedded tissue section of a specimen of a carcinoid tumor of a human appendix which was fixed in neutral buffered 10% formalin. These artifacts occurred because the slide was not kept in motion during exposure to the ammonical silver solution employed in the technique. Such artifacts could be mistaken for bacteria or fungi by an inexperienced observer. (Sevier-Munger stain, X265) (AFIP Negative No. 72-5346)

Figure 40. *Walbach's Giemsa Stain* (see Figure 402, Chapter VIII). This is a tissue section of a specimen of human spinal cord which has been stained with Walbach's Giemsa stain which contains glycerin. The tissue section is observed with the condenser of the microscope being partially closed to produce oblique illumination. Beads of glycerin are clearly seen above the focal plane of the tissue section. When viewed by bright-field illumination the morphologic details of the tissue section will be obscured by this artifact which resulted from failure to properly wash the tissue section after application of the stain. (Walbach's Giemsa, X615) (AFIP Negative No. 73-4909)

Figure 41. *Wright's Giemsa Stain* (see Figure 403, Chapter VIII). The wavy linear structures seen in this photograph of a portion of a blood smear resemble a helminth. They are wrinkles of the dried plasma film which stained darkly because of the double staining of both surfaces by the Giemsa stian. (Wright's Giemsa, X145) (AFIP Negative No. 74-6328)

Figure 42. *Clearing* (see Figure 416, Chapter VIII). Alcohol and water droplets were retained in this stained, paraffin-embedded tissue section of a specimen of human liver. These artifacts, which obscure the morphological details of the underlying tissue section, resulted from the use of xylene which had become saturated by the dehydrating solutions used in the staining sequence prior to coverslipping. (Hemtoxylin, X400)

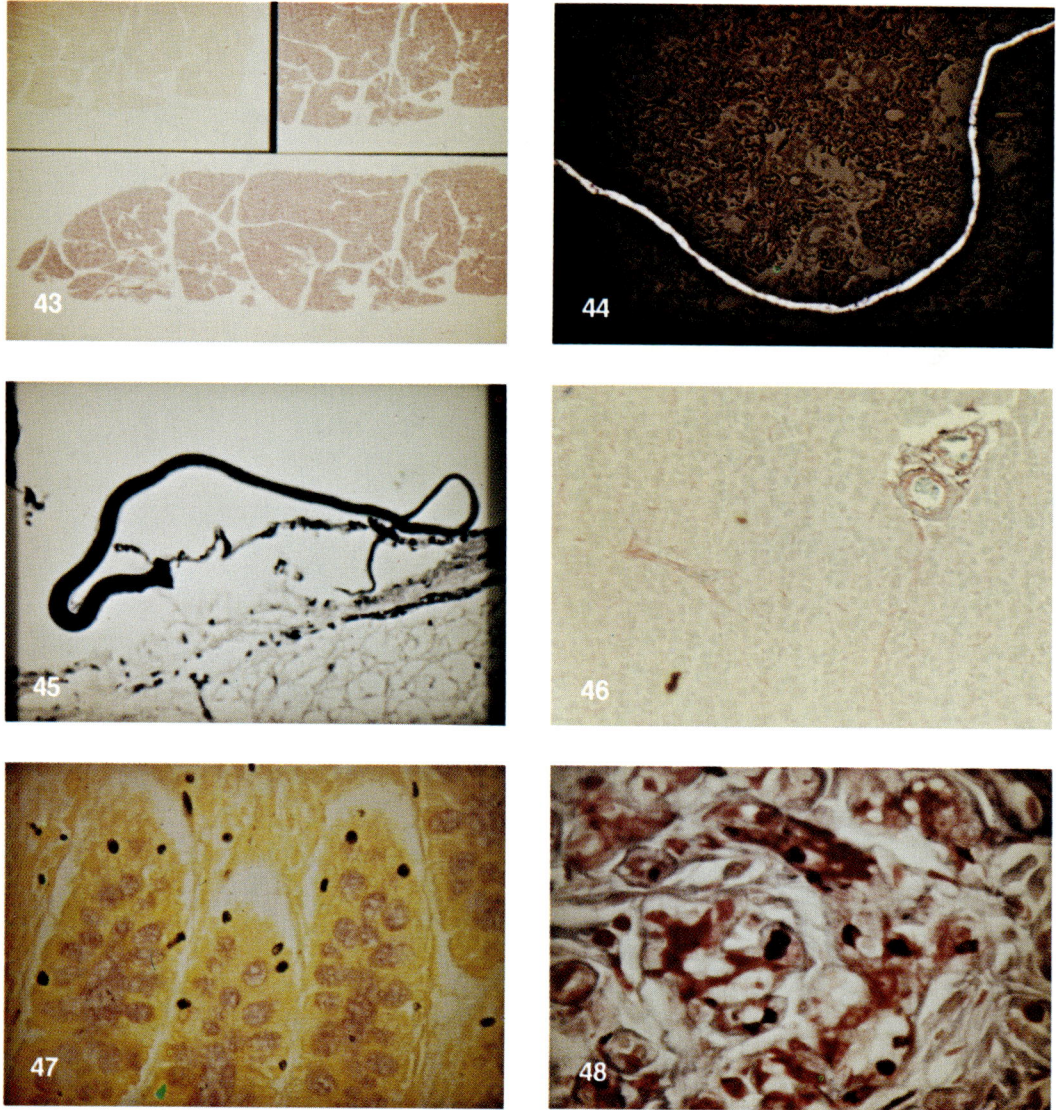

Figure 43. *Storage of Microscopic Tissue Sections* (see Figure 419, Chapter VIII). The slide shown at the bottom of the photograph was stored in a covered slide box at room temperature for eighteen days after being cut. The duplicate slide depicted at the upper right of the photograph was stored in a similar box held at 60°C for eighteen days. Macroscopically and microscopically, there was no detectable difference between these two duplicate tissue sections. The duplicate section seen at the upper left of the photograph was exposed to sunlight during the daylight hours for a period of eighteen days. The stain faded to the extent that microscopically it appeared to be unstained. (H&E, X3)

Figure 44. *Lint Fibers* (see Figure 423, Chapter IX). As depicted in this photomicrograph of a paraffin-embedded tissue section of a specimen of the lung of a human being, lint and/or other debris may be deposited on stained tissue sections at the time of coverslipping. While lint fibers maybe difficult to detect by means of bright-field microscopy, when viewed by means of partial polariscopy they are strongly anisotropic as depicted by the white fiber seen here. (H&E, X50) (AFIP Negative No. 72-18039)

Figure 45. *Lint Fibers* (see Figure 424, Chapter IX). The artifact depicted in this photograph consists of a fragment of fine linen thread which was left as a residue on a coverslip at the time it was cleaned. The tissue section is from a specimen of the spinal cord of a goat. The artifact seen within the meninges was originally mistaken by several observers for a nematode. (H&E, X125) (Contributed by Dr. J. R. M. Innes)

Figure 46. *Glass Coverslip Substitutes* (see Figure 431, Chapter IX). Many stains are soluble in the solvent phase of plastic solutions which are used as substitutes for glass coverslips and are leached from the tissue section as the plastic dries. The colored product of the condensation of Schiff's reagent was leached from this paraffin-embedded tissue section of a specimen of rat pancreas and diffused throughout the synthetic coverslip. (PAS, X125) (Contributed by Dr. F. Sigler)

Figure 47. *Entrapped Air* (see Figure 435, Chapter IX). This is a paraffin-embedded tissue section of a specimen of human intestinal mucosa, stained by Gridley's method for the demonstration of fungi. The small brown-to-black spherules seen within the section are not fungi. They are artifactitious interstitial air bubbles caused by permitting the tissue section to become dry before the application of the mounting medium and coverslip. (Gridley's fungi stain, X265) (AFIP Negative No. 73-4145)

Figure 48. *Entrapped Air* (see Figure 437, Chapter IX). Air bubbles entrapped in interstitial spaces will resemble crystalline materials, such as the dark reddish-black particles observed in this tissue section of a specimen of a human mammary gland. They can best be visualized by lowering the substage condenser of the microscope. Such artifacts could be confused with normal and abnormal tissue pigments. (Masson's trichrome stain, X440) (AFIP Negative No. 73-4146)

V

Artifacts Resulting from Embedding Procedures

INTRODUCTION

*V*IRTUALLY ALL OF THE ARTIFACTS which may be observed in microscopic tissue sections that are the result of embedding procedures are the fault of the histotechnologist. Most of the errors that occur in the embedding procedures can be attributed to a failure to appreciate the purpose of embedding tissue in paraffin or plastic media. The sole purpose of such procedures is to provide support to the tissue so that it can be sectioned on a microtome. Any factor which reduces the ability of the media to support the tissue specimen will result in artifacts being produced during microtomy. Examples of such faulty embedding procedures included in this chapter are:

- Multiple embedding of hard-tissue specimens
- Improper orientation of specimens
- Entrapped air around specimens
- Prolonged exposure to molten paraffin
- Exposure to overheated molten paraffin
- Use of excessively hard media in relation to the consistency of the specimen
- Multiple embedding of specimens of varied consistencies
- Some unusual effects of plasticized embedding media

Figure 217. *Venetian Blind Effect.* These tissue sections of the human uterus were prepared from multiple embedded-tissue specimens. With hard tissues such as the myometrium, multiple-embedding should be avoided since it reduces the amount of paraffin which surrounds the specimen and therefore provides inadequate support for hard tissues. The venetian blind effect observed in these tissue sections is characterized by alternately thick and thin zones in the tissue section. Such effects can also result from a loose screw on the specimen or knife chuck of the microtome (see Chapter VI). However, in this instance it resulted from the vibration of the tissue specimen within the paraffin block when the hard tissue became loose within the block because of inadequate support resulting from multiple embedding of the specimens in a single block. (H&E, ×3) (AFIP Negative No. 68-2180)

Figure 218. *Improper Orientation.* These tissue sections of human skin were prepared from multiple-embedded tissue specimens. Since the skin is a relatively hard tissue, multiple-embedding is best avoided for the same reasons as described for Figure 217. In this instance, not only was multiple-embedding employed, but the specimens were improperly oriented resulting in the specimens being mutilated as they were being cut on the microtome. Regardless of the nature of the infiltrating and embedding medium used, it is extremely important that the specimen of skin and attached hair be positioned horizontally to the knife at the time it is embedded. This is necessary so that when the block is trimmed and mounted in the microtome, the specimen can be oriented so that the hair and epidermis is presented to the knife last and the skin presents less resistance to the knife at any part of the cut, and the hairs are supported by the skin during sectioning. (H&E, ×4) (AFIP Negative No. 68-2181)

Figure 219. *Entrapped Air.* At times, air may be entrapped about the specimen during the embedding procedure. Noted here, white starry foci within the paraffin of the tissue block, adjacent to the embedded specimens. Such crevices and hairline separations between the tissue and paraffin may permit the specimens to fall out or vibrate within the paraffin block at such time as one attempts to cut tissue sections on a microtome (see also Figure 217). Such defects in the paraffin block may result from a failure to utilize vacuum procedures in embedding and/or by the slow transfer of specimens from the container of infiltrating paraffin to the embedding mold. Such faulty paraffin blocks should be melted down in molten paraffin and the specimens reembedded taking care to avoid entrapped air about the specimens again. (AFIP Negative No. 67-2652)

Figure 220. *Venetian Blind Effect.* If air is entrapped about the tissue specimen during the embedding procedure (see Figure 219) the specimen, if it does not fall out of the paraffin block, can vibrate within the paraffin block at such time as one attempts to cut tissue sections on a microtome (see also Figure 217). As the improperly embedded block of tissue is cut, the tissue sections will usually contain an artifact that resembles a venetian blind in that compressed zones of tissue are separated by open spaces as seen in this paraffin-embedded tissue section of a specimen of an adrenal gland of a dog. Such effects can also result from a loose screw on the knife or specimen chuck of the microtome (see Chapter VI). (H&E, ×75) (Contributed by Mr. L. E. Schellhammer)

Figure 221. *Embedding.* After tissue specimens have been processed and infiltrated with paraffin they are embedded in molten paraffin. A variety of modern devices and molds are available for this purpose. The method depicted here is still one that is commonly employed for large specimens. With all devices it is possible to overheat the molten paraffin used for embedding owing to a variety of factors such as faulty adjustment or mechanical failure of modern embedding devices or faulty judgment when employing simple devices such as the one depicted in this photograph.

Figure 222. *Dehydration.* If the paraffin used for embedding is overheated, the tissue specimen may become dehydrated by heat (cooked) during the embedding procedure. This tissue section was prepared from a specimen of human liver which was embedded in paraffin that was held at too high a temperature during the embedding procedure. The artifact seen at the top of the photograph is a subcapsular zone which stains gray and yellow with hematoxylin and eosin (see Color Plate 3, Figure 16). It is a zone of coagulated liver tissue produced by cooking in hot molten paraffin (see also Chapters I and IV). (H&E, ×145) (AFIP Negative No. 72-7029)

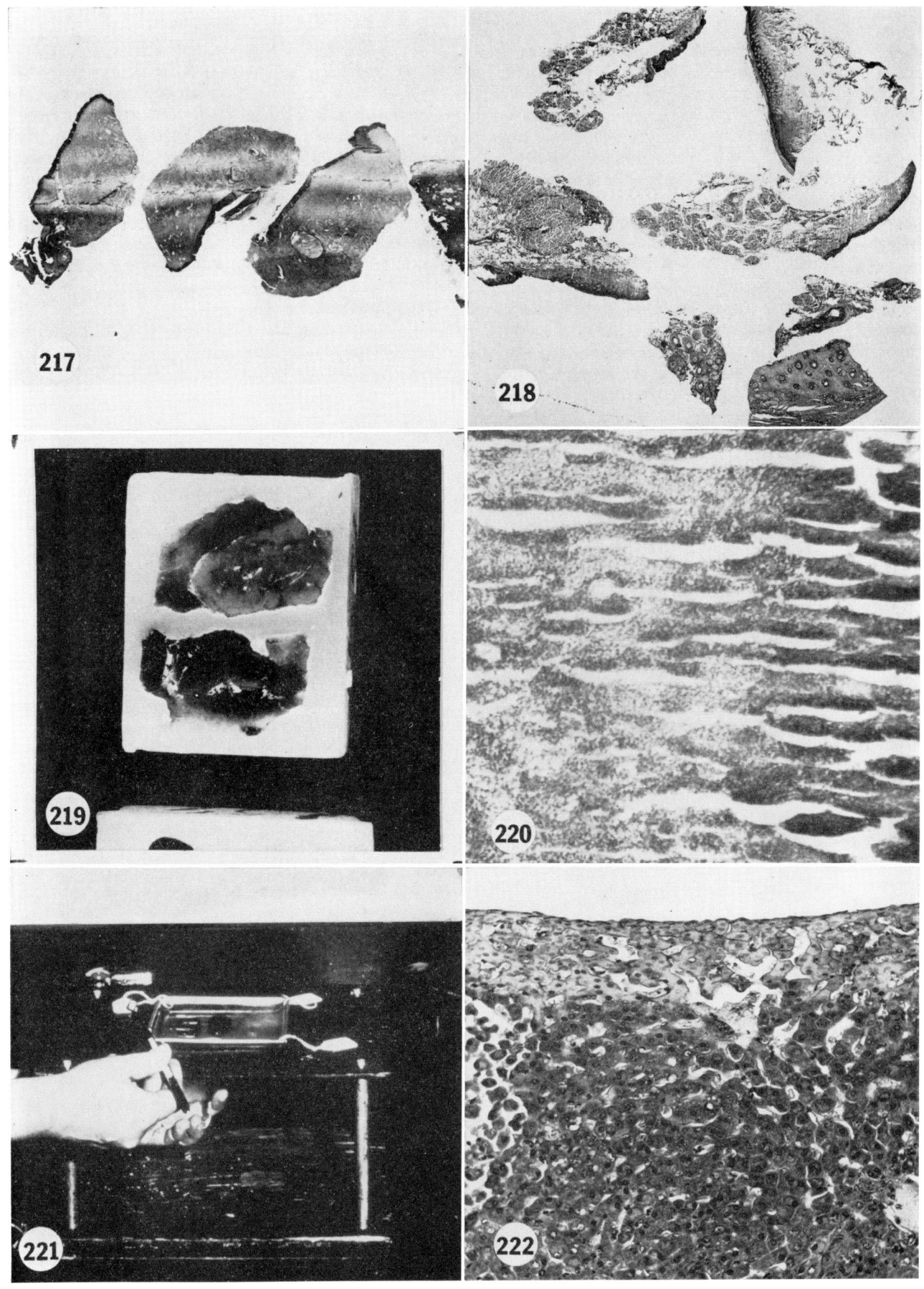

Figure 223. *Dehydration*. This is a paraffin-embedded tissue section of an adrenal gland of a rat. It is a common practice with rodent tissues to embed multiple tissues in a single small tissue block. This necessitates that the paraffin be held in the molten state for longer periods of time than when single tissue specimens are embedded separately. As a result, the first tissues to be embedded in a block of multiple tissues must be held at the temperature of molten paraffin for relatively long periods of time. Also, the need to hold the paraffin in the molten state for longer periods of time may easily result in exposure of some of the tissue to excessively high temperatures and the tissue will become dehydrated by heat (cooked) during the embedding procedure. The artifact seen at the top of the photograph is a subcapsular zone which stains inadequately. It is a zone of coagulated adrenal cortex produced by cooking in hot molten paraffin (see also Chapter I and IV). (H&E, ×40) (Contributed by Dr. W. L. Wooding)

Figure 224. *Dehydration*. This is a higher magnification of a portion of the tissue section depicted in Figure 223. In sections of a block of multiplicate embedded tissues one may observe that the majority of the tissues do not exhibit dehydration artifacts since only the first tissues embedded and held in molten paraffin for the longest period of time may exhibit such artifacts. This occurs when the paraffin is overheated at the beginning of the embedding procedure in an effort to have the paraffin remain molten long enough to complete the multitudinous specimen embedding procedure. As depicted here, the subcapsular zone of cooked tissue acts as a shell and prevents adequate rehydration of the section during tissue flotation subsequent to microtomy. This results in compression and disorientation of the cortical tissue beneath the zone of cooked tissue. (H&E, ×170) (Contributed by Dr. W. L. Wooding)

Figure 225. *Wrinkled Tissue Sections*. If the embedding medium is harder than the processed and infiltrated tissue specimen, either due to the inherent nature of the specimen, or the inherent nature of the embedding medium, or the temperature at which the sectioning procedure is carried out, any of the following defects may be encountered in the tissue sections: cracks in the section parallel to the cutting edge of the knife, the section is curved or rolled up upon itself, or ribbons fail to form or the section exhibits pin cushion distortion. The latter two problems were encountered in the cutting of tissue sections from this block of embedded tissue of a specimen of a kidney from a rat. The section contains both types of artifacts one may expect to encounter in such a situation. (H&E, ×40) (Contributed by Dr. W. L. Wooding)

Figure 226. *Wrinkled Tissue Sections*. This is a higher magnification of the central portion of the tissue section depicted in Figure 225. The type of wrinkles one may encounter due to residues of processing and clearing fluids being present in the embedded block of tissue (see Chapter IV) are different in appearance from those which one may encounter when the embedding medium is simply harder than a properly processed and infiltrated specimen. In the latter instance, if sections are obtained they may exhibit excessive wrinkling as depicted here, which cannot be corrected by flattening on a waterbath or microscope slide. The cause of such wrinkling of the section, as pointed out by Richards (Microtomy. In Glasser, O. (Ed.): *Medical Physics*. Chicago, The Year Book Publishers Inc., vol. 1, 1944, pp. 750-759) is related to the fact that: "Warm paraffin shrinks as it cools and compresses the tissue in the block. Tissue harder than paraffin withstands this pressure, but soft or spongy tissue may be under considerable strain. When sectioned, the tissue tends to expand to the shape and size it had before compression and, if confined by the paraffin around it, pleating or wrinkling results." (H&E, ×170) (Contributed by Dr. W. L. Wooding)

Figure 227. *Multiple Embedding*. This paraffin-embedded tissue section of specimens of a human spinal cord and gastrointestinal tract illustrates some of the problems related to embedding different tissues together. The muscular coats of the gastrointestinal specimen exhibit numerous wrinkles which were produced by the variable consistency between the two types of tissue embedded in this single block. The variance in consistency provided inadequate support to the gastrointestinal specimen and allowed it to vibrate within the block as it was being cut. The problem was compounded by the obvious nicks which were produced on the edge of the microtome knife by the vibrating denser specimen. In this instance, the section would have been of considerably better quality if the paraffin block had contained only the three segments of the specimen of spinal cord tissue. (H&E, ×4) (AFIP Negative No. 74-3307)

Figure 228. *Plasticized Paraffin*. A variety of proprietary mixtures of plastic and paraffin are currently being utilized for the embedding of fixed tissue specimens. If such media are inadequately removed from the tissue section prior to commencing the staining procedure, artifacts may be encountered which are dissimilar to those observed when paraffin-embedded tissues are inadequately decerated. Paraffin-embedded tissues which are inadequately decerated usually fail to stain in those portions of the section in which the paraffin is retained (see Chapter VIII). The plastic components of some proprietary plasticized paraffins are weakly anionic and stain faintly with cationic dyes used in many staining procedures. As depicted in this photograph of a formalin-fixed specimen of the brain of a Rhesus monkey embedded in plasticized paraffin embedding medium retained within the Virchow-Robin spaces is stained faintly by cationic dye (see Chapter VIII). This material was initially interpreted as mucin (mucocytes). (H&E, ×220) (Contributed by Mr. L. E. Schellhammer)

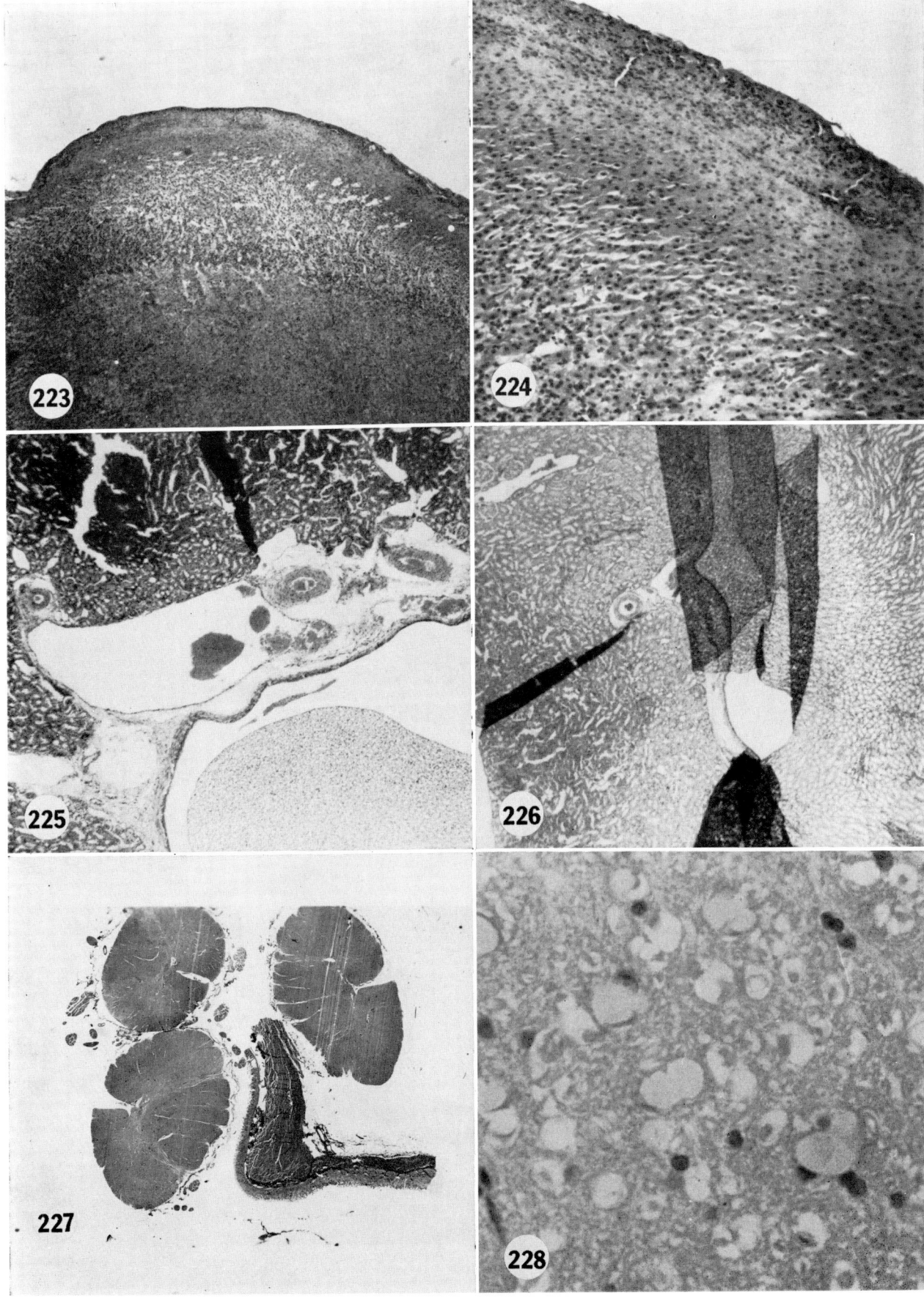

VI

Artifacts Resulting from Microtomy Procedures

INTRODUCTION

*V*IRTUALLY ALL ARTIFACTS which may be observed in microscopic tissue sections that are the result of microtomy procedures may be attributed to faulty techniques practiced by the histotechnologist. With but one possible exception, such artifacts cannot be attributed to malfunction of the microtome. Examples of artifacts resulting from faulty microtomy included in this chapter are:

    Freezing of surface of paraffin block
    Improper knife angulation
    Loose screws of knife or specimen chuck
    Contamination of cutting edge of the microtome knife
    Use of dull knives
    Use of knives of inadequate thickness
    Inadequate hydration
    Extraneous tissue debris

Figure 229. *Freezing Artifacts.* A practice which has become popular in the last several years is to use an aerosol spray of a mixture of fluorinated hydrocarbons for chilling the specimen surface of blocks of paraffin-embedded tissue rather than using ice. Such preparations are frequently used for the rapid freezing of fresh tissue prior to sectioning procedures on clinical microtomes or in cryostats. While such procedures have proven to be practical for the chilling of paraffin prior to sectioning, if the exposed specimen surface of the embedded tissue is exposed to such aerosols for more than a period of moments the embedded tissue may become excessively dehydrated at its surface and fissures will form along natural lines of cleavage as observed in this paraffin-embedded tissue section of a specimen of human adrenal gland. (Lendrum's stain, ×77) (AFIP Negative No. 73-4885)

Figure 230. *Freezing Artifacts.* This is a higher magnification of the central portion of the tissue section depicted in Figure 229. The fracture lines in the tissue section produced by freezing the specimen surface of the embedded tissue with dichlorotetrafluoromethane prior to sectioning are more clearly discernable. (Lendrum's stain, ×140) (AFIP Negative No. 71-11420)

Figure 231. *Compression.* If the microtome knife is set at too acute an angle, the knife compresses the tissue specimen as it is being cut. The effects of this compression as seen within this tissue section of a paraffin-embedded specimen of a human kidney is most pronounced at normal points of weakness. The firm tissue components such as the arteries seen here are pushed ahead as they are cut and compress the adjacent parenchyma. Note that the tissue surrounding the artifacts is not affected which indicates that the knife was sharp. The cutting clearance angle should be between 5° and 10° for most types of tissue although hard, fibrous tissue such as uterus and bone may require an angle of 15°. (H&E, ×100) (AFIP Negative No. 72-7027)

Figure 232. *Venetian Blind Effect.* If the screws which secure the knife on the microtome are not adequately tightened, the entire knife will move or vibrate as tissue sections are being cut. The tissue sections obtained with such a knife will usually contain an artifact that resembles a venetian blind in that compressed zones of tissue are separated by open spaces as seen in the trabeculae in this tissue section of a specimen of human spleen. The effect is usually more noticeable or limited to the more dense (hard) components of the specimen as depicted here. Note that the parenchymal tissue surrounding the collagenous trabeculae is unaffected which indicates that the loose knife was sharp. (H&E, ×40) (AFIP Negative No. 72-7019)

Figure 233. *Venetian Blind Effect.* In this tissue section of the human spleen, venetian blind artifacts are noted within the trabeculae. The artifact is identical to that which may be caused by failure to adequately tighten the screws which secure the knife on the microtome (see Figure 232). However, in this instance, the knife was properly secured, but the screws on the specimen chuck of the microtome were not adequately tightened. Instead of the knife, it is the specimen which moves or vibrates as it is being cut. As the specimen changes its orientation, on some strokes the angle at which the surface of the specimen meets the knife may be too acute and in addition to a venetian blind artifact the knife may compress the specimen as it is being cut as depicted here. (H&E, ×35) (AFIP Negative No. 72-2665)

Figure 234. *Focal Venetian Blind Effect.* This is a tissue section of a portion of a lymph node of a dog. The small area of alternating compressed tissue and open spaces simulates the venetian blind effect but actually results from contamination of the cutting edge of the microtome knife with lint or hair. (H&E, ×75)

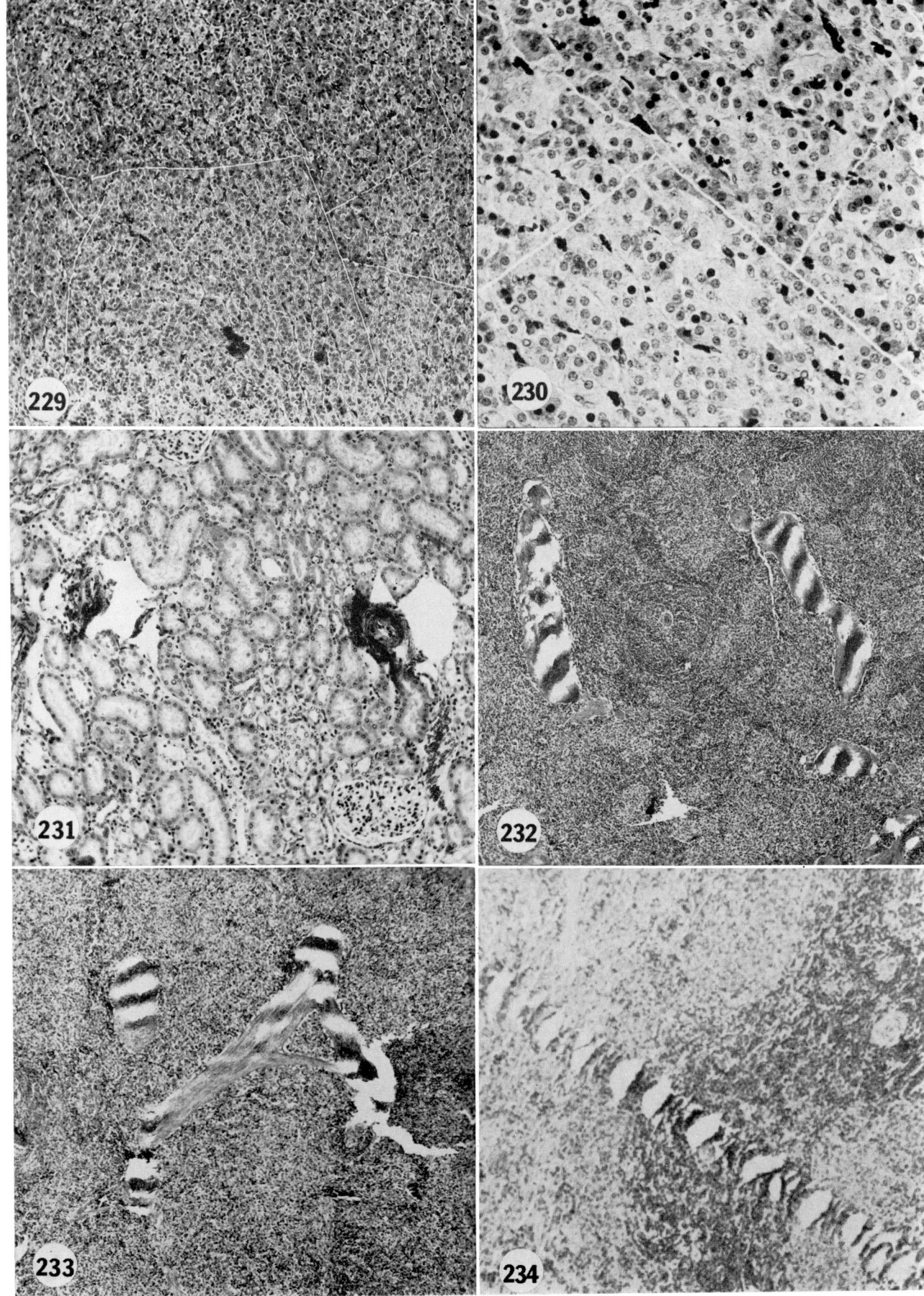

Figure 235. *Dull-knife Distortions.* This paraffin-embedded tissue section of a specimen of a human pituitary gland was prepared with a sharp microtome knife. Compare this with Figure 236. (H&E, ×245) (AFIP Negative No. 72-4059)

Figure 236. *Dull-knife Distortions.* This tissue section was prepared from the same block of paraffin-embedded pituitary gland tissue as the tissue section depicted in Figure 235. The sharp microtome knife was exchanged for a dull one. Note the numerous compression artifacts which render the tissue section useless for microscopic study. (H&E, ×245) (AFIP Negative No. 72-4060)

Figure 237. *Dull-knife Distortions.* If the cutting edge of the knife is dull or blunt any of a number of different forms of distortion of the tissue section may be encountered. As depicted in this photomicrograph of a paraffin-embedded tissue section of a specimen of liver tissue of a rat, cracks in the tissue section which are parallel with the edge of the knife can be produced with a dull or blunt knife. (H&E, ×40) (Contributed by Dr. W. L. Wooding)

Figure 238. *Dull-knife Distortions.* This is a higher magnification of a portion of the tissue section depicted in Figure 237. The cracks in the tissue section are seen at the edge of the section which was presented parallel to the edge of the knife. As the edge of the dull knife passed through the tissue block it pushed portions of the shattered tissue ahead of it so that they came to overlay portions of the tissue section. Although they may remain affixed to the slide at one extremity (arrow), these fragments stain more intensely than the tissue which they overlay since the stain has access to both surfaces of these fragments except where they remain attached to the microscope slide. (H&E, ×170) (Contributed by Dr. W. L. Wooding)

Figure 239. *Dull-knife Distortions.* If the cutting edge of the knife is dull or blunt a variety of distortions may be noted in the tissue sections. If only small portions of the knife edge are dull one may obtain sections which resemble this paraffin-embedded tissue section of the spleen of a rat. Such tissue sections are quite small, yet cracks which are parallel with the edge of the knife are seen in a portion of this small tissue section adjacent to relatively normal appearing tissue. The knife edge was dull in a relatively small zone of its entire length, resulting in localized dull-knife artifacts in the tissue section. The sharpening of microtome knives has been stated by some authorities to be an art (De Groat, A.: *Am J Med Tech, 24*:93-98, 1958 and Richards, O. W.: *Medical Physics,* vol. 1, 1944, pp. 750-759). It is certain that it is one of the most important steps in the preparation of any type of tissue section since there is no way in which one can improve the quality or value of a tissue section which has been prepared with an improperly sharpened knife. (H&E, ×30) (Contributed by Dr. W. L. Wooding)

Figure 240. *Dull-knife Distortions.* This is an enlargement of the focal artifact depicted in Figure 239 which resulted from a small zone of bluntness in the edge of the microtome knife. In addition to cracks which are parallel to the blunt edge of the microtome knife, in the lower central portion of the photograph a compression artifact can be seen. Such compression artifacts result from the blunt knife edge pushing soft parenchymal tissue against firmer tissue components such as arteries. The actual mechanics of knife sharpening are well covered in the references cited in the legend for Figure 239, as well as in the texts of Gray (*Handbook of Basic Microtechnique,* New York, Blakiston Company, 1952), Luna (*Manual of Histologic Staining Methods of the Armed Forces Institute of Pathology,* New York, McGraw, 1968) and Steedman (*Section Cutting In Microscopy,* Springfield, Thomas, 1960). (H&E, ×60) (Contributed by Dr. W. L. Wooding)

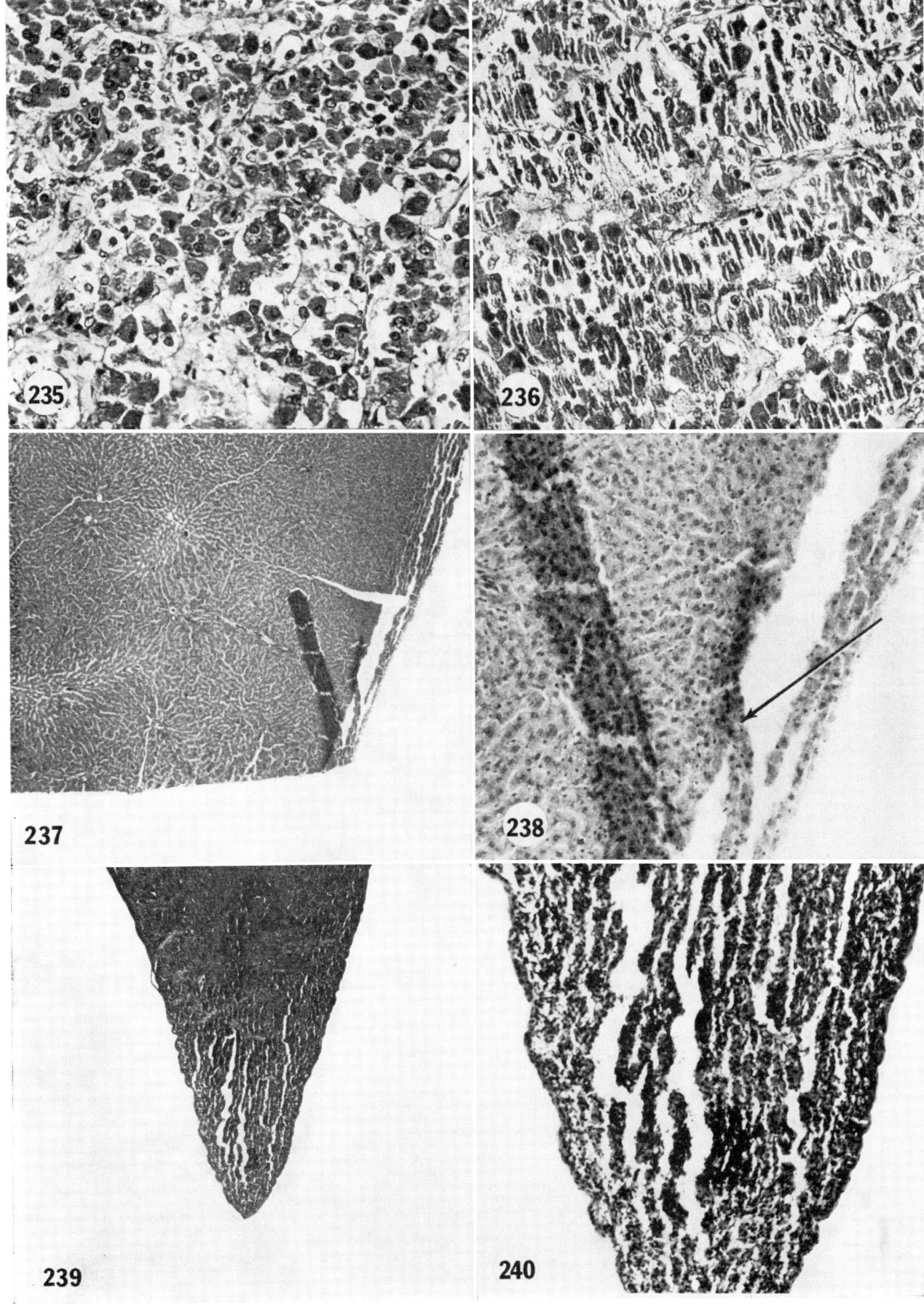

Figure 241. *Dull-knife Distortions.* This paraffin-embedded tissue section of a specimen of human lymph node was cut with a dull microtome knife. The compression artifacts which resulted are similar to those depicted in Figures 236, 249, and 250. The trabecular and arterial vascular components of the lymph node were firmer than the surrounding parenchyma. The compression of soft tissue components and the pushing of firm tissue components by the edge of a dull knife will, in effect, shatter the tissue section as depicted here. (H&E, ×35) (AFIP Negative No. 71-11704)

Figure 242. *Dull-knife Distortions.* This paraffin-embedded tissue section of a specimen of the lymph node of a human being was cut on a microtome knife which had a long blunt area on its edge. Cracks which are parallel with the edge of the microtome knife are seen throughout the tissue section. Although knife sharpening techniques will not be discussed in this text, there are several factors which should be borne in mind in the sharpening of knives, and which are frequently disregarded, that are worthwhile to consider. *Microtome knives are supplied commercially with a tubular device, referred to as a "honing (stropping) back" and a handle.* These are for use in sharpening and honing the knife. The honing back is specifically fitted to the back side of the knife so that it can be removed, but when in place it properly positions the facets of the knife edge for sharpening. In sharpening, the knife should be fitted with its *own* properly designed honing back or its beveled edge will not be properly sharpened and the shoulder of the bevel will be damaged, resulting in a long blunt edge of the knife. (H&E, ×60) (AFIP Negative No. 72-18033)

Figure 243. *Dull-knife Distortions.* This is a higher magnification of the central portion of the field depicted in Figure 242 which more clearly depicts the parallel cracks in the tissue section which are produced by a dull knife. As pointed out by Richards (reference cited in the legend for Figure 239), *"If a knife is well sharpened, stropping will add nothing to the process."* However, the stones available for hand honing or the automatic sharpening devices used in many laboratories are of such quality that perfect honing is not possible. Therefore, stropping, by the methods presented in the references cited in the legend for Figure 240, is required after honing in most instances. One should be cautious about excessive stropping since this may curve the edge of the knife and/or round the bevel of the knife resulting in a blunt edge. (H&E, ×175) (AFIP Negative No. 72-18034)

Figure 244. *Dull-knife Distortions.* This is a higher magnification of the central portion of the field depicted in Figure 243 which depicts not only the parallel cracks in the tissue section but also pinpoint foci of compression which may be produced by a dull knife. *After sharpening and/or honing, a knife should not be tested for sharpness with the fingernail, or a hair, or any other substance, prior to using it to prepare tissue sections.* Such practices only serve to dull or nick the knife and necessitates rehoning and/or stropping. The ultimate test for sharpness of a microtome knife is in cutting the tissue block. If a properly prepared block does not section satisfactorily, assume that the knife is dull and resharpen it. (H&E, ×485) (AFIP Negative No. 72-18035)

Figure 245. *Dull-knife Distortions.* Two of the various types of distortions which may result if the cutting edge of the microtome knife is dull or blunt are depicted in this paraffin-embedded tissue section of a specimen of liver from an animal (species unknown). Streaks or corrugations across the section may be produced by a dull knife. In addition, some tissue components may be compressed as seen in the dark stained areas surrounding segments of the hepatic artery. *Knives may be "touched up" after short periods of use by stropping on a strap impregnated with diamond dust or by sharpening on the finest grade of crocus paper.* However, as pointed out by De Groat (*Am J Med Tech*, 24:93-98, 1958), this means of "touching up" a dull knife should only be used a very few times between actual honing procedures. If a knife is stropped too frequently between honings, its bevel becomes rounded and its edge is dull. When such a knife is finally honed its edge does not position properly on the honing surface until a considerable portion of its shoulder and bevel has been ground away. (H&E, ×35) (AFIP Negative No. 73-3921)

Figure 246. *Dull-knife Distortions.* Severe compression artifacts such as observed in this paraffin-embedded tissue section of a specimen of intestine from an animal (species unknown) can be produced by a dull knife. In this instance, the knife was extremely dull. As a knife is used, its back side becomes worn and its honing back ceases to fit properly and therefore the edge ceases to be positioned properly against the honing surface. As this occurs, the bevel of the knife is increased in width and excessive amounts of metal must be removed in the sharpening procedure in order to get the knife edge sharp. (H&E, ×60) (AFIP Negative No. 73-4910)

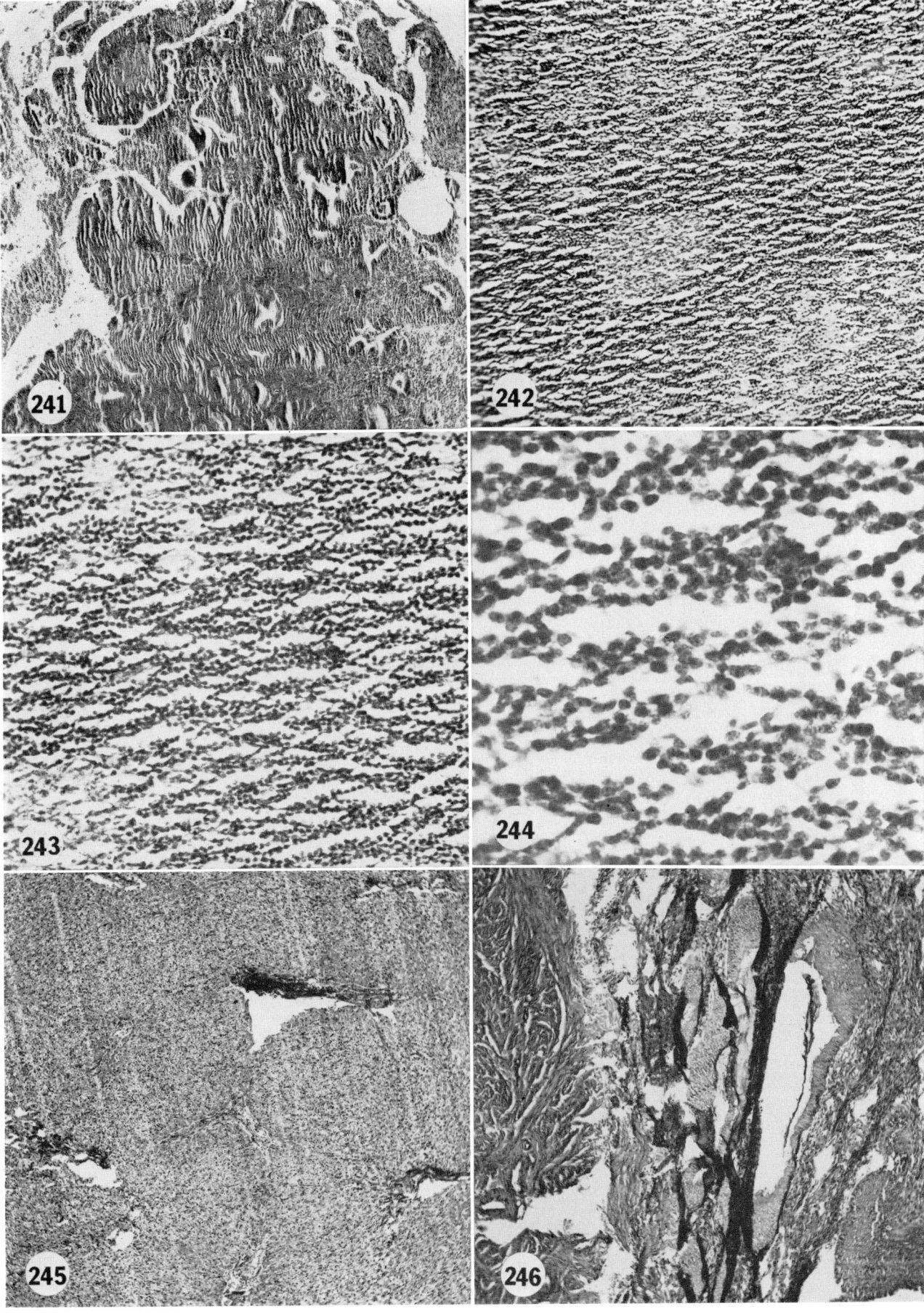

Figure 247. *Dull-knife Distortions.* The thick and thin zones observed in this paraffin-embedded tissue section of a specimen of intestine from a human being are the result of compression due to the use of a dull microtome knife. Notice the dramatic cellular alterations which result from the compression (compare with Figure 246). (H&E, ×350) (AFIP Negative No. 73-801)

Figure 248. *Dull-knife Distortions.* This tissue section was obtained from the same block of embedded tissue as the tissue section depicted in Figure 247. However, the tissue section depicted here was cut on a sharp microtome knife. (H&E, ×350) (AFIP Negative No. 73-802)

Figure 249. *Dull-knife Distortions.* Three important characteristics of a dull knife are that paraffin tissue sections will not ribbon when they are cut; the sections adhere to the block during the upstroke of the microtome; and tissue components are compressed as observed under a microscope. Noted here paired paraffin-embedded tissue sections of a specimen of human intestine and pancreas. The section on the left was cut with a sharp knife and is free of artifacts. The section on the right was cut from the same block of embedded tissue using a dull knife. The lamina propria of the intestine and the attached portion of the pancreas exhibit compression artifacts. (H&E, ×7) (AFIP Negative No. 72-6816-3)

Figure 250. *Dull-knife Distortions.* These photomicrographs are higher power views of the pancreatic tissue observed in Figure 249. At the left is a portion of the specimen of pancreas which was cut with a sharp microtome knife, and at the right is a portion of the specimen from the same block of embedded tissue which was cut with a dull microtome knife. The section which was cut on a dull knife exhibits considerable disorientation due to compression of the soft tissue components. (H&E, ×50) (AFIP Negative No. 72-6816-4)

Figure 251. *Dull-knife Distortions.* The shrinkage of tissue specimens which results from fixation is known to vary from 2 percent to 20 percent depending upon the nature of the fixative. Such causes of tissue shrinkage are well known. However, very little consideration has been given in the literature to tissue shrinkage which can result from compression artifacts produced by a dull microtome knife. A great deal of shrinkage can take place in tissues during microtomy as depicted in this photograph of tissue sections of specimens of human skin which were cut with a dull knife (compare with Figure 252). (H&E, ×4) (AFIP Negative No. 73-3542)

Figure 252. *Dull-knife Distortions.* These tissue sections were cut from the same specimen of embedded tissue as the sections depicted in Figure 251. However, a sharp microtome knife was used rather than a dull one. Note the difference in the dimension of the various components of these sections as compared to those depicted in Figure 251. It is clearly evident that a great deal of shrinkage may occur in tissue sections due to compression artifacts that are produced by a dull knife. (H&E, ×4) (AFIP Negative No. 73-3543)

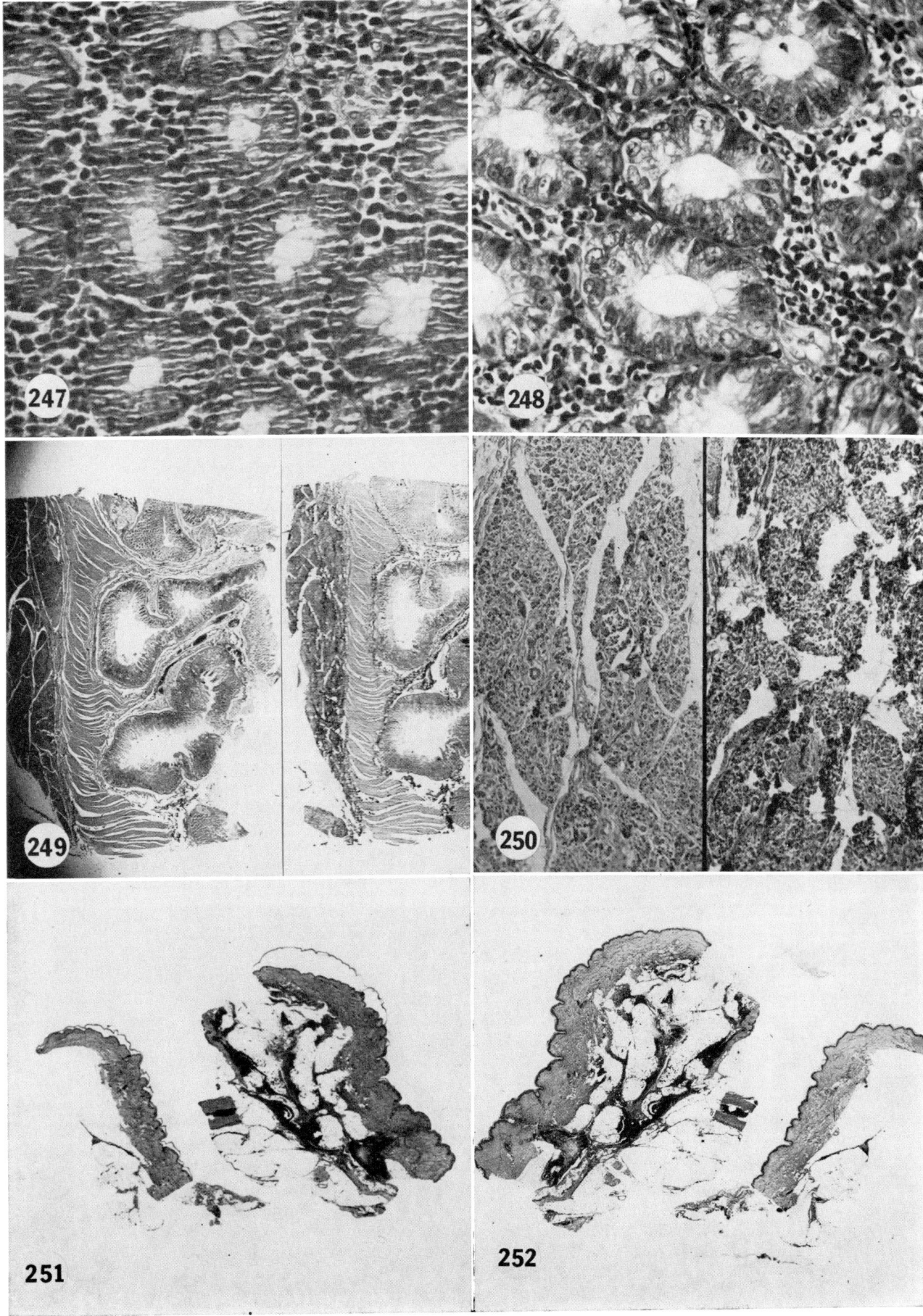

Figure 253. *Dull-knife Distortions.* This is a higher magnification of a portion of the microscopic field depicted in Figure 251 to illustrate the numerous folds throughout the epidermis which account for some of the shrinkage that resulted from sectioning with a dull microtome knife. Compression of the stroma of the dermis also accounted for some of the shrinkage. (H&E, ×70) (AFIP Negative No. 73-3540)

Figure 254. *Dull-knife Distortions.* In this tissue section of a specimen of a human lymph node numerous lepra bacilli have been displaced from a diseased site to the paraffin surrounding the tissue specimen. Such displacement of the bacilli can readily occur with a dull knife during microtomy. Similar artifacts are also encountered with pigment deposits within tissue specimens. With such faulty microtomy bacilli and/or pigment may be displaced and deposited elsewhere within the embedded specimen or its mounting media. Such displaced bacilli and/or pigment can readily contaminate the tissue flotation water bath and subsequently be picked up on subsequent tissue sections prepared from the same or different specimens. This problem can be reduced in large measure by the use of an extremely sharp knife during microtomy. Even when such precautions are undertaken, if the density of bacilli and/or pigment within the specimen is very abundant a minimal degree of displacement may be encountered. (Fite-Faraco stain, ×220) (AFIP Negative No. 69-1085)

Figure 255. *Alternate Thick and Thin Zones.* One of the defects observed in tissue sections, when the section being cut is thick and the knife employed is too thin, is depicted in this paraffin-embedded tissue section of a connective tissue tumor (fibroma) from a rat (see also Figure 256). The knife has a tendency to vibrate. This may readily occur in the cutting of thick sections when a knife of insufficient thickness or strength is used such as a razor mounted in a microtome holder or a new knife with a feather edge. In such instances, the knife bends back and forth numerous times as it passes through the tissue block. The resulting tissue section will contain a series of alternately thick and thin zones as depicted here, although other causes may also produce such an effect (see Figure 256). Such defects in tissue sections may be avoided by using properly sharpened knives of adequate thickness and strength. (H&E, ×26) (Contributed by Mr. L. E. Schellhammer)

Figure 256. *Alternate Thick and Thin Zones.* If the knife of the microtome is loose, or the specimen chuck is loose, or air bubbles or crevices surround the specimen in the paraffin block (see Chapter V), alternate thick and thin zones may be observed in the tissue section as depicted in this paraffin-embedded tissue section of a specimen of the human uterus. (H&E, ×40) (AFIP Negative No. 64-1681)

Figure 257. *Use of Quick-freeze Spray to Firm Paraffin Blocks.* This is a photomicrograph of an unstained glass microscope slide which has been sprayed with a quick-freeze aerosol spray. Such sprays have become very popular in the last few years for the preparation of frozen tissue sections. They are composed of a mixture of fluorinated hydrocarbons. When used for the preparation of frozen tissue sections, the spray may leave an oil-like residue on the surface of the tissue section similar to the droplets depicted here. These droplets do not disappear when the tissue section is mounted in water or glycerine mounting medium and may cause some confusion in the microscopic examination of fresh-frozen or fixed-frozen tissue sections which have been stained for the demonstration of lipid (Kohlmeyer, J.: *Trans Am Micros Soc, 91:*4, 607-608, 1972). (Unstained, ×350) (AFIP Negative No. 73-4137)

Figure 258. *Use of Quick-freeze Spray to Firm Paraffin Blocks.* The paraffin-embedded tissue section of a specimen of the adrenal gland of a human being depicted in this photomicrograph was cut from a tissue block which was chilled with an aerosol spray of dichlorotetrafluoromethane after rough cutting and prior to sectioning. The spray was applied for too long a period of time and the surface of the embedded tissue became excessively dehydrated and fissures formed along natural lines of cleavage (arrow). (Lendrum's stain, ×63) (AFIP Negative No. 71-10730)

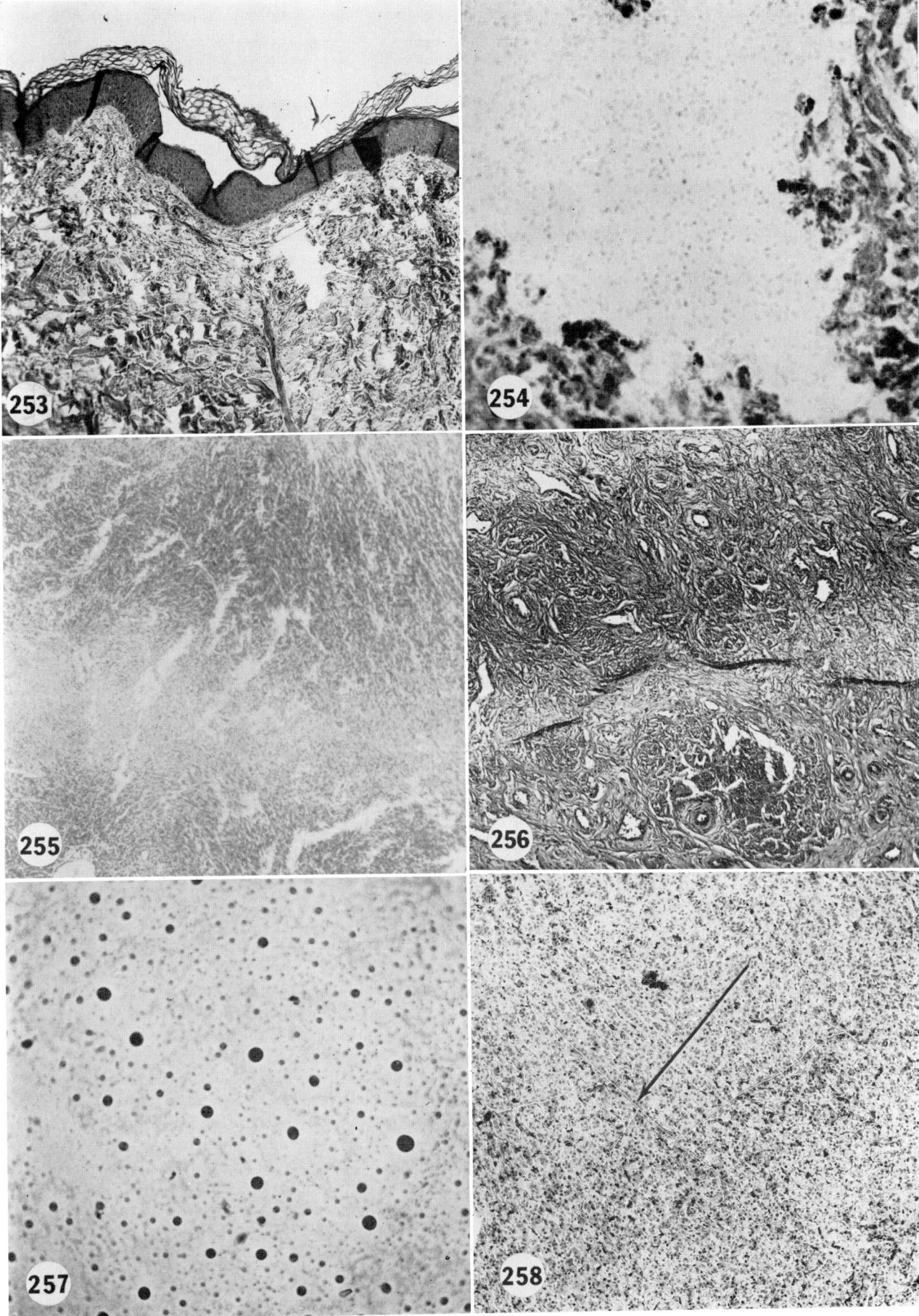

Figure 259. *Hydration.* Prior to commencing to cut dry or bloody paraffin-embedded tissue sections on a microtome, it is helpful to soak the face of the mounted tissue block with a pad of cotton which has been moistened in lukewarm water as depicted in this photograph. The block and the specimen surface of the knife may then be chilled with an ice cube immediately prior to sectioning. The purpose of these two techniques is to soften the specimen within the paraffin and to chill the paraffin so that it will be firm rather than soft when one attempts to cut tissue sections. (AFIP Negative No. 71-12088)

Figure 260. *Hydration.* If the soaking of the tissue block is not uniformly applied (see Figure 259) for an adequate period of time, the more hydrophilic components or areas of the embedded specimen will be softened and the denser hydrophobic components or areas will still be inadequately hydrated. With such a tissue block, the tissue sections may shatter as they are cut (see Figure 263) or have holes in their surfaces (moth-eaten effect) as depicted in this paraffin-embedded tissue section of a specimen of human liver. The inadequately hydrated hard tissue components resisted the knife more than the surrounding hydrated tissue components and were pushed or punched out of the section rather than being cut by the knife. The moth-eaten effect can also occur in tissue sections which are prepared from embedded tissue blocks, which are soaked for a period of time that is adequate for properly processed specimens, prepared from specimens which were improperly processed (see Chapter IV). (H&E, ×40) (AFIP Negative No. 64-1672)

Figure 261. *Hydration.* The alternately thick and thin horizontal bands noticed in this paraffin-embedded tissue section of a specimen of lung from a human being who died of pneumonia are the result of excessive dehydration of the specimen during tissue processing (see also Chapter IV). This problem can be eliminated by soaking the faced-off surface of the embedded specimen with a pledget of cotton which has been soaked with lukewarm water as depicted in Figure 259. Compare with Figure 262. (H&E, ×60) (AFIP Negative No. 73-1992)

Figure 262. *Hydration.* This tissue section was obtained from the same block of embedded tissue as the tissue section depicted in Figure 261. The faced-off surface of the embedded specimen had been soaked for several minutes with a pledget of cotton which had been soaked with lukewarm water. The block and the specimen surface of the knife were then chilled with an ice cube immediately prior to sectioning. Compare to Figure 261. (H&E, ×60) (AFIP Negative No. 73-1993)

Figure 263. *Hydration.* As previously mentioned, if the soaking of the tissue block is not uniformly applied (see Figure 259) for an adequate period of time, the more hydrophilic components or areas of the embedded specimens will be softened and the denser hydrophobic components or areas will still be inadequately hydrated. This is exemplified by the paraffin-embedded tissue section of the adrenal gland of a dog depicted in this photograph. The cortex of the gland was less hydrophilic than the medulla and the time period allowed for soaking the specimen surface of the block was inadequate to properly hydrate the cortical tissue. When the tissue section was cut the cortex of the gland shattered, although the knife was sharp, while the medulla remained intact. (H&E, ×40)

Figure 264. *Hydration with 10% Ammonium Hydroxide.* This photograph depicts one of the types of shattering artifacts that may frequently be encountered when tissue specimens containing large areas of hemorrhage are subjected to microtomy. Hemorrhagic areas within tissue specimens dry excessively during the processing and embedding procedures. This drying effect makes it difficult, if not impossible, to obtain good sections during microtomy unless special precautions are taken. The problem can be solved by the use of a 10% aqueous solution of ammonium hydroxide. The block is rough-cut to expose the entire surface of the specimen and then a piece of cotton soaked with the 10% ammonium hydroxide is placed on the surface of the specimen for fifteen to twenty seconds. The time allowed for soaking may have to be varied depending on the extent of the area of hemorrhage and the severity of the drying effect produced during processing and embedding procedures. (H&E, ×6.5) (AFIP Negative No. 74-5755)

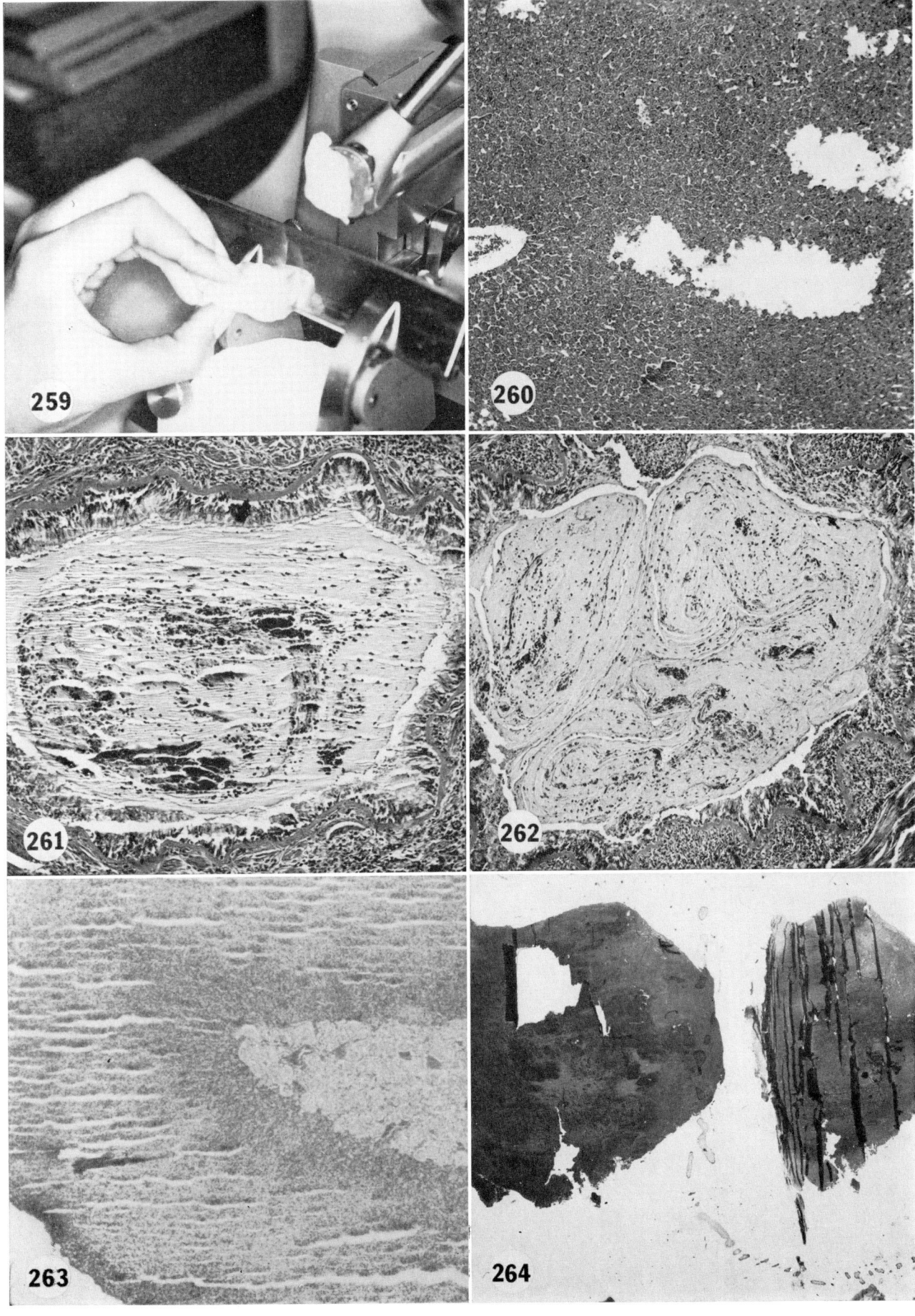

Figure 265. *Extraneous Debris.* Epithelial cells are frequently rubbed off from the technician's fingers during microtomy or shed on the knife surface as dandruff. These epithelial cells frequently end up on microscope slides of finished tissue sections as depicted in this paraffin-embedded tissue section of a specimen of liver from a human being. Tinctorially, the cells are eosinophilic after H&E staining. (H&E, ×70) (AFIP Negative No. 73-717)

Figure 266. *Extraneous Debris.* This is a higher magnification of a portion of the field of view depicted in Figure 265. The epithelial cells from the technician's fingers or dandruff can be identified by the characteristic nuclei which can be found in some of the cells. The acidophilic epithelial cells are difficult to remove and/or eliminate. Control of dandruff by the histotechnologist will materially lessen the occurrence of this type of artifact. (H&E, ×165) (AFIP Negative No. 73-718)

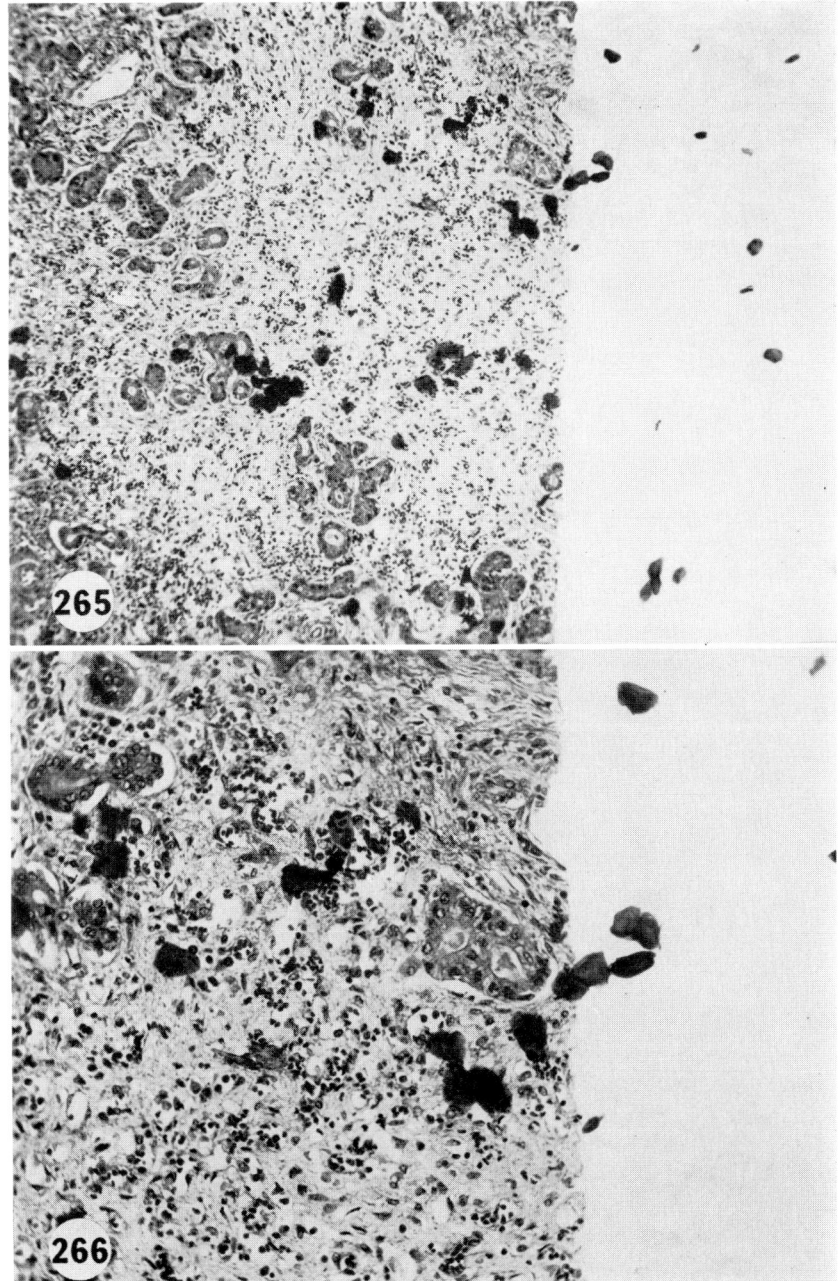

VII

Artifacts Resulting from the Mounting of Tissue Sections on Glass Slides

INTRODUCTION

*V*IRTUALLY ALL OF THE ARTIFACTS which may be observed in microscopic tissue sections that are the result of techniques employed in the mounting of tissue sections on glass microscope slides can be attributed to carelessness on the part of the histotechnologist. Examples of such artifacts that are included in this chapter are:

Contamination of glass slides by molds
Use of contaminated gelatin
Use of excessive quantities of adhesives
Use of tap water for tissue flotation
Failure to remove tissue debris from tissue flotation waterbath
Contamination of tissue flotation waterbath with cigarette, cigar, or pipe ashes
Wrinkling of tissue sections
Air bubbles beneath tissue sections
Elevation of temperature of tissue flotation waterbath
Improper drying of mounted tissue sections

Figure 267. *Mold Contaminants on Glass Slides.* The glass microscope slides which were used to mount the tissue sections depicted in Figures 268 through 271 were obtained from this box. Splotchy, gray-colored areas of mildew are seen between the cellophane wrapper and the slide box. The exterior surfaces of the box were also mildewed and the slides which it contained had a glazed appearance. Slides contained in mildewed boxes should be cleaned extremely well with 1% acid alcohol prior to being used.

Figure 268. *Mold Contaminants on Glass Slides.* This photomicrograph is of a portion of a glass microscope slide which had become contaminated by molds within the laboratory. The area depicted is adjacent to the tissue section which was mounted on this slide (see Figures 270 and 271). This artifact occurs most frequently when microslides are stored in humid, damp storerooms or when the slides are exposed to heat or sunlight which causes the cellophane wrapper to sweat. (Periodic acid-Schiff reaction, ×115) (AFIP Negative No. 72-6162)

Figure 269. *Mold Contaminants on Glass Slides.* This is a higher power view of a portion of the microscopic field shown in Figure 268. The mold which had contaminated the surface of the glass slide is not dissimilar in appearance from several forms of pathogenic molds. (Periodic acid-Schiff reaction, ×305) (AFIP Negative No. 72-6161)

Figure 270. *Mold Contaminants on Glass Slides.* This is the same preparation depicted in Figures 268 and 269. A paraffin-embedded tissue section of a specimen of human kidney has been mounted on the moldy surface of the glass microscope slide depicted in Figures 268 and 269. The mold is intensely basophilic and while it is not in the same focal plane as the tissue section it can be detected while examining the tissue section under the microscope (see Color Plate 3, Figure 17). If the focal plane is adjusted so that one focuses on the surface of the glass slide beneath the tissue section, the mold is readily detectable as depicted here. (Periodic acid-Schiff reaction, ×115) (AFIP Negative No. 72-6163)

Figure 271. *Mold Contaminants on Glass Slides.* This is a higher power view of a portion of the microscopic field shown in Figure 268. The conidia, vesicle, and hyphae of the mold are readily discernable as strongly basophilic structures. (Periodic acid-Schiff reaction, ×265) (AFIP Negative No. 72-6164)

Figure 272. *Mold Contaminants on Glass Slides.* Mildew fungi had contaminated the glass microscope slides which were stored in the box shown in Figure 267. Stains were applied to some of the blank slides which were stored in the box and fungi were readily demonstrated as contaminants on both surfaces of each slide. At the bottom, a slide has been stained with hematoxylin and eosin which demonstrates anionic and cationic components of the fungi. At the top left-hand side, a slide has been stained with Gomori's methenamine silver (GMS) technique and at the top right-hand side by the periodic-acid-Schiff reaction (PAS). If a tissue section was mounted on such a glass microscope slide, such fungi could perhaps be mistaken for pathogenic fungi by the inexperienced observer. It is interesting to note that different portions of the fungi yield positive reactions with the GMS and PAS techniques. The PAS reaction demonstrates those components of the fungi which yield aldehydes upon oxidation with periodic acid (polysaccharides). These same tissue components yield aldehydes upon acid hydrolysis in the GMS reaction and are blackened when the silver of the methenamine-silver complex is reduced by the aldehyde of the hydrolyzed polysaccharide. However, aldehydes alone do not account for all the reduced silver observed with the GMS technique since various reducing substances that the fungi apparently possess can also reduce the silver of the methenamine-silver complex. (×165) (AFIP Negative No. 73-5051-2)

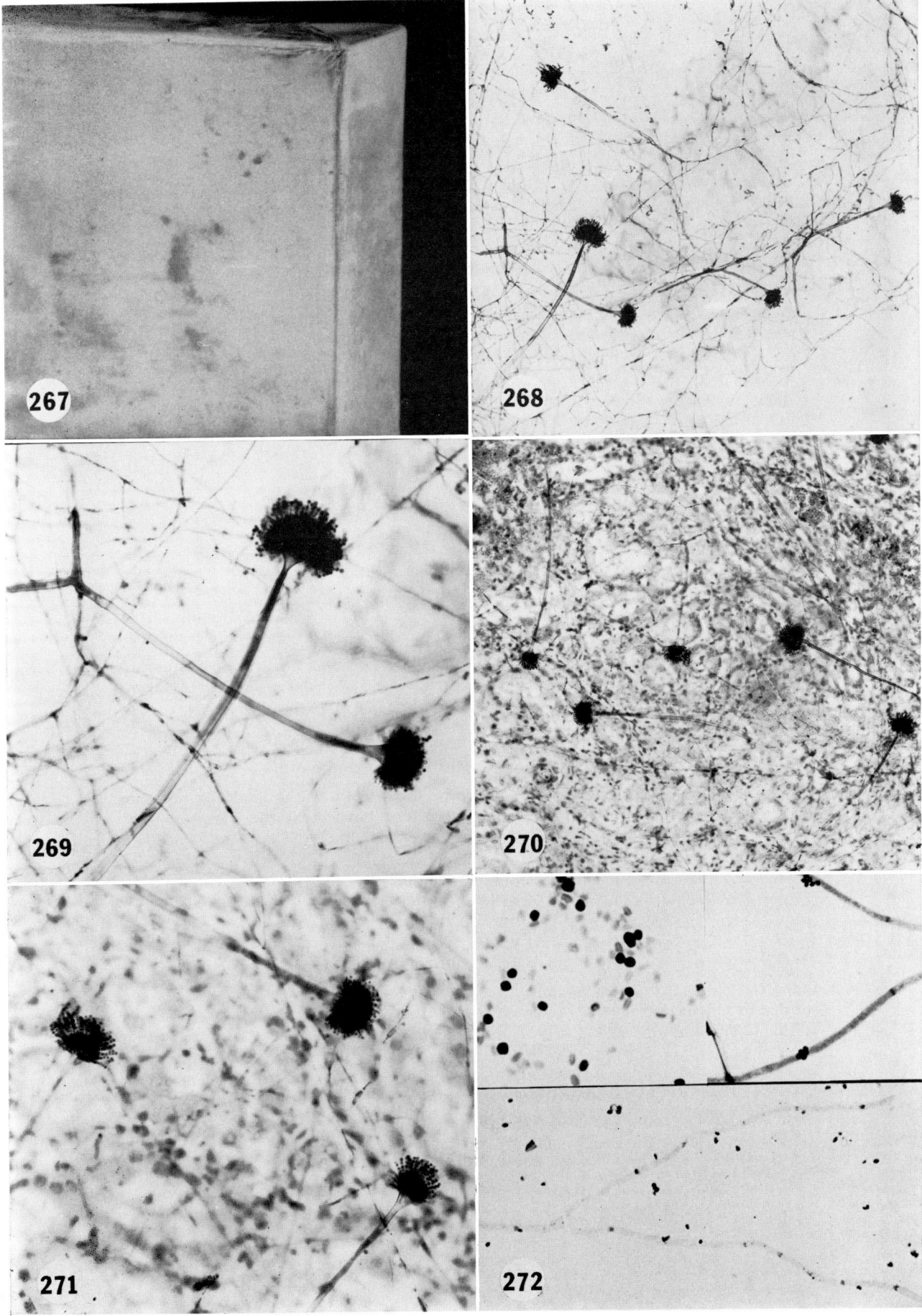

Figure 273. *Bacterial Contamination of Gelatin.* Virtually all of the proteins used to cause tissue sections to adhere to glass microscope slides are excellent media for bacteria. In this photograph, two bottles are observed, each containing a 2% aqueous solution of gelatin. On the right, the solution is clear and obviously is not contaminated. However, with little effort, such stock solutions can become contaminated in which case the growth of bacteria will ultimately cause the solution to become cloudy as depicted by the contents of the bottle on the left. Such solutions should not be used in the preparation of tissue sections.

Figure 274. *Tissue Flotation Waterbath.* As tissue sections are cut, they are removed from the specimen surface of the microtome knife and are flattened. The most common method used for flattening such tissue sections is to float them on water as depicted here. As the tissue sections are flattened, they are picked up on glass microscope slides. In order for the tissue sections to adhere to the microscope slide, it is necessary to either coat the specimen surface of individual slides with adhesive or add a small quantity of gelatin, either in solution (see Figure 273) or in dry form, to the waterbath. If the latter technique is used, it is not necessary to apply a film of such adhesive to the microscope slides which are used to pick up the floating tissue sections.

Figure 275. *Bacterial Contaminants.* The rod-shaped structures seen in the center of this tissue section of a specimen of human splenic tissue are waterbath bacterial contaminants which simulate acid-fast bacilli in both morphology and staining characteristics (see Color Plate 3, Figure 18) (also see Figures 276 through 278). Every effort should be made to avoid such waterbath contaminants since this type of bacteria may be confused with pathologic acid-fast bacilli. (Kinyon's acid-fast stain, $\times 80$) (AFIP Negative No. 67-8645)

Figure 276. *Bacterial Contaminants.* This specimen is a smear on a glass microscope slide of the contaminated gelatin solution from the bottle depicted at the left in Figure 273. Numerous rod-shaped bacteria are present throughout the smear. (H&E, $\times 500$) (AFIP Negative No. 64-1673)

Figure 277. *Bacterial Contaminants.* If contaminated adhesive (see Figures 273 and 276) is used to coat the microscope slides to be used for mounting tissue sections, the bacteria continue to thrive. In succession, they can contaminate the waterbath (see Figure 274) used for floating the tissue sections, and the tissue sections which are affixed to the surface of the slide as shown in this paraffin-embedded tissue section of a specimen of human liver. The bacteria seen in this section are artifacts although an inexperienced observer might mistake them for pathogens. (H&E, $\times 500$) (AFIP Negative No. 73-5051-5)

Figure 278. *Bacterial Contaminants.* Bacteria in the water of the tissue flotation bath due to contamination of the water with contaminated gelatin (see Figures 273 and 276) or due to failure to maintain the bath in a clean condition may contaminate the tissue sections. The coccoid bacteria seen in this paraffin-embedded tissue section of a specimen of human liver are artifacts. The bacteria were derived from the water on which the tissue section was flattened. Such artifacts can be prevented by daily washing of the waterbath and utensils, such as camel's hair brushes and forceps used to tease sections onto slides, with a good detergent. (Brown & Brenn stain, $\times 500$) (AFIP Negative No. 67-2659)

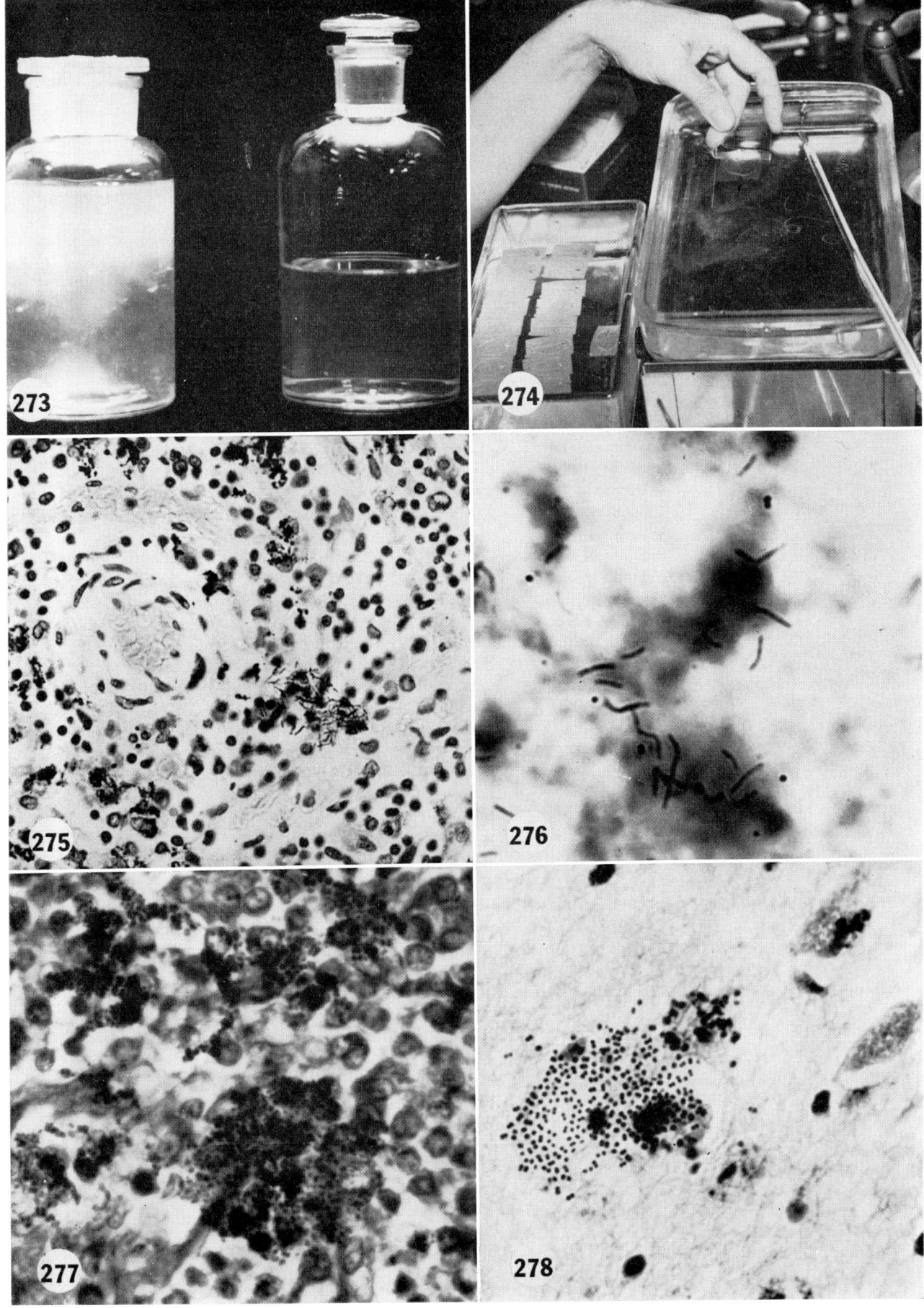

Figure 279. *Excessive Adhesive.* When excessive quantities of section adhesives are used to coat glass microscope slides or are added to the water of the tissue flotation waterbath, strands or clumps of gelatin may adhere to the tissue sections. Basophilic strands and clumps of such gelatin are the artifacts noted (arrow) in this paraffin-embedded tissue section of a specimen of human lung. However, adhesive artifacts on microscope slides may appear as basophilic or acidophilic strands or splotches depending on how well the hematoxylin was differentiated in the staining of the tissue section. (H&E, ×125)

Figure 280. *Contamination of Tissue Sections During Flotation.* Distilled water is recommended for use in tissue flotation waterbaths (see Figure 274) but it is not unusual to find conventional tap water being used for this purpose. At times, the water from such sources has a high mineral content, particularly of iron (see Chapter IV). If unfiltered water from such sources is used for tissue section flotation the section may become contaminated on one or both surfaces with iron particulate matter. The dark-colored material distributed across the surface of this paraffin-embedded tissue section of a formalin-fixed specimen of brown adipose tissue from a rat yields a positive Prussian blue reaction for iron. The section was contaminated during flotation on unfiltered tap water (see also Figures 281 and 282). Unlike similar contamination of specimens during postfixation washing (see Chapter IV) the iron particulate matter is not in the same focal plane as the tissue section but is observed to be above as well as below the focal plane of the tissue section. (H&E, ×35) (Contributed by Dr. W. L. Wooding)

Figure 281. *Contamination of Tissue Sections During Flotation.* As mentioned previously (see Figure 280), if unfiltered tap water from a source which has a high mineral content is used for tissue section flotation the section may become contaminated on one or both surfaces with iron particulate matter. The dark-colored material observed as seemingly attached to this paraffin-embedded tissue section of a formalin-fixed specimen of a rat's uterus yields a positive Prussian blue reaction for iron. The section was contaminated during flotation on unfiltered tap water (see also Figure 279). (H&E, ×35) (Contributed by Dr. W. L. Wooding)

Figure 282. *Contamination of Tissue Sections During Flotation.* This is a higher magnification of the central portion of the tissue section depicted in Figure 281 to better demonstrate that the iron particulate matter artifact is beneath the focal plane of the tissue section per se. Only a small portion of the contaminate underrides the tissue section. (H&E, ×175) (Contributed by Dr. W. L. Wooding)

Figure 283. *Contamination of Tissue Sections During Flotation.* This paraffin-embedded tissue section of a specimen of rat kidney was contaminated with iron particulate matter during flotation on unfiltered tap water in the same fashion as described for Figures 280 through 282. In addition, due to sloppy technique, fragments of tissue sections cut from previously sectioned blocks of embedded tissue were not removed from the surface of the water and such a tissue fragment has adhered to the tissue section while it was being flattened on the waterbath. (H&E, ×40) (Contributed by Dr. W. L. Wooding)

Figure 284. *Contamination of Tissue Sections During Flotation.* This is a higher magnification of a portion of the tissue section depicted in Figure 283. Three iron particles are seen in the upper left hand portion of the photomicrograph. The tissue fragment overlaying the section contaminated the tissue section per se after the section had been picked up on the microscope slide since it is above the focal plane of the section per se. The fragment stains more intensely than the underlaying section since, except for points of firm adhesion, both surfaces of the fragment are exposed to the stain. (H&E, ×170) (Contributed by Dr. W. L. Wooding)

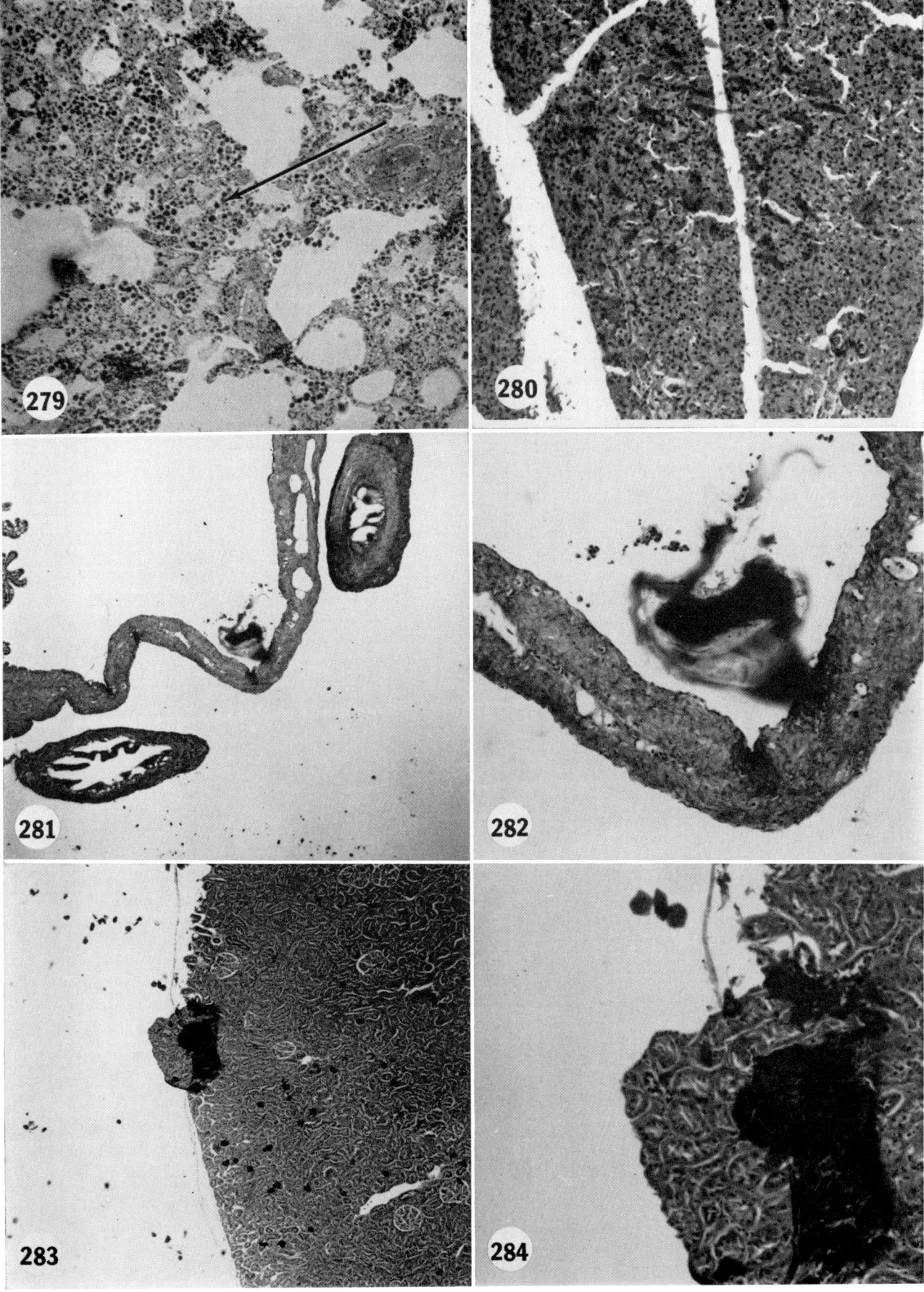

Figure 285. *Contamination of Tissue Sections During Flotation.* Technicians should not smoke cigarettes, cigars, or pipes while coverslipping finished tissue sections. The artifact observed above the focal plane of this paraffin-embedded tissue section of a specimen of skin from a human being is cigarette ash which the technician spilled on the wet stained slide prior to the application of mounting medium. (H&E, ×80) (AFIP Negative No. 73-2494)

Figure 286. *Contamination of Tissue Sections During Flotation.* Technicians should not smoke cigarettes, cigars, or pipes while cleaning glass microscope slides, picking up tissue sections on microscope slides, or staining tissue sections. The cigarette ash observed on this photomicrograph of an unstained glass microscope slide has a different pattern than that depicted in Figure 285. (Unstained, ×150) (AFIP Negative No. 73-2495)

Figure 287. *Contamination of Tissue Sections During Flotation.* This paraffin-embedded tissue section of a specimen of the spleen of a rat was flattened on distilled water in a tissue flotation waterbath. The technique was sloppy in that fragments of previous sections which had been flattened on the same waterbath had not been removed from the surface of the water. A section of an artery was picked up on the microscope slide at the time it was submerged to pick up the section of splenic tissue. As a result, the section of the artery came to partially underlay the section of splenic tissue and is beneath the focal plane of the splenic tissue section. The section of the artery does not stain more intensely than the tissue which it underlays because it is firmly affixed to the microscope slide on its bottom surface and the stain only had access to its upper surface. The underlaying tissue stretches the overlaying tissue and a rent is seen in the overlaying section of splenic tissue in the vicinity of the underlaying tissue section of the artery. The overlaying section of splenic tissue stains more intensely in the area adjacent to the underlaying tissue because the rent and the elevation of the margin of the splenic tissue section in this focal area permitted the stain to have access to both surfaces of the overlaying tissue section. (H&E, ×70) (Contributed by Mr. L. E. Schellhammer)

Figure 288. *Contamination of Tissue Sections During Flotation.* This paraffin-embedded tissue section of a specimen of the oviduct of a rat was flattened on distilled water in a tissue flotation waterbath. In the same fashion as described in the legend for Figure 287 the technique was sloppy. Unidentified fragments of a previous tissue section which had been flattened on the same waterbath had not been removed from the surface of the water. The debris was picked up on the microscope slide at the time it was submerged to pick up the section of the oviduct. As a result, the debris came to underlay one of the longitudinal mucosal folds and overlay the adjacent mucosal fold. The fold which overlays the debris is also folded upon itself since it was not affixed to the surface of the microscope slide. This fold also stains more intensely since the stain had access to both surfaces of the tissue section in this area. (H&E, ×66) (Contributed by Mr. L. E. Schellhammer)

Figure 289. *Contamination of Tissue Sections During Flotation.* One of the techniques which is frequently employed to cause tissue sections to adhere to glass microscope slides consists of coating the individual slides with a thin film of albumin or gelatin on the surface to be used to pick up the section from the waterbath. One means employed for spreading adhesive on the slide consists of using a finger or the palm of the hand. The debris noted adjacent to this tissue section of the cornea of a human eye are epithelial cells from the hand of the technician who coated the slide with albumin. Most of these cells stain light pink with hematoxylin and eosin and are devoid of nuclei. However, occasionally distinct nuclei can be identified (see Figure 290). (H&E, ×35) (AFIP Negative No. 71-11016-1)

Figure 290. *Contamination of Tissue Sections During Flotation.* This is an enlargement of a portion of Figure 289 which depicts a single epithelial cell from the hand of the technician who coated the slide with albumin. Such artifacts can be avoided by spraying the adhesive on the slide or by using uncoated slides and adding the gelatin directly to the waterbath used for tissue flotation. One should keep in mind that the contamination of tissue sections with human epithelial cells during flotation can also result from the shedding of dandruff by histotechnologists (see Chapter VI). (H&E, ×750) (AFIP Negative No. 71-11016-2)

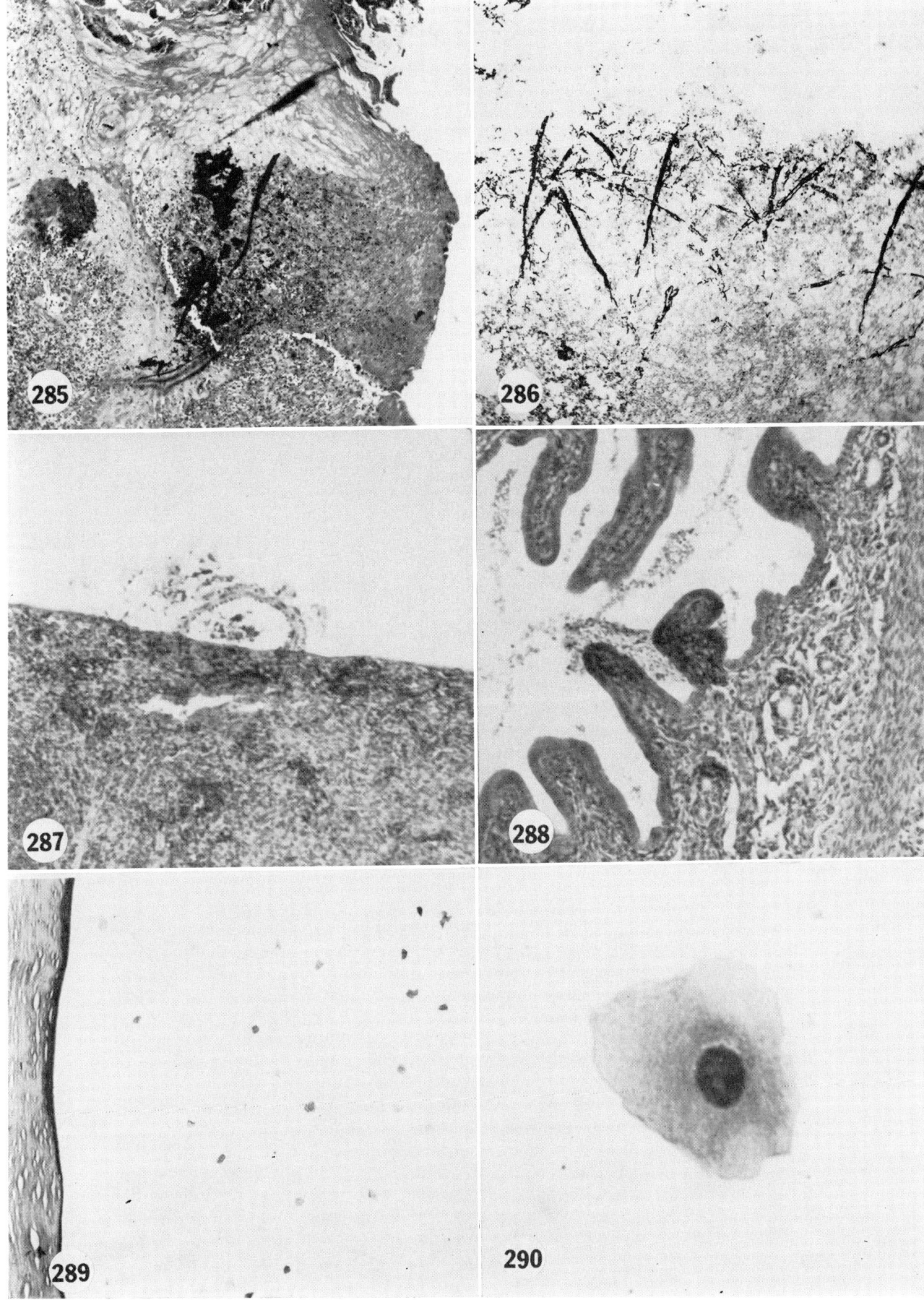

Figure 291. *Wrinkled Tissue Sections.* Tissue sections may become wrinkled as they are being cut on the microtome. The causes for such alteration of the tissue sections are varied: (1) the paraffin may be softer than the processed and infiltrated tissue specimen; (2) the paraffin may be much harder than the processed and infiltrated tissue specimen; or (3) the cutting edge of the microtome knife may be dull or blunt. Frequently, tissue sections which are wrinkled can be flattened on a waterbath. However, it is not always possible to adequately flatten wrinkled tissue sections or, if possible, the technician may fail to do so. The lines seen in this paraffin-embedded tissue section of a specimen of human liver are artifacts due to wrinkles in the tissue section which could not be flattened. The wrinkles permitted the stain to flow beneath the wrinkled portion of the tissue section and the wrinkled area stains much more intensely than the surrounding tissue because the dye stained both surfaces of the tissue section at these points. (H&E, ×125)

Figure 292. *Wrinkled Tissue Sections.* The causes for wrinkling of tissue sections have been discussed in the legend for Figure 291. At times, the wrinkles may assume bizarre patterns since the paraffin in the lumina of ducts, glands, and vessels is removed prior to staining and although it originally composed part of the wrinkle it is not apparent in the stained tissue section. In this paraffin-embedded tissue section of a specimen of the epididymis of a dog seemingly unrelated small wrinkles are seen in the walls of the tubules. (H&E, ×125)

Figure 293. *Air Bubbles.* As tissue sections are flattened in a tissue flotation waterbath, bubbles of air may become entrapped beneath them. These can be and should be removed at the time the tissue section is picked up on a glass microscope slide. Frequently, such air bubbles are not detected by the histotechnologist and remain beneath the tissue section on the dried slide. When such a tissue section is stained, an artifact develops such as depicted in this paraffin-embedded tissue section of a specimen of human liver. The air bubble is broken and the overlaying tissue is shattered. The tissue which overlaid the air bubble is stained more intensely than the surrounding tissue since the stain accumulated on both surfaces of the tissue section at the site of the artifact. (H&E, ×80) (AFIP Negative No. 64-1670)

Figure 294. *Air Bubbles.* As mentioned in the legend for Figure 293, as tissue sections are flattened in a tissue flotation waterbath, bubbles of air may become entrapped beneath them. If they are not removed prior to picking the tissue section up on a glass microscope slide an artifact develops such as depicted in this paraffin-embedded tissue section of the brain of a rat. From the tissue section depicted in Figure 293 one might gain the impression that such air bubbles are relatively large and are readily detectable. Such is not always the case. The air bubbles may be extremely minute and difficult to detect and/or remove from beneath the tissue section on the flotation waterbath. The air bubble responsible for the small artifact depicted here was of pinpoint size, yet it seriously damaged the tissue section. (H&E, ×40) (Contributed by Mr. L. E. Schellhammer)

Figure 295. *Air Bubbles.* This is a higher magnification of the central portion of the tissue section depicted in Figure 294 to better illustrate the shatter pattern of the tissue which formerly overlaid a minute air bubble. Unlike the circumferential shattering depicted in Figure 293, tissue that overlays a very small bubble more frequently shatters from the center to the periphery of the affected portion of the tissue section which overlaid the air bubble. The tissue which overlaid the air bubble is stained more intensely than the surrounding tissue since the stain accumulated on both surfaces of the tissue section at the site of the artifact. (H&E, ×175) (Contributed by Mr. L. E. Schellhammer)

Figure 296. *Air Bubbles.* One might gain the impression that it is only with sizable tissue sections, such as those depicted in Figures 294 and 295, that difficulty might be expected in the detection of a minute air bubble entrapped beneath the section on a tissue flotation waterbath. However, this is not the case. This is a paraffin-embedded tissue section of the pituitary gland of a rat. Such tissue sections are routinely small. Yet a minute air bubble remained undetected beneath this very small tissue section on the tissue flotation waterbath and produced the artifact seen here. (H&E, ×100) (Contributed by Mr. L. E. Schellhammer)

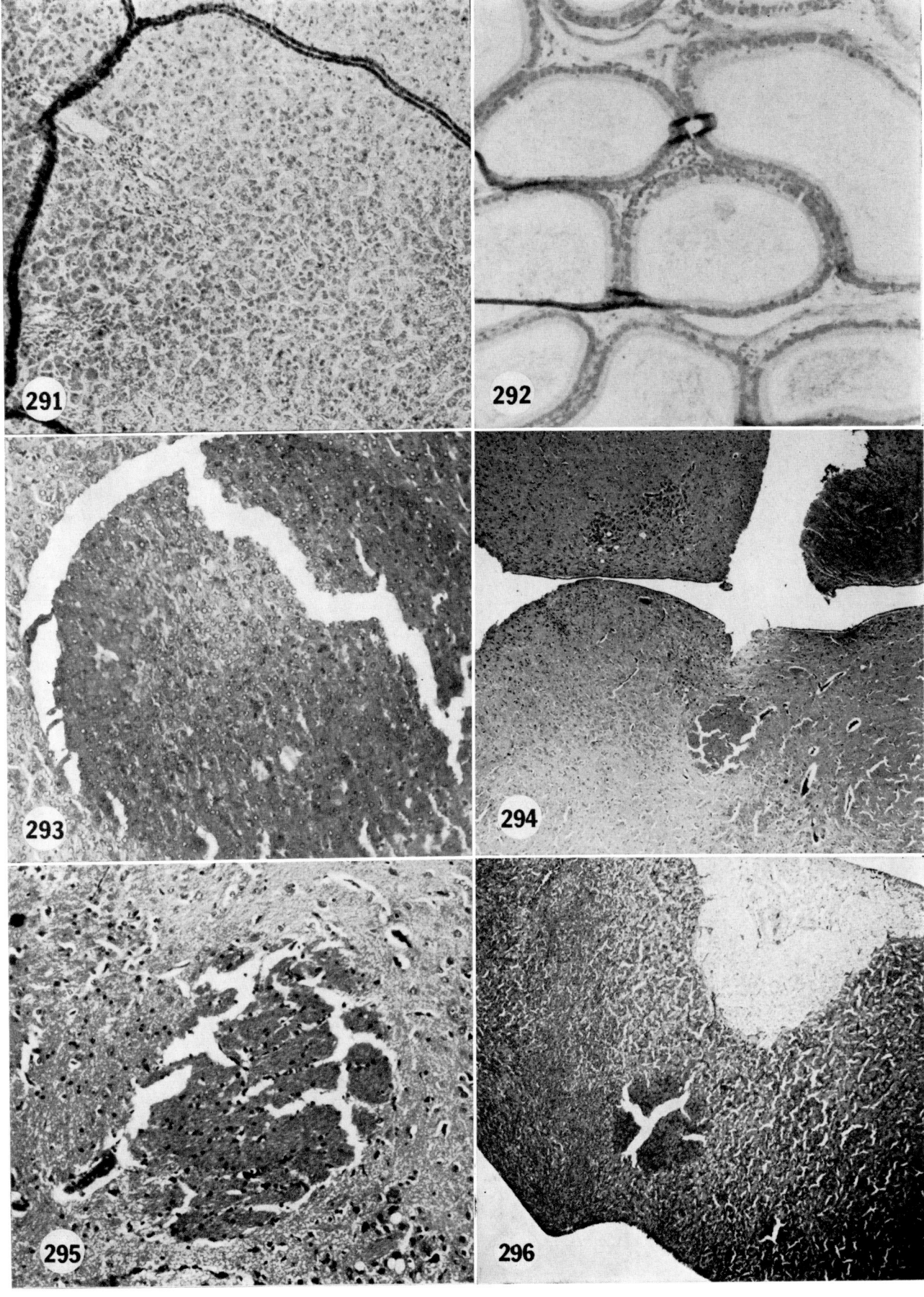

Figure 297. *Overexpansion of Tissue Sections.* This same illustration has been utilized in the chapter on tissue processing procedures since it was inadequately impregnated with paraffin during processing (see Chapter IV). It is utilized in this chapter since it is a good example of a common problem encountered with the tissue flotation waterbath. The temperature of the waterbath is critical from several standpoints: (1) if it is not warm enough the tissue will not spread out sufficiently and will develop wrinkles when picked up on the glass slide; (2) if it is too hot the tissue can expand excessively and when picked up on the glass slide it will be overexpanded. In the latter instance, upon drying, the tissue section will attempt to shrink to its original size. In this attempt to return to its original size the bonds between the tissue and the slide adhesive can be broken and the section will fall off of the slide during staining. If the tissue section does not fall off of the slide during staining one may see the artifact illustrated in this photograph of a tissue section of a specimen of human cardiac muscle in which the muscle bundles are separated. Once a tissue section has expanded to the degree shown here there is nothing that can be done to correct the individual problem with the affected tissue section. If the embedded tissue specimen is properly impregnated with paraffin (see Chapter IV), one must adjust the temperature of the waterbath to approximately 42°C and prepare an additional section. If the embedded specimen has not been adequately impregnated with paraffin during tissue processing, and duplicate wet tissue specimens are available, a new specimen can be processed and embedded. (H&E, ×4) (AFIP Negative No. 72-3732)

Figure 298. *Parched-earth Effect.* The parched-earth effect is depicted in this paraffin-embedded tissue section of a specimen of human brain tissue. The specimen was inadequately impregnated with paraffin during processing (see Chapter IV). However, the cracks resulted from using a tissue flotation waterbath which was excessively hot. This caused the floating tissue section to expand beyond its normal size and to crack during the staining procedure. (H&E, ×50) (AFIP Negative No. 74-5748)

Figure 299. *Parched-earth Effect.* This photograph of a paraffin-embedded tissue section of a specimen of human brain tissue illustrates the most severe effects of improper processing and impregnation procedures (see Chapter IV). During the staining procedure, as the cracking of the tissue takes place (parched-earth effect) the various solutions used in deceration, dehydration, hydration, staining, and clearing of the tissue section are able to get between the tissue section and the slide. These solutions working beneath the tissue section affect the adhesive properties of the mounting medium and break tissue away from the slide. The net result is that much of the tissue section falls off of the slide as depicted in this photograph. (H&E, ×13) (AFIP Negative No. 74-5754)

Figure 300. *Drying of Tissue Sections.* This is a paraffin-embedded tissue section being picked up on a glass microscope slide as the tissue section is abstracted from the surface of a tissue flotation waterbath (left). The mounted tissue section is subsequently allowed to air dry for a brief period of time on a slide drying block (center) before being placed on a slide warming table (right), oven or slide dryer. These simple mounting procedures must be adhered to if one is to avoid the splotchy staining effects depicted in Figures 301 and 302.

Figure 301. *Drying of Tissue Sections.* The splotchy staining effect depicted in this tissue section of a soft tissue specimen from a human being also resulted from inadequate drying of the section after being picked up from the tissue flotation waterbath. Compare with Figure 302. Inadequately dried tissue sections will stain with irregular red- and gray-colored zones. (H&E, ×130) (AFIP Negative No. 73-5051-1)

Figure 302. *Drying of Tissue Sections.* In order to obtain satisfactory staining results it is imperative that paraffin-embedded tissue sections be exposed to heat of some sort soon after they have been picked up on microscopic slides from the tissue flotation waterbath. The lack of proper drying (room temperature) of mounted tissue sections produces erratic staining results as seen in the epidermis of this paraffin-embedded tissue section of a specimen of human skin. (H&E, ×575) (AFIP Negative No. 68-1268)

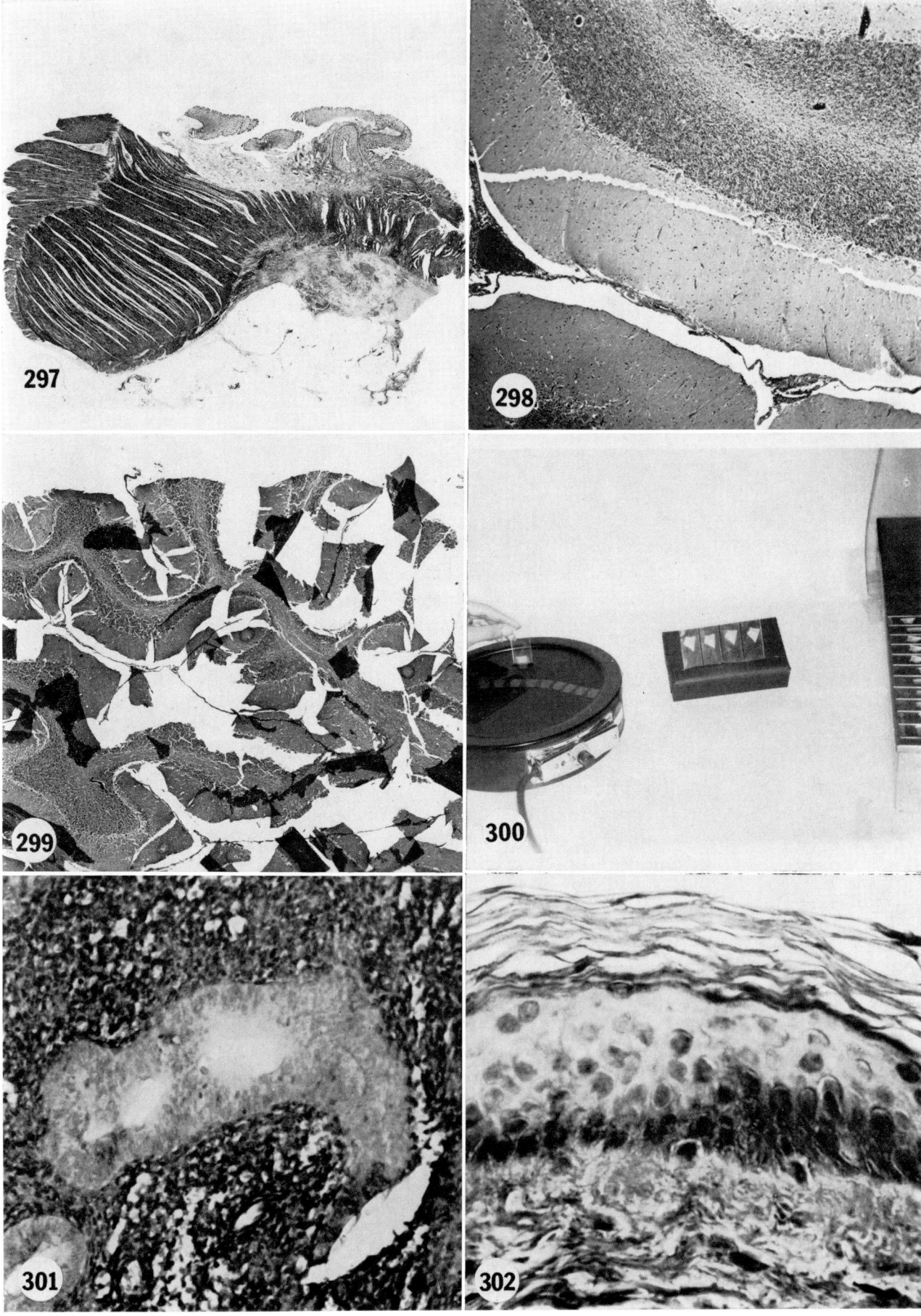

VIII

Artifacts Encountered in Staining Procedures

INTRODUCTION

THE ARTIFACTS which may be observed in microscopic tissue sections that are encountered in staining procedures may have their origin in the choice by the prosector of a fixative which is inappropriate for the staining procedure which he later requests from the histotechnologists. However, the cause of most artifacts encountered in staining procedures can be found in the manner in which the procedure was performed. Examples of such staining artifacts included in this chapter are:

- Adverse effects encountered upon storage in paraffin following fixation in Bouin's fluid
- Effect of Bouin's fluid fixation on the colloidal iron stain
- Adverse effect of acid-formalin fixation on aldehyde-fuchsin staining
- Adverse effect of Zenker's-fixation on stains for the demonstration of copper
- Adverse effect of Zenker's-fixation on Von Kossa stain
- Effect of delayed fixation on H&E staining
- Faulty deceration
- Artifacts due to faulty technique in the performance of the:
  - Aldehyde-fuchsin stain
  - Alizarin blue stain
  - Best's carmine stain
  - Bodian's silver protein reaction
  - Congo red stain
  - Cresyl echt violet stain
  - Crystal violet stain
  - Eosin counterstain
  - Fite-Faraco acid-fast stain

- Hematoxylin (Harris')
- Hematoxylin (Mayer's)
- Hematoxylin (Phosphotungstic Acid)
- Hematoxylin and eosin
- Iron reaction (Mallory's)
- Kinyon's acid-fast stain
- Methenamine silver nitrate stain
- Mucicarmine (Mayer's) stain
- Nuclear fast red stain
- Oil red O
- Periodic acid-Schiff reaction
- Rubeanic acid stain
- Sevier-Munger silver method
- Thionin (Mallory's) stain
- Trichrome (Masson's) stain
- Walbach's Giemsa stain
- Wright's Giemsa stain

Effects of prolonged storage of specimens as wet tissue, or embedded tissue, or unstained tissue sections or stained tissue sections

Faulty clearing techniques

Figure 303. *General Effect of Fixation on Staining.* It is generally believed that, once a tissue specimen is embedded in paraffin, it makes little difference in the quality of the stained slides which will be obtained if one cuts the tissue sections immediately or later after a considerable time lapse. This may be the case with formalin-fixed tissue, but it is not the case with all types of fixed tissues. This photograph depicts a low- and a high-power magnification of a paraffin-embedded tissue section of a specimen of human liver which was fixed in Bouin's fluid. The tissue section was cut and stained within twenty-four hours after it was embedded in paraffin. The result is an excellent tissue section. (H&E, ×125 and 375) (AFIP Negative No. 64-2667)

Figure 304. *General Effect of Fixation on Staining.* This tissue section seen at both a low- and high-power magnification was cut from the same paraffin-embedded block of liver tissue as the tissue section depicted in Figure 303. What has happened? All things are identical to the procedures used with the tissue section depicted in Figure 303 with the exception that this tissue section was cut twelve weeks after the specimen had been embedded in paraffin. The stains are diffused. Some cellular boundaries are indistinct and the cytoplasm of some hepatocytes has a hyalin appearance. The picric acid within Bouin's fluid, is rarely completely removed during the processing of gross specimens. Some picric acid remains in the embedded tissue to be finally removed from the exceedingly thin tissue section during the actual staining procedure. This picric acid continues to act upon the tissue components, adjacent to its site of deposition, even in the embedded tissue specimen. The longer one waits to cut and stain the tissue section, the greater is the influence exerted by the picric acid residues in the embedded tissue specimen. To be certain, not all fixatives leave residues in the embedded tissue specimen which can be likened to the picric acid of Bouin's fluid. However, all other factors being equal, it can be generalized that the sooner the tissue sections are cut and stained from any embedded specimen, fixed in any fashion, the better will be the quality of the tissue sections which one can obtain. (H&E, ×125 and 375) (AFIP Negative No. 67-2654)

Figure 305. *Effects of Fixation on Colloidal Iron Staining.* Duplicate blocks of tissue from this specimen of human skin were fixed in (1) Bouin's fluid and (2) neutral buffered 10% formalin. The specimens were subsequently processed and embedded in paraffin. A modification of Hale's colloidal iron stain, for the demonstration of acid mucopolysaccharides, was subsequently applied to tissue sections which had been fixed in each fixative (see Color Plate 4, Figure 19). The fixatives recommended for use with the colloidal iron stain are neutral buffered 10% formalin, absolute alcohol, Carnoy's fluid, cetylpyridinium chloride (0.5% in 4% aqueous formaldehyde) or 5-aminoacridine hydrochloride (0.4% in 50% ethyl alcohol). Acid mucopolysaccharides are not demonstrable by the colloidal iron stain in tissues fixed in Bouin's fluid. The tissue shown at the left was fixed in Bouin's fluid and no colloidal iron positive material is observed, whereas the tissue shown at the right was fixed in neutral buffered 10% formalin and yields a positive staining reaction. (Colloidal iron stain, ×145) (AFIP Negative No. 71-12159-1)

Figure 306. *Effect of Fixation on Aldehyde Fuchsin Staining.* Both of these paraffin-embedded tissue sections of a specimen of human skin have been stained by Gomori's aldehyde fuchsin technique for the demonstration of Paget cells (see Chapter III). The tissue section on the left was prepared from a portion of the specimen after forty-eight hours of exposure to unbuffered acid 10% formalin. Although unbuffered formalin is not recommended as a fixative the short period of exposure did not adversely effect the specimen to the extent that the Paget cells were not demonstrable by aldehyde fuchsin staining. The tissue section on the right was prepared from a portion of the specimen which was stored in the unbuffered acid formalin for four months. Due to the prolonged exposure of the tissue to acid formalin, the Paget cells cannot be demonstrated by means of aldehyde fuchsin staining. (Gomori's aldehyde fuchsin, ×125) (AFIP Negative No. 70-10870)

Figure 307. *Effect of Fixation on the p-Dimethylaminobenzylidene Rhodanine Stain for Copper.* This technique is recommended (Lindquist, R. R.: *Arch Path, 87*:370-379, 1969) for the cytochemical localization of copper (CU I and CU II). As shown in this paraffin-embedded tissue section of a specimen of liver fixed in neutral buffered 10% formalin from a human being with hepatolenticular degeneration, the granular precipitates of copper yield a red-colored reaction product. In tissue sections which have low concentrations of copper, the reaction product may be golden in color (see Color Plate 4, Figure 20). Slight fading of the color of the reaction product may occur after dehydrating and mounting in Permount® of tissue sections which contain low concentrations of copper. (Rhodanine, ×575) (AFIP Negative No. 72-5667)

Figure 308. *Effect of Fixation on the p-Dimethylaminobenzylidene Rhodanine Stain for Copper.* This tissue section was prepared from a specimen of the same liver as depicted in Figure 307 which was fixed in unbuffered rather than buffered formalin. The specimen was stored in unbuffered formalin for a period of six months prior to being embedded in paraffin. The tissue section was subjected to the p-dimethylaminobenzylidene rhodanine to technique. The prolonged period of storage in acid formalin results in a negative reaction for copper (see Color Plate 4, Figure 21). Such effects of unbuffered formalin fixation may possibly account for the invariable failure of this method which has been reported by some workers (Lindquist, R. R.: *Arch Path, 87*:370-379, 1969). (Rhodanine, ×575) (AFIP Negative No. 72-7022)

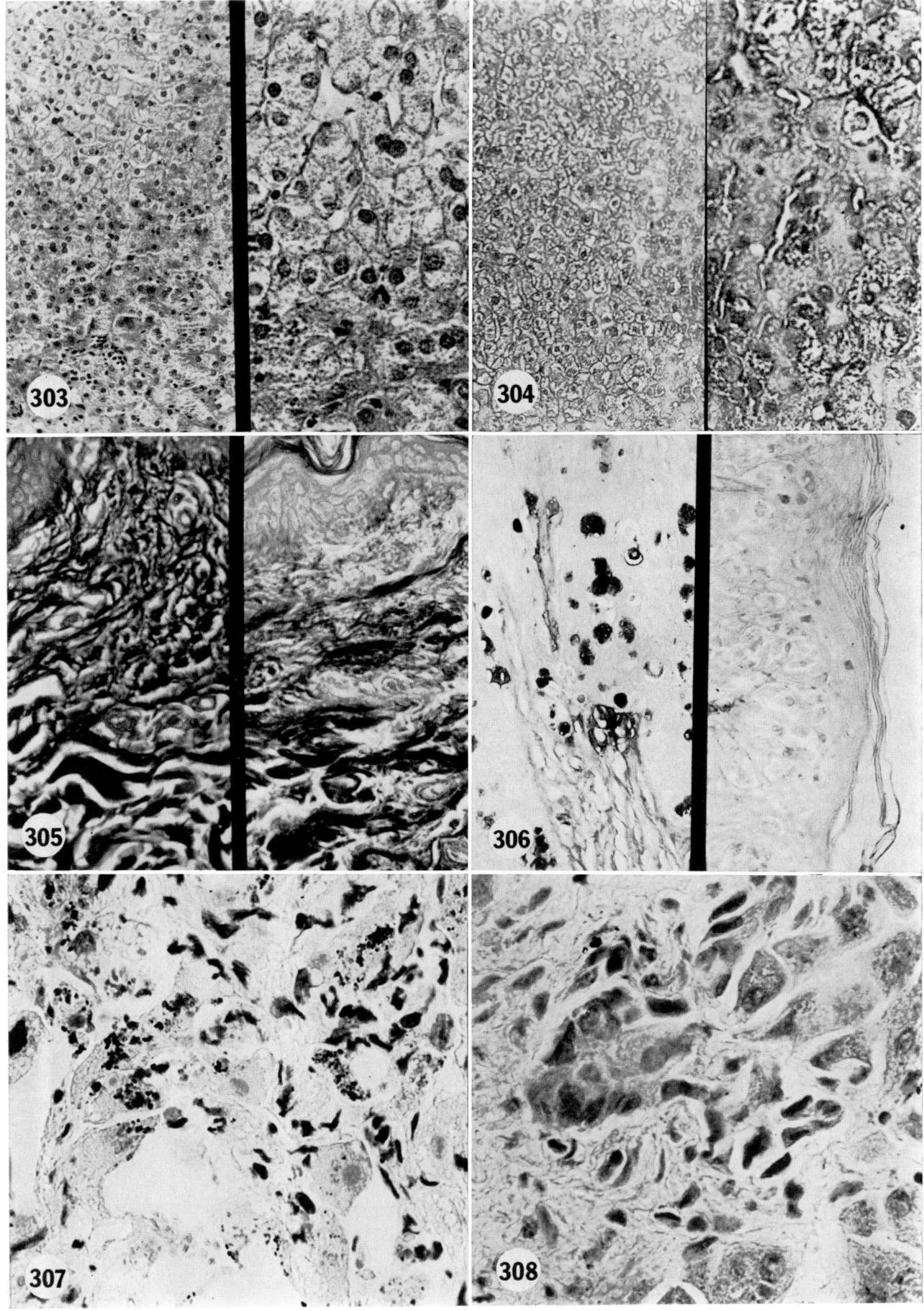

Figure 309. *Effect of Fixation on the p-Dimethylaminobenzylidene Rhodanine Stain for Copper.* This Zenker's-fixed biopsy specimen of human liver tissue was properly washed prior to processing. Although Zenker's fixation does not result in a false positive rhodanine reaction (see Figures 311 and 312) if the specimen has been properly washed, this form of fixation consistently results in the oxidation and/or removal of copper from the tissue section and a negative reaction even if copper was present in the unfixed specimen. Microscopically, the tissue section appears to be light yellow in color. (Rhodanine, ×115) (AFIP Negative No. 72-13671)

Figure 310. *Effect of Fixation on the p-Dimethylaminobenzylidene Rhodanine Stain for Copper.* This tissue section was prepared from a portion of the same biopsy specimen depicted in Figure 309 with the exception that it was fixed in 10% neutral buffered formalin rather than Zenker's fluid (see Figure 307). Macroscopically, the section appears to be blue in color. Although this case did not contain copper within the specimen, if deposits had been present they would have appeared red (heavy concentrations of copper) to golden yellow or yellow colored (light concentrations of copper) against a blue background. Since Zenker's fixation results in a yellow background it would be exceedingly difficult to detect small deposits of copper that might remain in Zenker's-fixed tissue that had been properly washed (see Figure 308). (Rhodanine, ×115) (AFIP Negative No. 72-13672)

Figure 311. *Effect of Fixation on the p-Dimethylaminobenzylidene Rhodanine Stain for Copper.* Although one of the most useful methods for the histochemical demonstration of copper is the p-dimethylaminobenzylidene rhodanine technique (see Figures 307 and 308), this technique cannot be used on tissue specimens which have been fixed in Zenker's fluid or solutions containing mercuric chloride or potassium dichromate. This paraffin-embedded tissue section of a specimen of liver from a human being was fixed in Zenker's fluid. It was subjected to the p-dimethylaminobenzylidene rhodanine technique. Beside the fact that copper is oxidized and/or removed from the tissue specimen by Zenker's fluid, such mercurial sublimate fixatives also result in a positive rhodanine reaction when the tissue has not been properly washed. The reddish-orange rhodanine reaction product can be seen as the dark area in the lower left portion of this section. Such reaction sites in Zenker's-fixed tissue specimens may be confused with a positive reaction for copper. (Rhodanine, ×10) (AFIP Negative No. 73-3918)

Figure 312. *Effect of Fixation on the p-Dimethylaminobenzylidene Rhodanine Stain for Copper.* This is a higher magnification of a portion of the tissue section depicted in Figure 311. Notice the dark-staining area in the hepatic tissue adjacent to Glisson's capsule. This positive rhodanine reaction was due to Zenker's fixation rather than the presence of copper within the specimen. (Rhodanine, ×35) (AFIP Negative No. 73-3925)

Figure 313. *Effect of Fixation on the Von Kossa Stain.* Mercurial sublimate crystals are scattered throughout this tissue section of a Zenker's-fixed specimen of human cardiac muscle. The fine black granules seen throughout the section are mercurial sublimate crystals which are present in all Zenker's-fixed tissue but are seldom seen unless a silver stain, like the Von Kossa, is performed. The large circular forms in the center of the field are also mercurial sublimate crystals of uncommon shape which appear coffee brown in color when stained by the Von Kossa technique. Such forms might conceivably be interpreted as calcific granules by the casual observer. (Von Kossa, ×395) (AFIP Negative No. 73-5170)

Figure 314. *Effect of Fixation on Hematoxylin and Eosin Staining.* Tissue sections of optimal quality are only possible if each step of the fixation, processing, microtomy, and staining procedures is followed with meticulous care. This and the following three figures (Figures 315 through 317) illustrate the variable effects of delayed fixation on the quality of hematoxylin and eosin-stained tissue sections. The specimen used in each example is an experimentally grown reticulum cell sarcoma. For each example half of the specimen was placed in the fixative of choice at the time it was removed from the host. The other half of the specimen was placed in a household refrigerator (4°C) in the unfixed state and held for sixteen hours before it was placed in the fixative of choice. The specimen depicted in this photograph was fixed in 10% unbuffered formalin. On the left is the tissue section prepared from the portion of the specimen which was placed in the fixative immediately. On the right is the identical preparation from that portion of the specimen which was subjected to delayed fixation. Notice the distinct variation in the staining of nuclear chromatin in the tissue section prepared from the immediate versus the delayed fixation specimens. The section from the immediately fixed specimen has more cytoplasmic and nuclear detail than the section from the delayed fixation specimen which contains pyknotic nuclei and very poor cytoplasmic detail. (H&E, ×500)

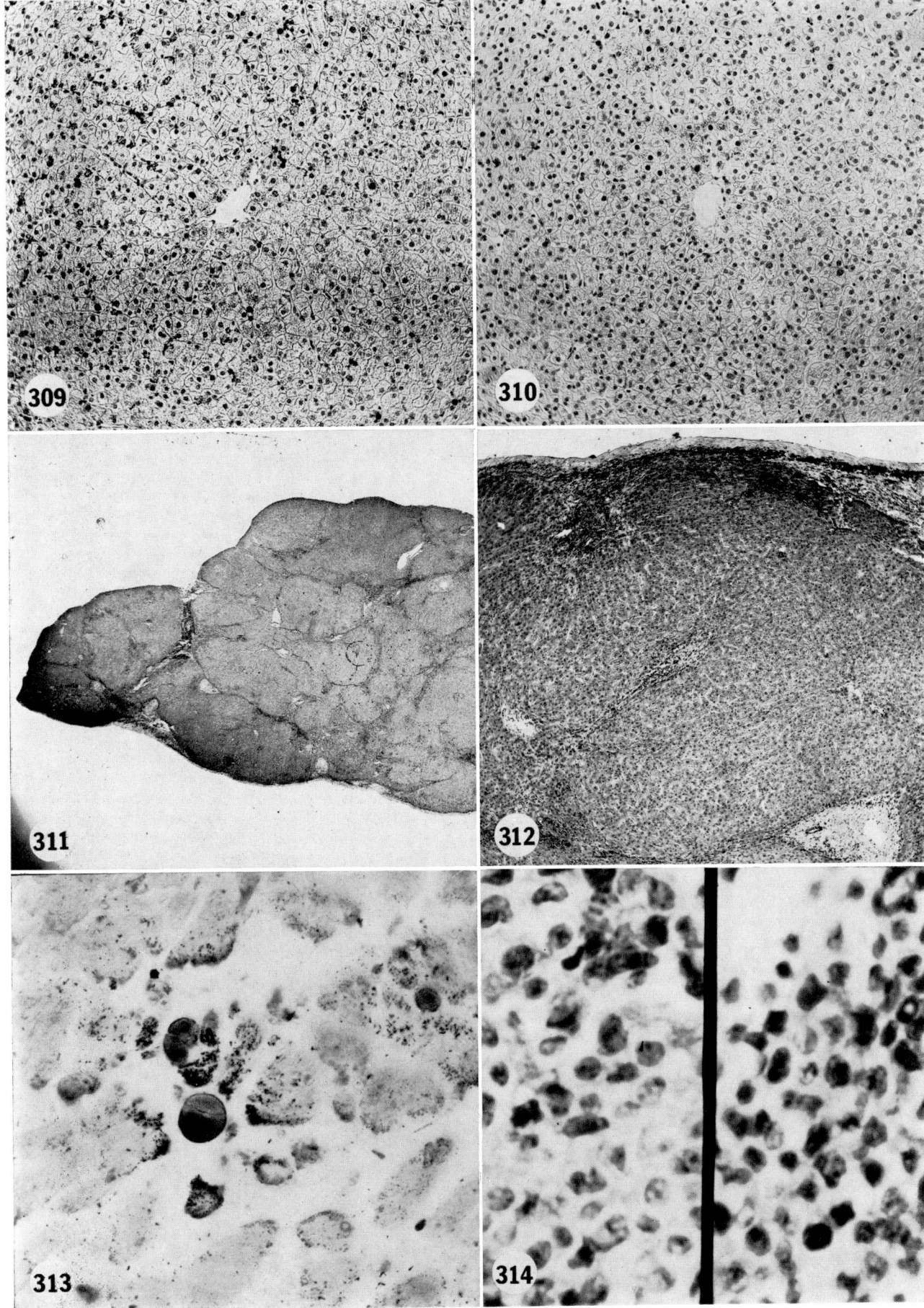

Figure 315. *Effect of Fixation on Hematoxylin and Eosin Staining.* The specimens from which the tissue sections depicted in this photomicrograph were derived were handled in the same fashion as described in the legend for Figure 314 with the exception that they were fixed in Carnoy's fluid. The results achieved are similar to those described for Figure 314. The tissue section prepared from the specimen (left) which was placed in Carnoy's fluid immediately after removal from the host exhibits considerably better detail than the tissue section (right) from the specimen which was held in the fresh state for sixteen hours at 4°C before it was placed in Carnoy's fluid. Notice that a large number of the nuclei in the latter specimen (right) exhibit distinct shrinkage artifacts. (H&E, ×500) (AFIP Negative No. 73-4288-6)

Figure 316. *Effect of Fixation on Hematoxylin and Eosin Staining.* The specimens from which the tissue sections depicted in this photomicrograph were derived were handled in the same fashion as described in the legend for Figure 314 with the exception that they were fixed in Zenker's formol fluid. The tissue section prepared from the specimen (left) which was placed in Zenker's formol fluid immediately after removal from the host exhibits considerably better detail than the tissue section (right) from the specimen which was held in the fresh state for sixteen hours at 4°C before it was placed in the fixative. Again, the pyknotic nuclei in the specimen which was subjected to delayed fixation (right) are very evident. (H&E, ×500) (AFIP Negative No. 73-4288-4)

Figure 317. *Effect of Fixation on Hematoxylin and Eosin Staining.* The specimens from which the tissue sections depicted in this photomicrograph were derived were handled in the same fashion as described in the legend for Figure 314 with the exception that they were fixed in Zenker's acetic fluid. The specimen on the left was placed in the fixative immediately after removal from the host and the cytoplasm and nuclear chromatin stain distinctly. Notice that in the specimen on the right, which was subjected to delayed fixation after sixteen hours at 4°C, the nuclear chromatin is disarrayed and nuclear detail is lacking. (H&E, ×500) (AFIP Negative No. 73-4288-8)

Figure 318. *Deceration.* In the staining of tissue sections, the first step consists of decerating the tissue section in a lipid solvent such as xylene. If the xylene is already saturated with wax or has been contaminated with water or tissue processing fluids, its efficiency as a solvent is materially reduced. In such instances, the paraffin or other embedding medium may not be adequately removed from the tissue section prior to commencing the staining procedure. The paraffin was not adequately removed from this tissue section of a specimen of human liver, fixed in neutral buffered 10% formalin, and the tissue was not capable of binding the stain which was used. Frequently, such an artifact can be corrected by destaining the tissue section in acid-alcohol, treating it with a fresh supply of xylene and restaining. (H&E, ×75)

Figure 319. *Deceration.* The anisotropic material demonstrated in and on this tissue section of a specimen of human skin, by means of polariscopy, is residual paraffin (see Color Plate 4, Figure 22). The paraffin was not removed properly during deceration of the tissue section prior to staining. Failure to totally remove all paraffin from tissue sections prior to staining adversely affects the staining reactions. Deceration should be accomplished by exposing 5- or 6-micron thick tissue sections to three (3) changes of fresh xylene for a minimum of two (2) minutes per change. (H&E, ×130) (AFIP Negative No. 73-6274)

Figure 320. *Deceration.* This is a higher magnification of a portion of the microscopic field depicted in Figure 319 to better illustrate the appearance of residual paraffin within a tissue section as observed by polariscopy. Compare with Figure 322. (H&E, ×305) (AFIP Negative No. 73-5172)

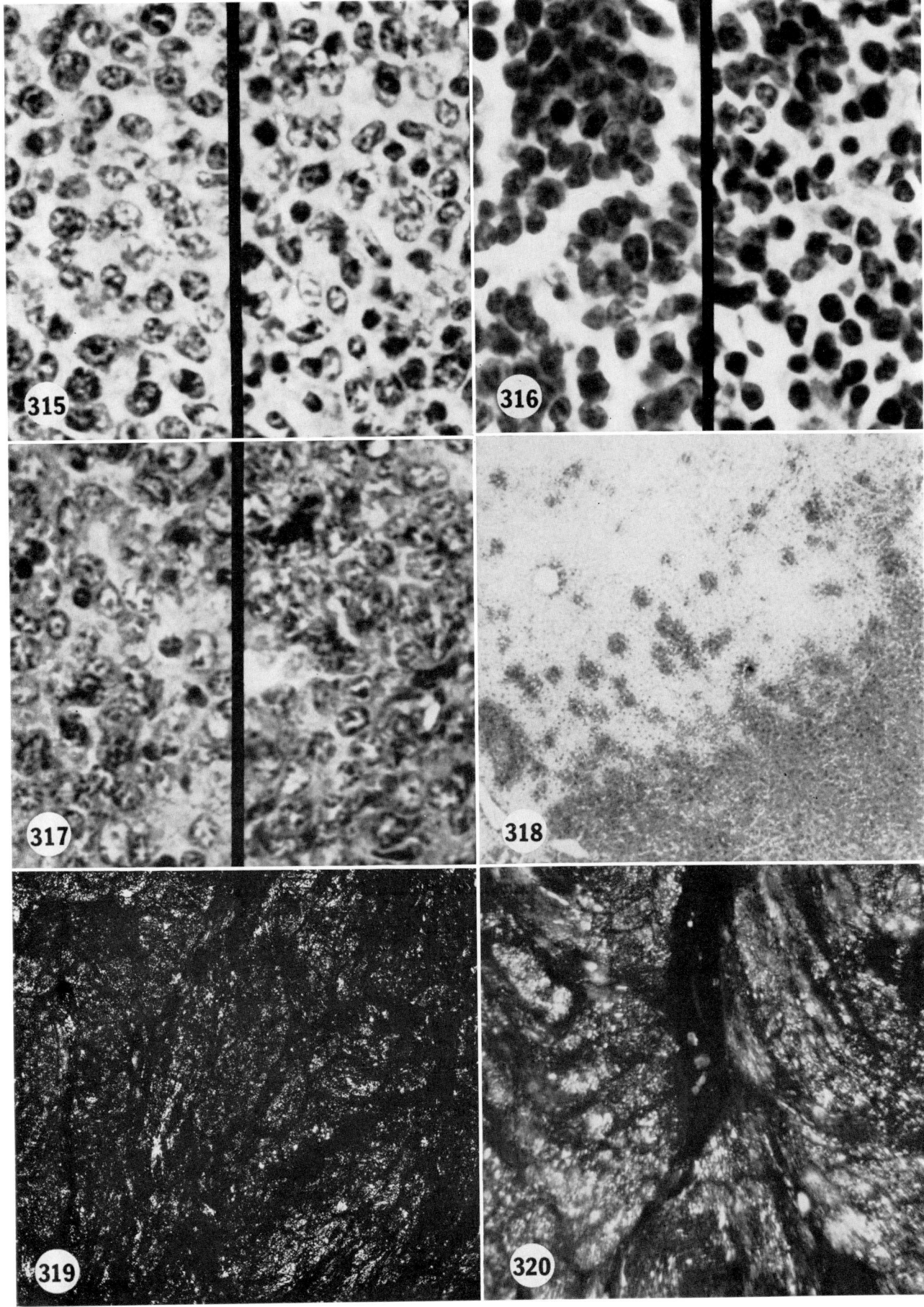

Figure 321. *Deceration.* This is the same microscopic field as depicted in Figure 319 as viewed by partial polariscopy to demonstrate the anistropic residual paraffin and the adverse staining effect which results from inadequate deceration. (H&E, ×80) (AFIP Negative No. 73-3926)

Figure 322. *Deceration.* This is a higher magnification of a portion of the microscopic field depicted in Figure 319 viewed by conventional bright field microscopy. This unpolarized section illustrates that inadequate deceration is difficult to detect without polariscopy. One may realize that a problem exists if the tissue section stains unevenly. However, unless one has had previous experience with the problem or can specifically identify residual paraffin as the cause for the lack of adequate staining, one will have a tendency to attribute the poor staining to a breakdown of the staining solutions or other factors. (H&E, ×305) (AFIP Negative No. 73-5173)

Figure 323. *Deceration.* This is the same microscopic field as depicted in Figure 321, as viewed by conventional bright field microscopy, to demonstrate the inadequate staining that results from residual paraffin within the tissue section. (Leder stain, ×80) (AFIP Negative No. 73-3924)

Figure 324. *Deceration.* A variety of proprietary mixtures of plastic and paraffin are currently being utilized for the embedding of fixed-tissue specimens. The plastic components of such embedding media are sometimes weakly anionic and will bind cationic dyes to a limited extent. As depicted in this photograph of a "Paraplast"-embedded, formalin-fixed specimen of the brain of a Rhesus monkey, embedding medium retained within the Virchow-Robin spaces is stained faintly by cationic dye. This material was initially interpreted as mucin (mucocytes). The retained embedding medium resulted from shortening the prescribed period of deceration in xylene. When the tissue sections were decerated in xylene by the prescribed exposure of two periods of five minutes each, the embedding medium was not retained within the tissue sections. (H&E, ×220) (Contributed by Mr. L. E. Schellhammer)

Figure 325. *Aldehyde-Fuchsin Stain.* This technique is recommended for the demonstration of aldehyde groups and sulfuric acid groups in tissue sections (presumably components of, or derived from, certain acid mucopolysaccharides, and possibly cystine). However, the most common use is for the staining of elastic tissue. In this tissue section of a paraffin-embedded specimen of a human salivary gland, fixed in neutral buffered 10% formalin, the technique was utilized to demonstrate acid mucopolysaccharides. In the performance of the staining procedure, it is essential that the tissue section be rinsed in 95% ethyl alcohol before and after an exposure to the solution. If the excess aldehyde-fuchsin is not rinsed off quickly in 95% ethyl alcohol, it will precipitate as crystals on the tissue section as demonstrated in this photograph. (Aldehyde-fuchsin, ×130) (AFIP Negative No. 72-53420)

Figure 326. *Aldehyde-Fuchsin Stain.* This is a higher magnification of a portion of the field depicted in Figure 325. The precipitated crystals of aldehyde-fuchsin are more clearly depicted than in Figure 325. (Aldehyde-fuchsin, ×265) (AFIP Negative No. 72-3736)

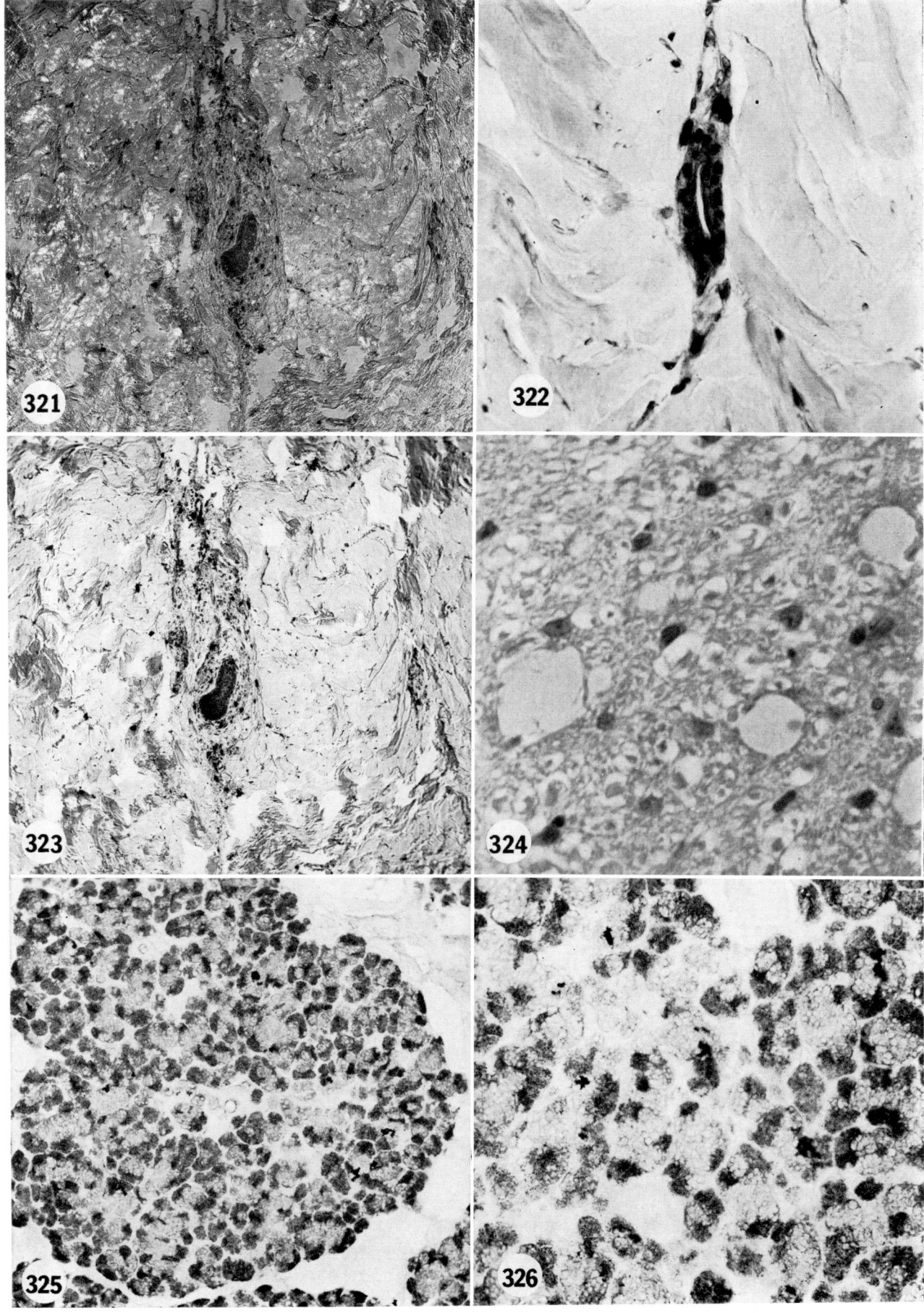

Figure 327. *Aldehyde-Fuchsin Stain.* This is a higher magnification of a portion of the field depicted in Figure 326. The precipitated crystals of aldehyde-fuchsin are observed to be out of focus since they are above the focal plane of the tissue section. (Aldehyde-fuchsin, ×485) (AFIP Negative No. 72-4767)

Figure 328. *Alizarin Blue S Stain.* Staining with Alizarin blue S is one of the techniques which is frequently employed for the demonstration of copper in tissue sections. The technique was employed with this paraffin-embedded tissue section of a specimen of human liver which had been fixed in Zenker's fluid. Note the numerous mercuric chloride crystals within the field of view (see also Figure 329). (Alizarin blue S, ×150) (AFIP Negative No. 73-4883)

Figure 329. *Alizarin Blue S Stain.* This is a higher magnification of the central portion of the field of view depicted in Figure 328. The Alizarin blue S stain reacts with the mercuric chloride crystals and colors them blue. The blue coloration of the crystals could add a potentially confusing factor to the interpretation of this reaction for the demonstration of copper. The photomicrograph illustrates the various forms and shapes in which mercuric chloride crystals may occur in Zenker's-fixed tissue. Zenker's fixation should never be used when the need for the demonstration of copper in tissue sections is anticipated. (Alizarin blue S, ×350) (AFIP Negative No. 73-4882)

Figure 330. *Best's Carmine Stain.* This technique is recommended for the specific histochemical demonstration of sites of glycogen deposition within tissue sections. As shown in this paraffin-embedded tissue section of a specimen of human liver, fixed in neutral buffered 10% formalin, one of the most commonly occurring difficulties encountered with this technique is the frequent adherence of precipitated dye to the sections. There is also a tendency for the tissue sections stained by this technique to develop a pink tinge throughout, even in the nuclei which, though stained with hematoxylin, may change color in the carmine. (Best's carmine with hematoxylin counterstain, ×100) (AFIP Negative No. 72-5666)

Figure 331. *Best's Carmine Stain.* Precipitated carmine dye is also observed in this paraffin-embedded tissue section of a specimen of human liver which was fixed in neutral buffered 10% formalin (see Figure 330). Note the dense and irregular diffusion of the stain into the tissue surrounding the site of deposition of the precipitated dye (see Color Plate 4, Figure 23). The tendency for tissue sections stained by this technique to develop a pink tinge within nuclei, even though counterstained with hematoxylin, is more apparent in this figure than in Figure 330. (Best's carmine with hematoxylin counterstain, ×100) (AFIP Negative No. 72-5668)

Figure 332. *Bodian's Silver Protein Reaction.* Many silver staining techniques result in the deposition of silver precipitate on and within the tissue section. The extent of such precipitation is unpredictable. In this tissue section of a specimen of human brain tissue, numerous black granular structures of variable sizes are shown in the middle portion of the photographic field. Such silver precipitates are frequently seen in vacuolated areas of the tissue section such as the lumens of blood vessels or vacuoles due to shrinkage artifacts. (Bodian's stain, ×305) (AFIP Negative No. 74-5747)

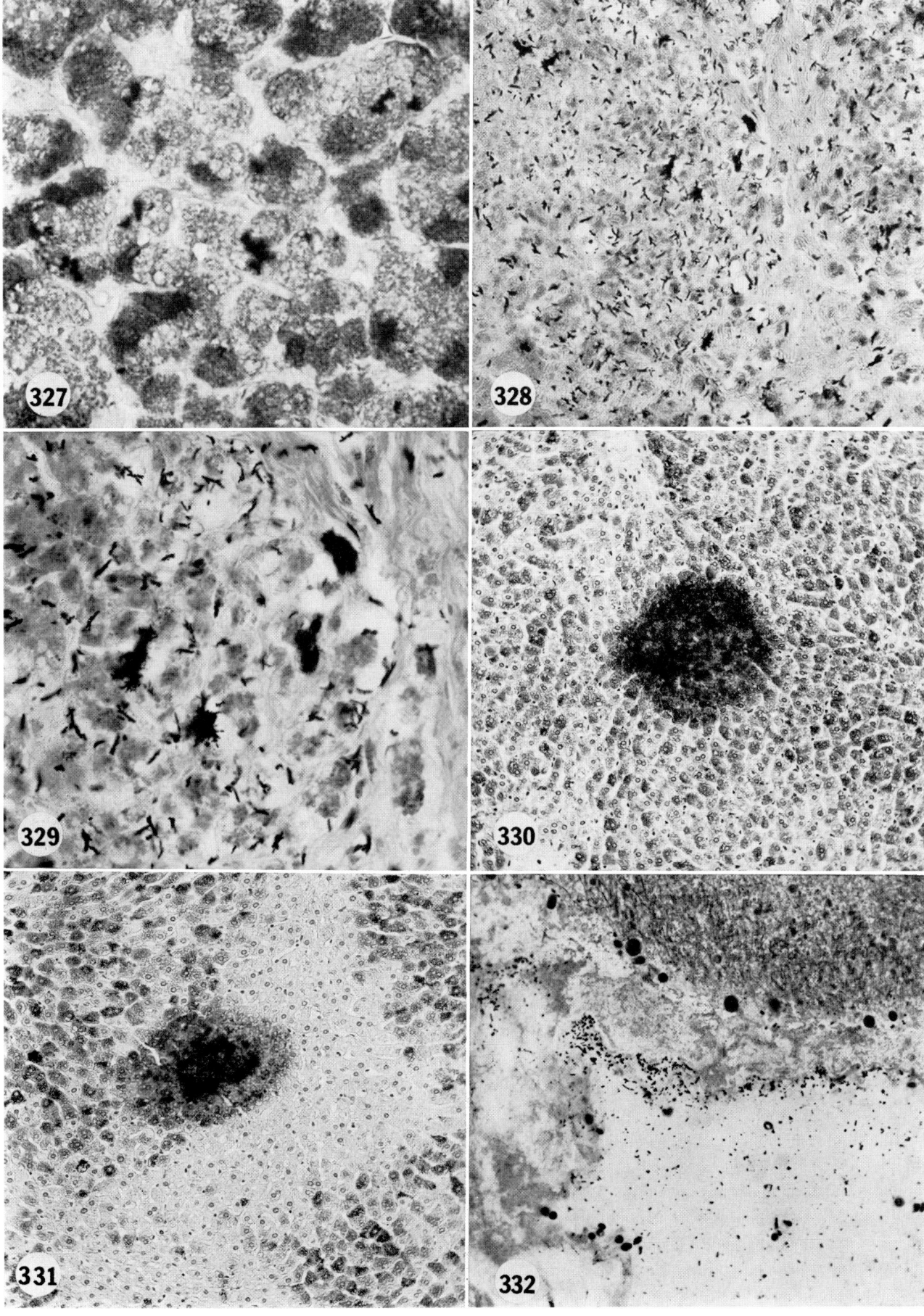

Figure 333. *Bodian's Silver Protein Reaction.* This is a higher magnification of a portion of the field depicted in Figure 332. The point of focus was at a level just above the focal plane of the nerve fibers to illustrate the minute silver granules that were deposited on the surface of the tissue section during the staining procedure. Such fine silver deposits will frequently go undetected if one focuses on the focal plane of the nerve fibers within the tissue section since they are usually deposited only on the surface of the tissue section. (Bodian's stain, ×675) (AFIP Negative No. 74-5745)

Figure 334. *Bodian's Silver Protein Reaction.* This is the same field depicted in Figure 333. The photograph was taken at the focal plane of the nerve fibers and the minute deposits of silver granules have seemingly disappeared. However, the microscopist will detect the silver precipitate if the slide is studied by continual focusing as is commonly done by most microscopists. (Bodian's stain, ×675) (AFIP Negative No. 74-5746)

Figure 335. *Congo Red Stain.* The usual procedure in the staining of frozen, fixed tissue sections or paraffin-embedded tissue sections with the Congo red technique for the demonstration of amyloid consists of exposure of the tissue section for thirty minutes to a 1% solution of the dye in distilled water. The stained tissue section should be examined by both bright-field microscopy and polariscopy since amyloid deposits stained by Congo red are anisotropic. If too concentrated a solution of the dye is used in the staining procedure, the dye will precipitate out of solution. The artifact noted in this tissue section of a specimen of a human kidney consists of recrystallized Congo red which precipitated out of solution during the staining procedure. On the right, the crystals are depicted as seen by means of bright-field microscopy and on the left as seen under partial polariscopy. (Congo red, ×395) (AFIP Negative No. 72-2329)

Figure 336. *Cresyl Echt Violet Stain.* The exact chemical nature of cresyl echt violet is unknown, and although it is frequently referred to as a metachromatic dye, it is more probably a mixture of two dyes. It is frequently used for making permanent stains of Nissl substance as in Vogt's method for nerve cell products which was employed with this paraffin-embedded tissue section of a specimen of neoplastic tissue from a human being which was fixed in neutral buffered 10% formalin. The actual procedure calls for staining in a working solution composed of 1 part of a 2% aqueous solution of the dye and 100 parts of a buffer solution (2 gm sodium acetate, 3 ml glacial acetic acid, 1000 ml distilled water). In this instance, the histotechnologist mistakenly prepared a 1% solution of the dye in the buffer as the working solution. The dye was relatively insoluble at this concentration and precipitated out of solution as needle-shaped greenish colored crystals which contaminated the tissue section (see Color Plate 4, Figure 24). (Vogt's cresyl echt violet method for nerve cell products, ×145) (AFIP Negative No. 72-7797)

Figure 337. *Cresyl Echt Violet Stain.* This photomicrograph is of the same tissue section depicted in Figure 336 taken with partially polarized light. Cresyl echt violet crystals are anisotropic (see Color Plate 5, Figure 25). When subjected to polariscopy, it is more readily apparent that the crystals are above the focal plane of the tissue section per se. (Vogt's cresyl echt violet method for nerve cell products, ×145) (AFIP Negative No. 72-7798)

Figure 338. *Crystal Violet.* This photomicrograph of a paraffin-embedded tissue section of a specimen of human intestinal tissue depicts crystal violet contaminant which is frequently seen in slides which have been stained with a procedure which requires crystal violet as one of the primary stains. The anisotropic crystals appear purplish-black in color when viewed by means of bright field microscopy. They are frequently depicted in such a pattern that it may be difficult to distinguish them from cellular organelles. However, the artifact can be readily distinguished from cellular organelles by means of polariscopy as demonstrated here (see also Figures 397 and 398). (Mallory's thionin stain, partial polariscopy, ×165) (AFIP Negative No. 72-6775)

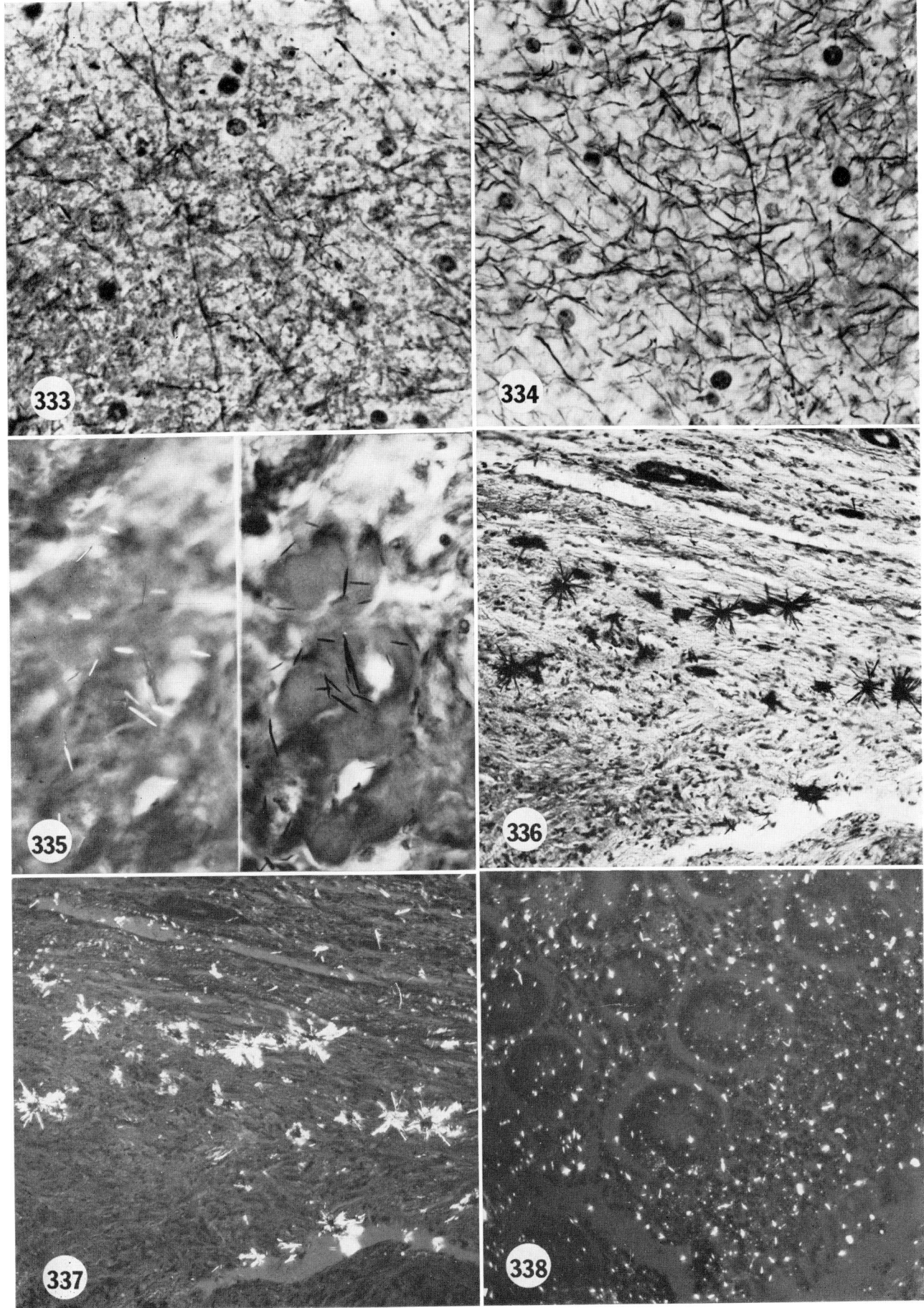

Figure 339. *Eosin.* Alcoholic solutions of Eosin Y or Ethyl Eosin are extensively used as counterstains. The solubility at 26°C of Eosin Y in alcohol is 2.18% and the solubility of Ethyl Eosin in alcohol is 1.13%. A flaky precipitate will form in stock solutions and working solutions of the dye as the alcohol evaporates. Stock solutions should be filtered prior to use and working solutions in staining dishes should be filtered frequently. This paraffin-embedded tissue section of a specimen of the brain of a rat was stained in a working solution of eosin which had been prepared from a stock solution that had not been filtered prior to use. The irregularly shaped flakes of foreign material seen above the focal plane of the tissue section is precipitated dye derived from the unfiltered stock solution. (H&E, ×66) (Contributed by Mr. L. E. Schellhammer)

Figure 340. *Eosin.* This is a higher magnification of a portion of the tissue section depicted in Figure 339 to better illustrate the variable configurations of the flaky precipitate of eosin observed in Figure 339 (see Color Plate 5, Figure 26). (H&E, ×266) (Contributed by Mr. L. E. Schellhammer)

Figure 341. *Eosin.* This is an example of poor staining technique in the application of an eosin counterstain. The uneven staining of this paraffin-embedded tissue section of a specimen of human skin, fixed in neutral buffered 10% formalin, resulted due to the failure of the histotechnologist to agitate the slide while it was in the solution of eosin. (Eosin, ×575) (AFIP Negative No. 68-1268)

Figure 342. *Fite-Faraco Acid-fast Stain.* This technique is recommended for the demonstration of acid-fast bacteria, particularly lepra bacilli, in paraffin-embedded tissue sections. In the procedure the deceration of the tissue section is carried out by using a mixture of xylene-peanut oil (2 : 1) or cottonseed oil or olive oil or paraffin oil. After deceration the slide is drained, the excess oil is drained off and the tissue section is blotted with filter paper until it is opaque. The artifact noted in this tissue section of a paraffin-embedded specimen of a human lymph node consists of intensely stained droplets of peanut oil which remained on the section due to inadequate blotting of the section prior to staining. (Fite-Faraco stain, ×50) (AFIP Negative No. 72-5667)

Figure 343. *Hematoxylin.* Solutions of oxidized hematoxylin are generally thought of as cationic dyes, although the active dye component of most solutions of hematoxylin is hematein, which is the oxidation product of hematoxylin. Hematein per se is an amphoteric dye and is not generally employed for the staining of tissues. However, when employed with suitable alum mordants it forms a dye-lake which functions as a cationic dye and stains anionic tissue components blue to blue-black. The most frequently employed mordants for hematein are aluminum ammonium sulfate or aluminum potassium sulfate. If the mordant is not properly dissolved, or is used in excessive quantities during the preparation of the hematein dye-lake, the alum will recrystalize and precipitate out of solution. The particles depicted here are alum crystals which were precipitated in the course of preparing a faulty batch of hematoxylin stock dye solution. They were recovered by filtering the stock solution prior to use. (Hematoxylin, ×4)

Figure 344. *Hematoxylin.* If alum crystals precipitate in the stock solution of hematoxylin (see Figure 343), they may contaminate the tissue sections which are stained in the working dye solution which is prepared from such a batch of unfiltered hematoxylin. The dark, granular pigments (arrow), seen in this photomicrograph of a paraffin-embedded tissue section of a specimen of human skin, fixed in neutral buffered 10% formalin, are alum crystals from improperly prepared hematoxylin. (H&E, ×145)

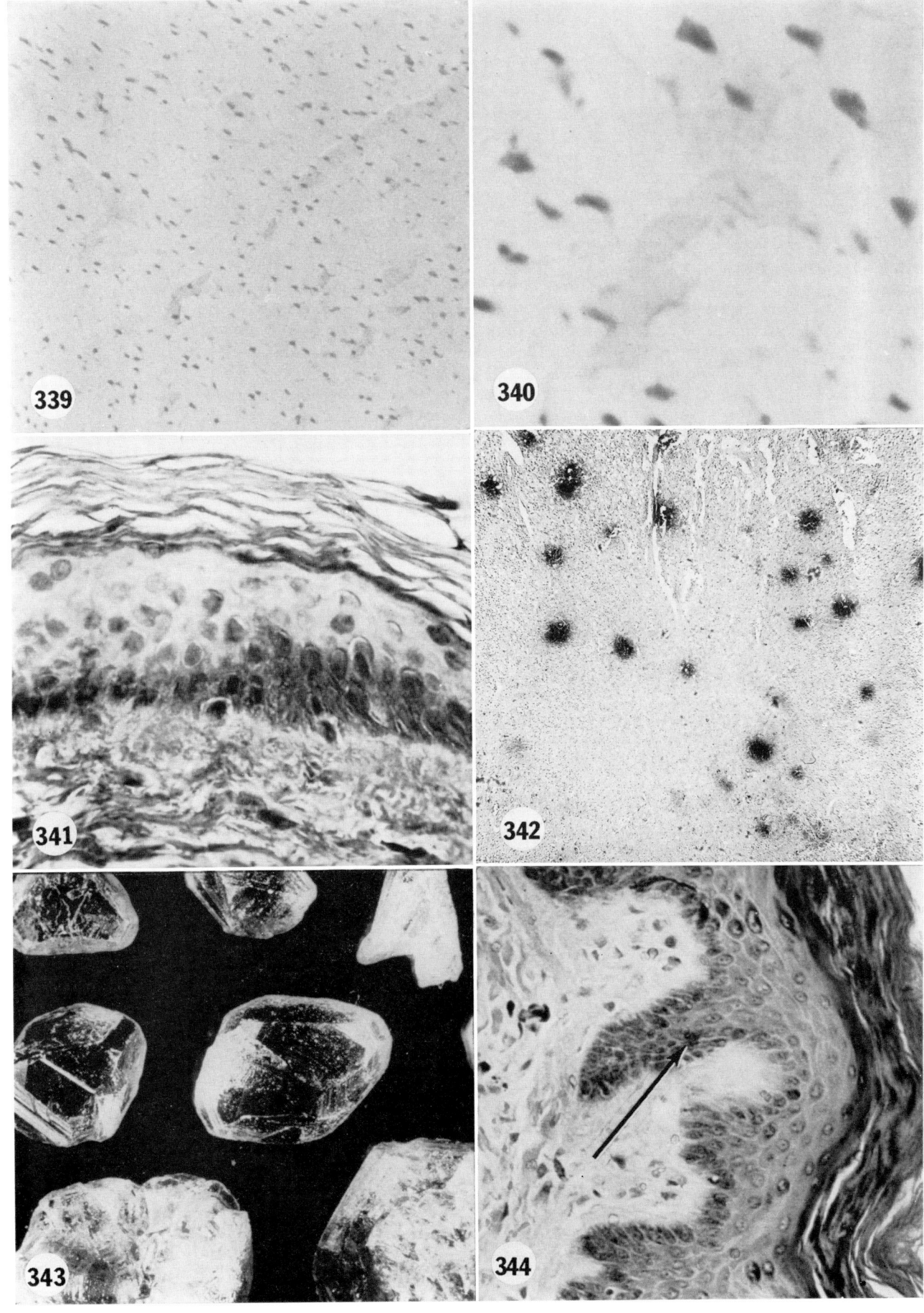

Figure 345. *Hematoxylin.* This is the same tissue section as depicted in Figure 344. The alum crystals which have been deposited upon the tissue section are anisotropic and are observed to be above the focal plane of the tissue section per se (see Color Plate 5, Figure 27). (H&E, partial polariscopy, ×145) (AFIP Negative No. 64-1678)

Figure 346. *Hematoxylin.* Hematein, which is derived by the oxidation of hematoxylin, is the active dye component of solutions of hematoxylin. However, hematein per se is comparatively unstable and undergoes fairly rapid oxidation to form products which function less well in the staining of tissue than hematein. Some of these oxidation products precipitate out of solution as hematein crystals. If the stock solution of hematoxylin is filtered prior to use such precipitates are removed. However, such hematein precipitates also form in working solutions of hemtoxylin and such solutions of hematoxylin must also be filtered at frequent intervals. If hematein crystals are present in the staining dish used for the working hematoxylin solution, they may contaminate the tissue sections which are stained with the dye as depicted in this paraffin-embedded section of a specimen of the small intestine which was fixed in neutral buffered 10% formalin. The hematein crystals are above the focal plane of the tissue section. (Hematoxylin, ×450)

Figure 347. *Hematoxylin.* The irregularly shaped granules seen in this tissue section of a paraffin-embedded specimen of a human liver are hematein crystals (see also Figure 346). (Periodic acid-Schiff reaction with a hematoxylin counterstain, ×100) (AFIP Negative No. 72-5665)

Figure 348. *Hematoxylin.* This is a higher magnification of the central portion of the tissue section depicted in Figure 347. Note the irregularly shaped hematein crystals which are particularly well visualized within the lumina of sinusoids and a central vein (see Color Plate 5, Figure 28). In such locations they may appear to be in the same focal plane as the cellular components of the tissue section. Where the crystals overlay hepatocytes they are clearly seen as being above the focal plane of the tissue components. (Periodic acid-Schiff reaction with hematoxylin counterstain, ×305) (AFIP Negative No. 72-6774)

Figure 349. *Hematoxylin.* Numerous hematein crystals can be seen on and within this paraffin-embedded tissue section of a specimen of human tissue of unknown origin. These artifacts appear as the dark staining granular precipitate seen throughout the field (see also Figures 347 and 348). (H&E, ×165) (AFIP Negative No. 74-5752)

Figure 350. *Hematoxylin.* In this paraffin-embedded tissue section of a specimen of the trachea of an animal, two distinct forms of hematein crystals are observed. Clumps of large hematein crystals are scattered on the peripheral surface of the specimen (left side). Between the displaced mucosa and tracheal cartilage the clumps of hematein crystals are composed of extremely minute particles. (H&E, ×115) (AFIP Negative No. 74-7442)

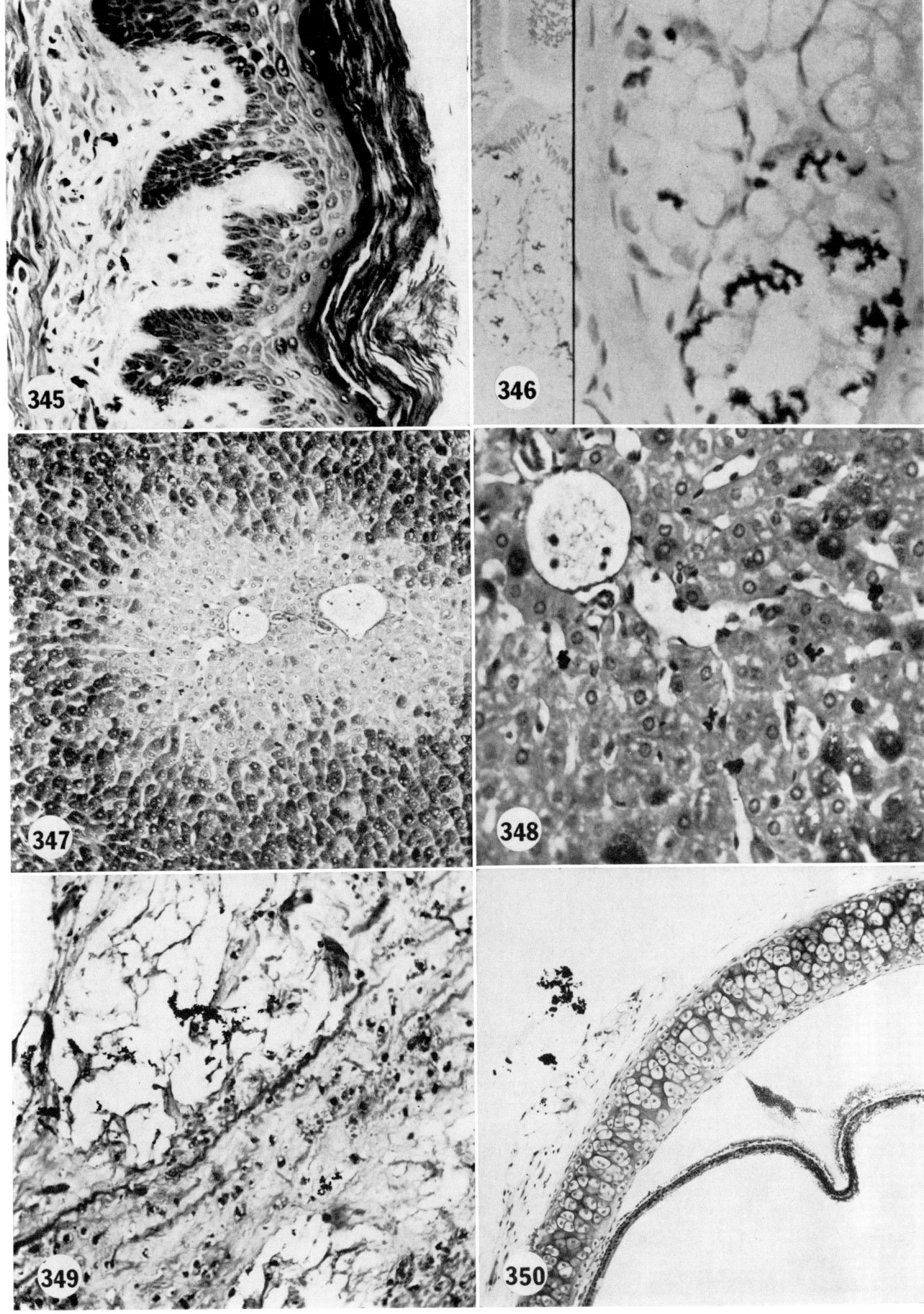

Figure 351. *Hematoxylin.* When a staining dish containing a working solution of hematoxylin is allowed to stand at room temperature for long periods of time, a metallic appearing scum accumulates on the surface of the solution. This scum forms more rapidly if the staining dishes are not covered when they are not in use. The scum consists of oxidized mordant and hematein and is referred to as hematoxylin surface oxidant. Such scum can contaminate tissue sections which are stained in the affected working dye solution. In this paraffin-embedded tissue section of a specimen of a spleen fixed in neutral buffered 10% formalin, the deep staining materials above the focal plane of the tissue section are hematoxylin surface oxidant artifacts. (H&E, ×75)

Figure 352. *Hematoxylin.* As mentioned previously (see Figure 346), the active dye component of hematoxylin is hematein. If the quantity of hematein available within the dye solution is inadequate, the tissue sections will not be adequately stained. Several reasons may account for the diminished hematein content of the solution of hematoxylin such as: (1) faulty formulation of the stock dye solution in that too little hematoxylin, mordant, or oxidant was employed; (2) if an oxidant was not employed, it may be that the stock dye solution was not sufficiently ripened before it was used; (3) or the stock solution may be old enough that its hematein content is drastically reduced. In respect to the latter possibility, it should be emphasized that hematein per se is comparatively unstable and undergoes fairly rapid oxidation to form products which function less well in the staining of tissue than hematein. Therefore, any solution of hematoxylin will gradually diminish in its staining quality. This paraffin-embedded tissue section of a specimen of glandular tissue, fixed in neutral buffered 10% formalin, was stained with a solution of hematoxylin which has lost much of its hematein content. The nuclei are not stained as intensely as they should be and other basophilic tissue components are poorly stained. (Hematoxylin, ×400)

Figure 353. *Hematoxylin.* This is a duplicate tissue section from the same specimen as depicted in Figure 352. It was stained with freshly prepared Harris' hematoxylin which had a high content of hematein. The basophilic tissue components are stained more intensely and the entire tissue section has a "crisper" appearance. (Hematoxylin, ×400)

Figure 354. *Hematoxylin.* The breakdown of hematoxylin is difficult to determine. The unavailability of methods for determining the end point of hematoxylin oxidation results in inadequate basophilic staining of tissue sections as demonstrated with this soft tissue specimen from a human being. This photograph illustrates the staining effect that results with the breakdown of hematoxylin. Notice that the nuclear chromatin within individual cells is not distinctly stained. Chromatically, this tissue section appears to be very lightly stained when examined microscopically. (H&E, ×220) (AFIP Negative No. 73-6312)

Figure 355. *Hematoxylin.* This is a higher magnification of a portion of the tissue section depicted in Figure 354 to better illustrate the poor nuclear staining effect that results with the breakdown of hematoxylin (see Color Plate 5, Figure 29). One might not be impressed with such an illustration and tend to be satisfied with the staining achieved. However, the inadequacy of the staining is more apparent if one compares this photograph to Figures 356 and 357. (H&E, ×350) (AFIP Negative No. 73-6313)

Figure 356. *Hematoxylin.* This tissue section was prepared from the same specimen depicted in Figure 354. The dramatic difference in the staining achieved with this tissue section results from using a fresh solution of hematoxylin. Notice that the nuclei appear to be well compacted with nuclear chromatin. Much of this nuclear chromatin did not stain with the solution of degraded hematoxylin used to stain the tissue section depicted in Figure 354. (H&E, ×220) (AFIP Negative No. 73-6310)

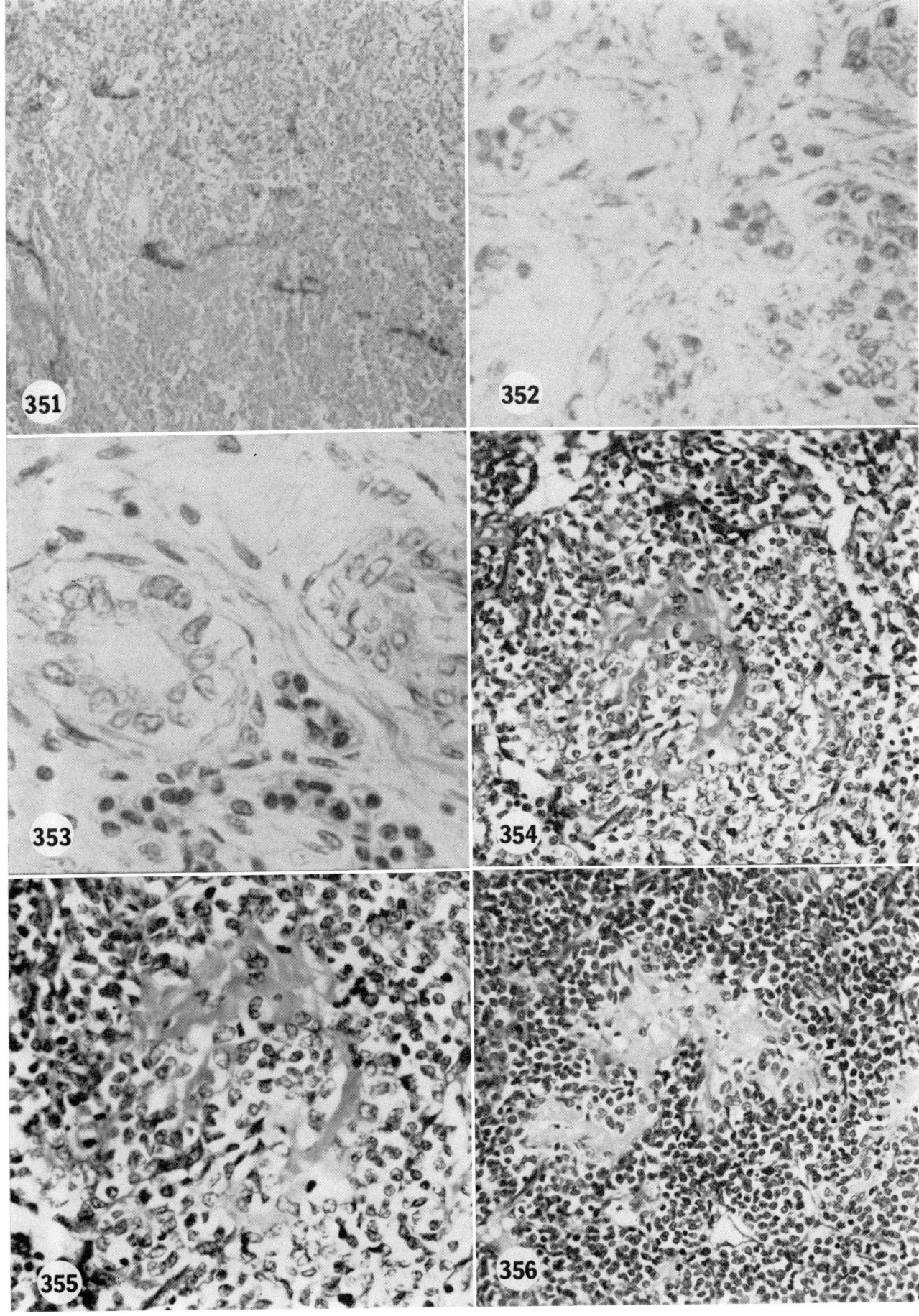

Figure 357. *Hematoxylin.* This is a higher magnification of the central portion of the microscopic field depicted in Figure 356 to better illustrate the good staining effect of a good working solution of hematoxylin. Compare to Figure 355 (see also Color Plate 5, Figure 30). Microscopically this tissue section appeared crisp and sharp and its cellular components were distinct. (H&E, ×350) (AFIP Negative No. 73-6311)

Figure 358. *Hematoxylin.* Inadequate exposure of tissue sections to hematoxylin and/or subsequent bluing frequently produces a finished tissue section which possesses a brownish tint when observed microscopically. Such an effect is noted in this paraffin-embedded tissue section of an unknown specimen from a human being. The brown coloration may be splotchy in its distribution and give the impression that certain portions of the tissue section have faded. Note the dark and light splotchy staining in this photomicrograph. (Hematoxylin, ×50) (AFIP Negative No. 73-5613)

Figure 359. *Hematoxylin.* This is a higher magnification of a portion of the field of view depicted in Figure 358. The lighter staining nuclei are those which appear brown when examined under the microscope (see Color Plate 6, Figure 31). This type of artifact can be prevented by longer exposure to hematoxylin and/or bluing agents such as lithium carbonate or ammonia water. Compare to Figure 360. (Hematoxylin, ×115) (AFIP Negative No. 73-5614)

Figure 360. *Hematoxylin.* This tissue section was prepared from the same block of paraffin-embedded tissue as depicted in Figures 358 and 359. Subsequent to staining with hematoxylin, it exhibited the same artifact as depicted in Figures 358 and 359. However, subsequent to staining with hematoxylin it was exposed to a bluing agent (see Color Plate 6, Figure 32). Note that by the simple addition of a bluing agent such as lithium carbonate or ammonia water to the staining train, the nuclear detail has been considerably improved compared to Figures 358 and 359. (Hematoxylin, ×115) (AFIP Negative No. 73-5618)

Figure 361. *Hematoxylin.* Bluing is necessary subsequent to staining with hematoxylin and prior to counterstaining with eosin. Bluing of tissue sections that have been stained with hematoxylin can be accomplished by submersion in (1) aqueous lithium carbonate, or (2) Scott's water, or (3) ammonia water, or (4) running tap water. Regardless of the method used, one should exercise every precaution to insure that the bluing is performed correctly. This photograph of a tissue section of a specimen of diseased kidney from a human being was not blued and illustrates achromatic staining. Microscopically, the entire section appeared to be stained a light pink color with a lack of adequate hematoxylin staining due to the omission of bluing subsequent to staining with hematoxylin. (H&E, ×180) (AFIP Negative No. 73-6272)

Figure 362. *Hematoxylin.* This is a higher magnification of a portion of the microscopic field depicted in Figure 361. Although some nuclei appear to be adequately stained by the hematoxylin, many nuclei did not retain the stain due to the omission of bluing. The overall effect produced by the omission of bluing was an overstaining effect produced by the eosin. Many tissue components which should normally appear to be basophilic were stained acidophilically. (H&E, ×575) (AFIP Negative No. 73-6273)

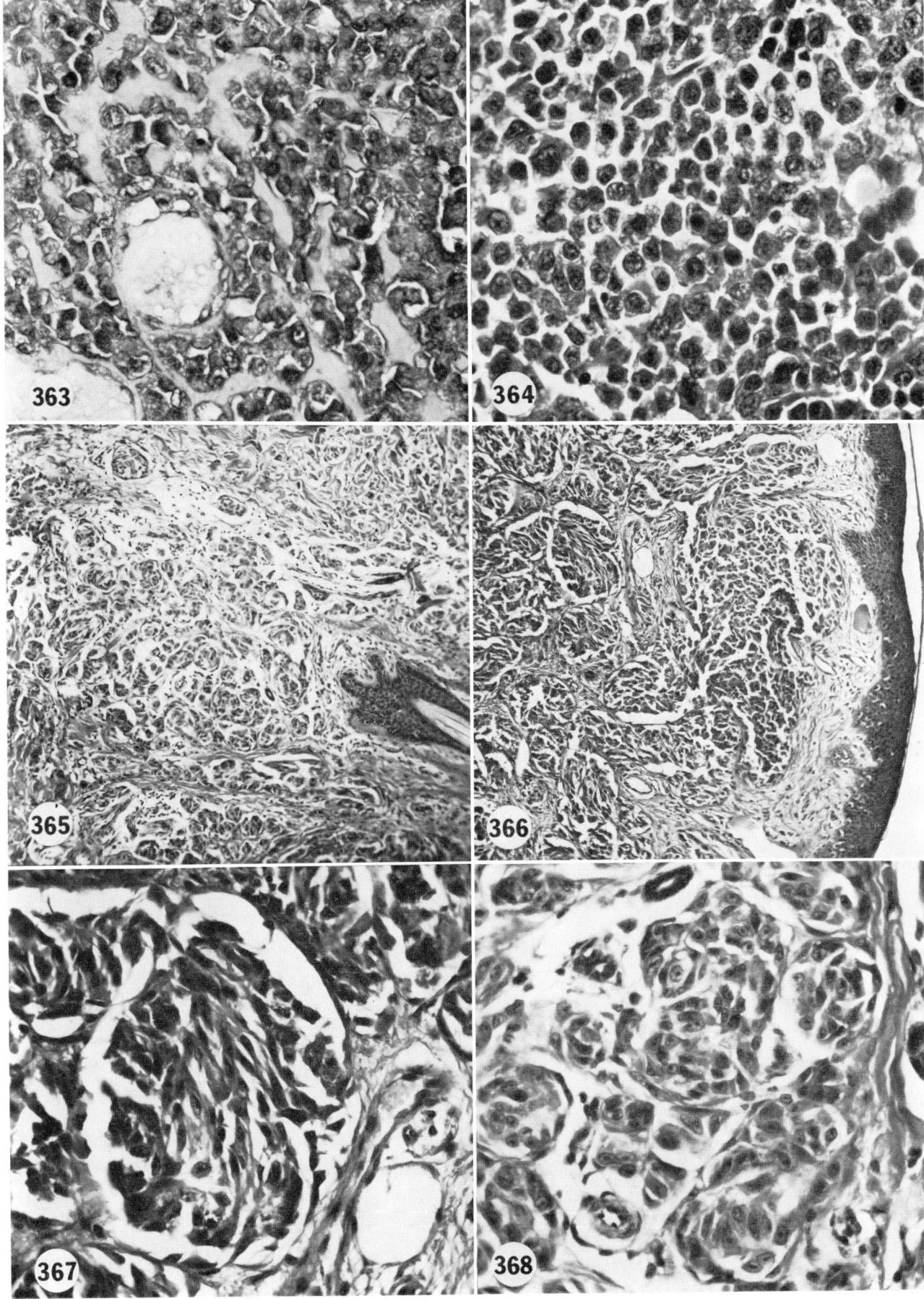

Figure 369. *Hematoxylin (Phosphotungstic Acid).* This photograph depicts a portion of a paraffin-embedded tissue section of a specimen of human brain which was stained with PTAH. Such a specimen which contains glial cells is the recommended control tissue for determining the staining quality of PTAH procedures. The staining quality depicted here was optimal. Notice the intensity of the staining of the glial cells. Microscopically, the glial cells should appear bright blue in color against a bluish-purple tint of the parenchyma. Compare with Figure 370. (PTAH, ×400) (AFIP Negative No. 74-8659)

Figure 370. *Hematoxylin (Phosphotungstic Acid).* This tissue section was prepared from the same paraffin-embedded specimen depicted in Figure 369. It was stained with a PTAH solution which had either broken down or was not adequately oxidized during its preparation. The staining quality is suboptimal. Although some glial cells appear dark in this black and white photograph they were stained purple rather than light blue. Also notice that the cell processes are shorter than those seen in Figure 369. The neuronal cytoplasm was stained pink rather than salmon colored and the parenchyma was unstained. (PTAH, ×400) (AFIP Negative No. 74-8657)

Figure 371. *Hematoxylin and Eosin.* Uneven staining with the eosin counterstain may occur in routine hematoxylin and eosin staining procedures, as demonstrated in this photograph of a paraffin-embedded tissue section of a specimen of intestine fixed in neutral buffered 10% formalin, if one fails to agitate the tissue section during the brief eosin staining period. This type of artifact can be avoided by repeatedly dipping the section in and out of the eosin during the staining period. (H&E, ×400) (AFIP Negative No. 67-2647)

Figure 372. *Hematoxylin and Eosin.* Eosin is frequently regarded as a counterstain which does not contribute to the diagnostic interpretation of a tissue section. However, as depicted in these paraffin-embedded tissue sections of the brain of a human being who died of rabies, eosin plays a very important role in the demonstration of acidophilic inclusion bodies. The three tissue sections depicted in this photograph illustrate two problems which may be encountered in the demonstration of such inclusion bodies. The section at the top of the photograph contains a well-stained Negri body within the cytoplasm of a neuron. This particular tissue section was well differentiated during the hematoxylin and eosin staining procedure. The section at the lower left depicts a similar observation; however, it is difficult to characterize the intracytoplasmic neuronal inclusion body as a Negri body. This tissue section is overstained with hematoxylin due to inadequate differentiation of the Harris' hematoxylin during the staining procedure. The tissue section at the lower right depicts a similar observation, and again it is difficult to characterize the intracytoplasmic neuronal inclusion body as a Negri body. In this instance, the differentiation of hematoxylin staining was adequate but the tissue section was overstained with eosin. When both of the lower tissue sections were examined under the microscope, the Negri bodies appeared very indistinct and almost undetectable. It would have been difficult to specifically identify them as Negri bodies although they appear to be distinct within these pictures due to the photographic technique. (H&E, ×500)

Figure 373. *Iron Reaction (Mallory's).* The paraffin-embedded tissue section depicted in this photomicrograph was prepared from human eye tissue which was fixed in a container which had a metal cap that was oxidized by the fixative (see Chapter III). The oxidized iron was deposited on the peripheral nerve and it subsequently yielded a positive reaction for iron when stained by Mallory's procedure (see Color Plate 6, Figure 33). Microscopically, the reaction was impossible to differentiate from true iron deposition. (Mallory's method for iron, ×115) (AFIP Negative No. 72-13669)

Figure 374. *Iron Reaction (Mallory's).* This paraffin-embedded tissue section of the cornea of a human eye was derived from the same specimen as depicted in Figure 373. The iron deposition in this instance was a little less well defined than in the segment of nerve tissue depicted in Figure 373 which made it easier to assume that the deposits which yielded a positive reaction to Mallory's procedure were artifacts. Metal caps which can be oxidized by fixatives should not be used on fixative containers. (Mallory's method for iron, ×305) (AFIP Negative No. 73-13670)

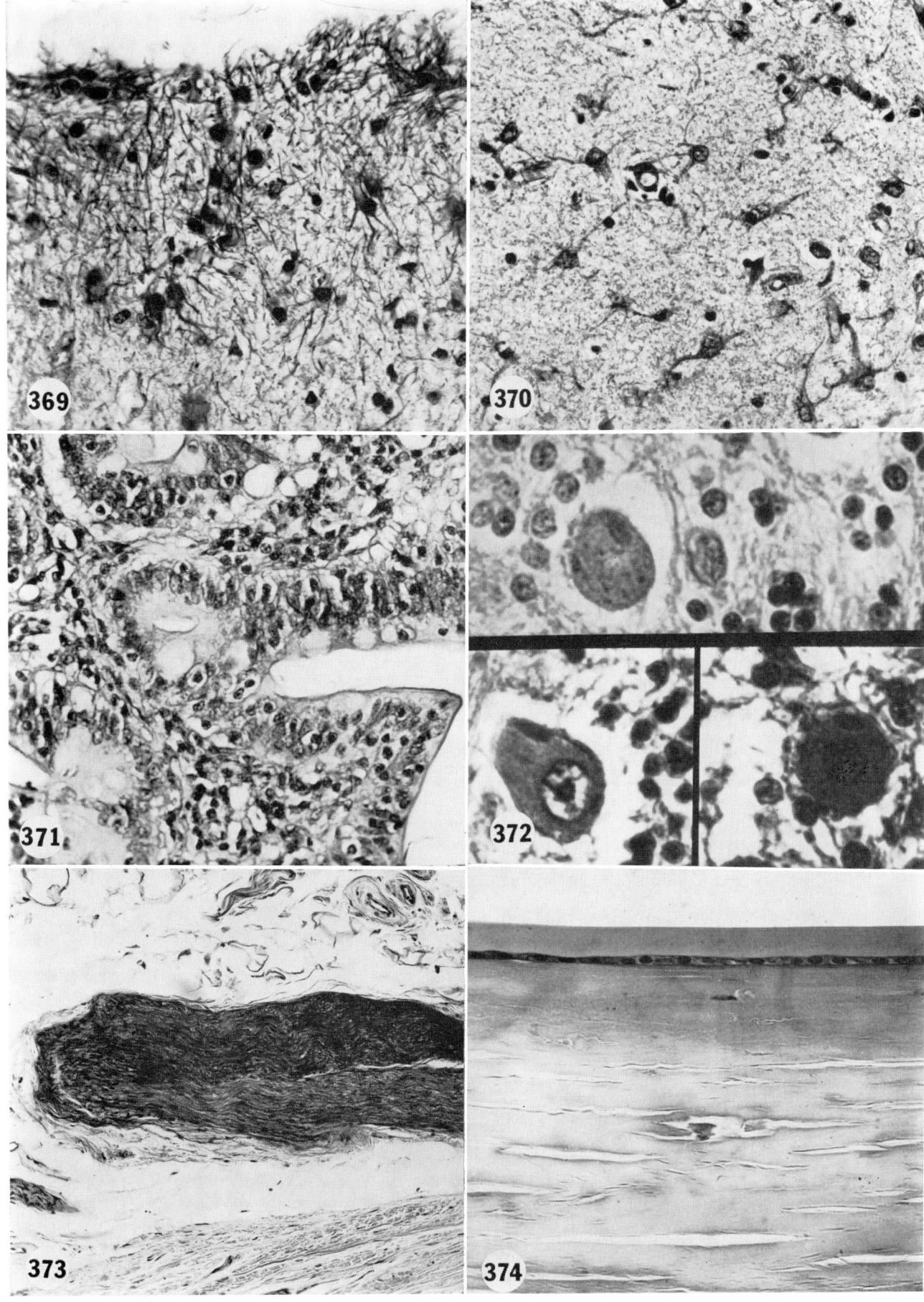

Figure 375. *Kinyon's Acid-fast Stain.* Both of the tissue sections depicted in this photograph were prepared from the same paraffin-embedded specimen of human lung tissue. The tissue section shown at the left was overstained with the methylene blue counterstain resulting in purple-stained tubercle bacilli being displayed against a deep blue background. The tissue section shown at the right is correctly stained by the Kinyon's procedure for the demonstration of acid-fast bacteria (bright red) against a light blue, evenly stained background. (Kinyon's stain, ×265) (AFIP Negative No. 67-8659)

Figure 376. *Methenamine Silver Nitrate Stain.* This technique is recommended for the demonstration of argyrophilic tissue components. It is widely used for the demonstration of certain fungi in tissue sections. When employed for this purpose with a light green counterstain, the procedure is frequently referred to as Grocott's method for the demonstration of fungi. The stock methenamine silver nitrate solution used in this procedure is stable for months but must be stored in a mechanical refrigerator. The stock solution may become contaminated with various forms of microorganisms and will support the growth of some fungi, particularly if it is not kept refrigerated. This paraffin-embedded tissue section of a specimen of dermis, fixed in neutral buffered 10% formalin, was stained with a working solution of stock methenamine silver nitrate solution and subsequently counterstained with a 0.2% aqueous solution of light green. The fibrillar and spherical contaminant observed above the focal plane of the tissue section is fungus which was deposited upon the surface of the section while it was in the working solution of methenamine silver nitrate. (Gomori's methenamine silver stain, ×265) (AFIP Negative No. 72-5345)

Figure 377. *Methenamine Silver Nitrate Stain.* The presence of acid formalin hematein pigment (see Chapter III) within tissue sections can, and frequently does, interfere with the interpretation of pathologic entities. This is well illustrated in this tissue section of the lung of a human being which is infected with *Pneumocystis carinii*. The tissue section is stained by Gomori's methenamine silver nitrate stain (Grocott's stain) which is recommended for the demonstration of argyrophilic tissue components. It is widely used for the demonstration of certain fungi in tissue sections. (×145) (AFIP Negative No. 72-18028)

Figure 378. *Methenamine Silver Nitrate Stain.* This is a higher magnification of the central portion of the field of view depicted in Figure 377. The *Pneumocystis carinii* organisms are demonstrated by the deposition of reduced silver nitrate upon their surface. They are visualized as small, round, black structures (arrows). However, the presence of acid formalin hematein pigment may cause some confusion because it is also capable of reducing silver nitrate. The large, black, centrally located structures are aggregates of acid formalin hematin pigment. The round to ovoid structures (arrows) are *Pneumocystis carinii* organisms (see Figures 379 and 380). (Gomori's methenamine silver nitrate stain, ×395) (AFIP Negative No. 72-18029)

Figure 379. *Methenamine Silver Nitrate Stain.* This is the same tissue section and field of view depicted in Figure 377 as observed by partial polariscopy. The stained *Pneumocystis carinii* organisms are isotrophic while the stained acid formalin hematin pigment is anisotropic (as is unstained pigment). The aggregates of the pigment are strongly anisotropic; however, individually discrete anisotropic granules of the pigment are also scattered over the tissue section (see Figure 380). (Gomori's methenamine silver nitrate stain, partial polariscopy, ×145) (AFIP Negative No. 72-18030)

Figure 380. *Methenamine Silver Nitrate Stain.* This is the same tissue section as depicted in Figures 377 through 379 and the same field of view as depicted in Figure 378 as observed by partial polariscopy. Note the isotrophic stained *Pneumocystis carinii* organisms (arrows) and compare their size to some of the minute anisotropic deposits of acid formalin hematin pigment. By comparing Figure 378 and this figure, it is evident that without the aid of polariscopy, such minute deposits of acid formalin hematin when stained with methenamine silver could be confused with the *Pneumocystis carinii* organisms. (Gomori's methenamine silver nitrate stain, partial polariscopy, ×145) (AFIP Negative No. 72-13031)

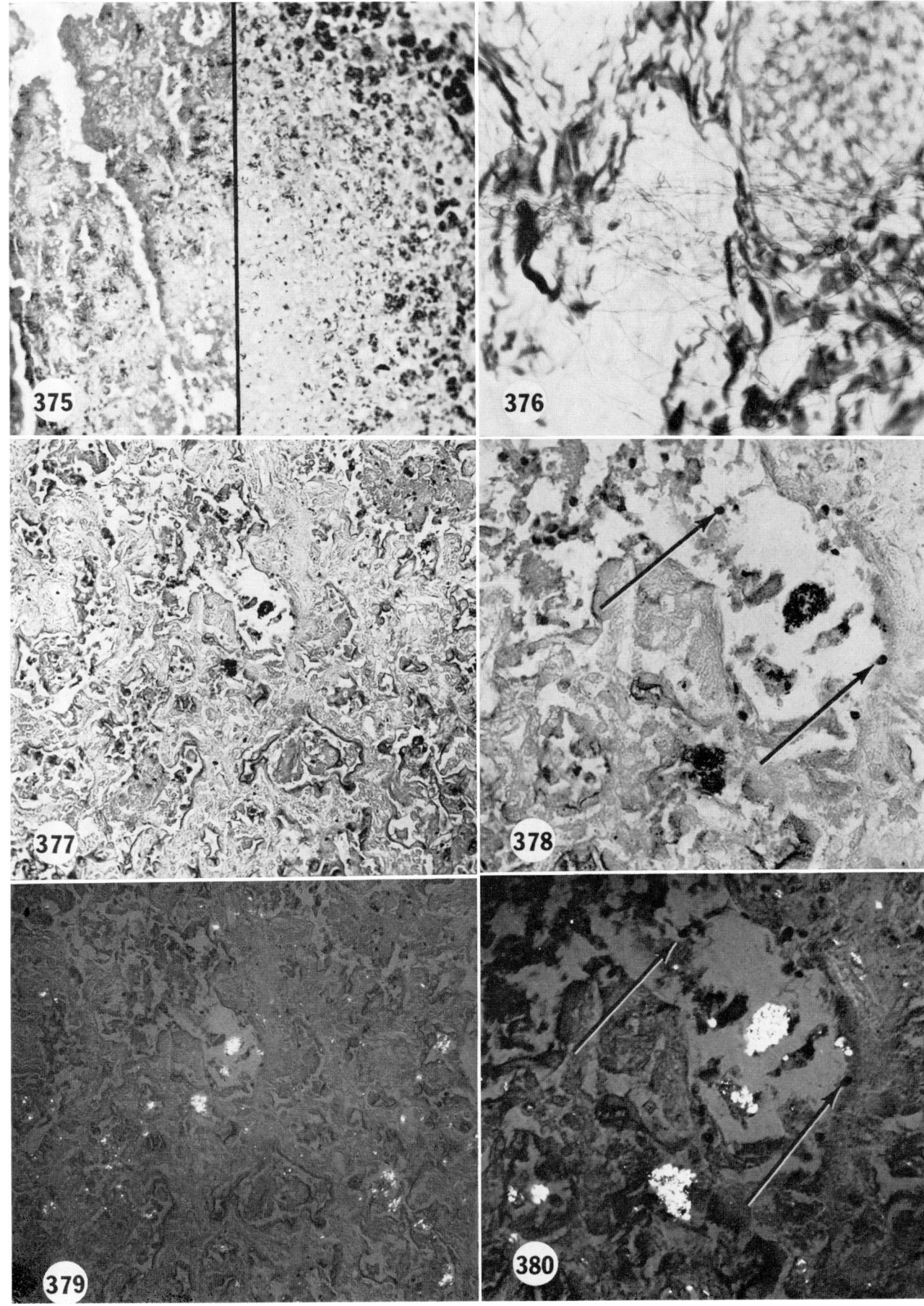

Figure 381. *Mucicarmine Stain (Mayer's)*. This technique is recommended for the histochemical demonstration of acid mucopolysaccharides (mucins) of epithelial origin in tissue sections. In the preparation of the carmine stock solution used in this staining procedure, carmine, aluminum chloride and water are heated in a crucible until they fuse and become dark red in color. The crucible and its contents are then dropped into a quantity of 50% ethyl alcohol and allowed to stand for twenty-four hours after which time the solution is filtered. Most of the fused material will dissolve in the alcohol. However, if the solution is not filtered prior to use, particles of undissolved fused material may precipitate on tissue sections which are exposed to the carmine stain. The particulate matter seen in this paraffin-embedded tissue section of a human lymph node fixed in neutral buffered 10% formalin is undissolved fused material. The particles resemble fungi and may be mistaken for such organisms by the inexperienced observer. (Mucicarmine, ×220) (AFIP Negative No. 72-5662)

Figure 382. *Mucicarmine Stain (Mayer's)*. In this higher magnification of a portion of the field depicted in Figure 381, the carmine stain precipitate can be seen more clearly. The particles of the precipitate resemble branching hyphae of fungi (see Color Plate 6, Figure 34). However, they are above the focal plane of the tissue section in most instances. (Mucicarmine, ×440) (AFIP Negative No. 72-5663)

Figure 383. *Nuclear Fast Red*. This smear of human blood was stained by the Prussian (Berlin, Perl's, Gomori's) blue reaction for the demonstration of iron with a nuclear fast (Kernechtrot) red counterstain. The staining reactions were carried out while the slide was held in a horizontal position. The linear structures seen throughout the smear were red in color. (Prussian blue reaction with nuclear fast red counterstain, ×305) (AFIP Negative No. 74-6509)

Figure 384. *Nuclear Fast Red*. This is the same view as depicted in Figure 383 as viewed by means of polariscopy. The linear artifacts are anisotropic. (Prussian blue reaction with nuclear fast red counterstain, ×305) (AFIP Negative No. 74-6510)

Figure 385. *Nuclear Fast Red*. This is a higher magnification of the field depicted in Figure 383 to more clearly depict the linear artifacts which were identified as deposits of crystalline, nuclear fast (Kernechtrot) red dye. These deposits of crystalline dye resulted from staining the slide in a horizontal position. (Prussian blue reaction with nuclear fast red counterstain, ×800) (AFIP Negative No. 74-5211)

Figure 386. *Nuclear Fast Red*. This is the same field depicted in Figure 385 as viewed by partial polariscopy to demonstrate the anisotropism of the crystalline dye artifacts. Excessive deposition of dye can usually be expected when tissue sections or smears are stained in the horizontal position by pouring the dye on their surfaces. Such artifacts can be avoided by staining the slide in a vertical position. (Prussian blue reaction with nuclear fast red counterstain, ×800) (AFIP Negative No. 74-5212)

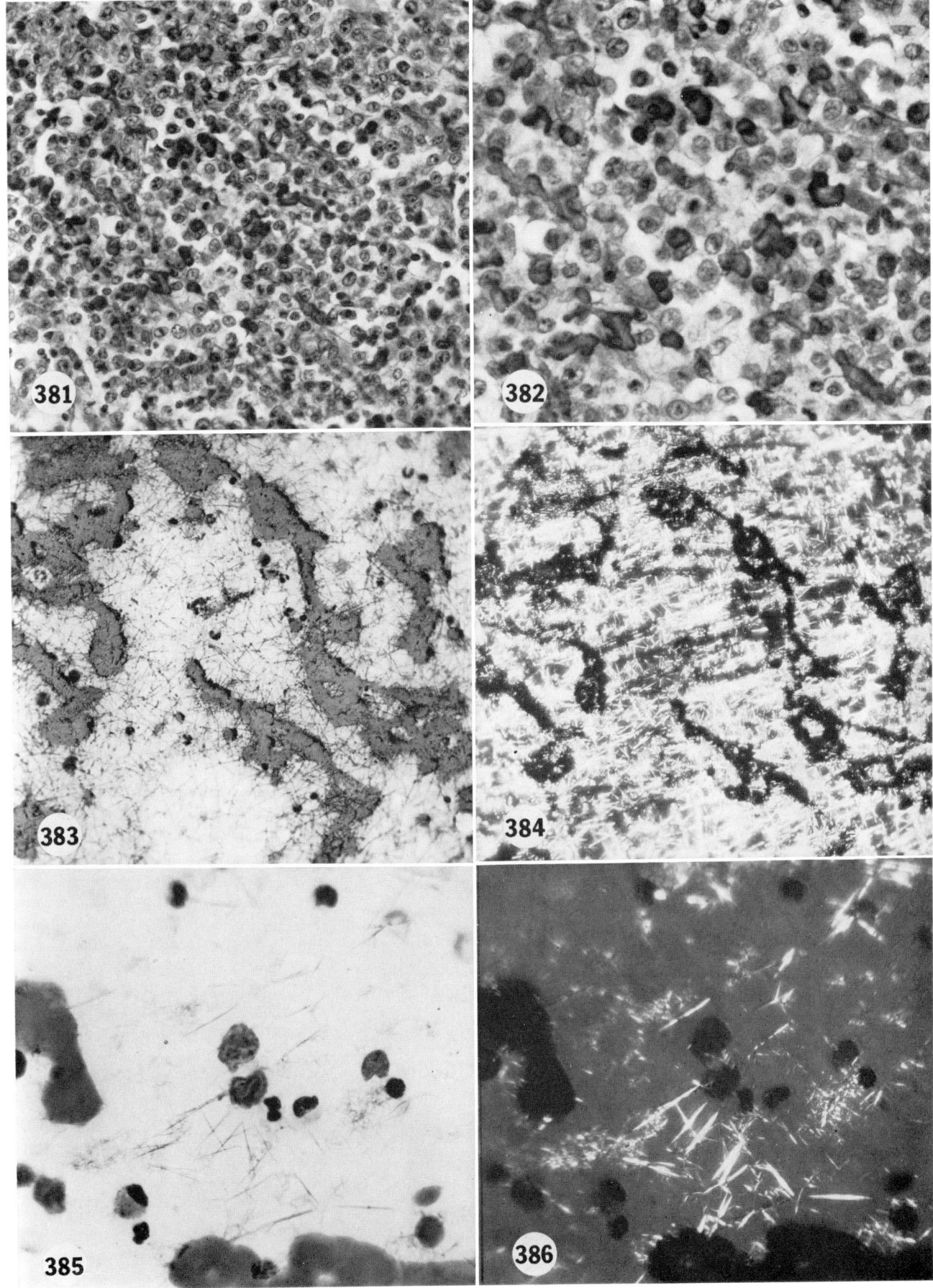

Figure 387. *Nuclear Fast Red (Kernechtrot) Stain.* The dark-to-clear crystalline materials seen throughout this paraffin-embedded tissue section of a fixed specimen of a human spleen are aluminum sulfate crystals. Such precipitates are retained on tissue sections which are counterstained with nuclear fast red (Kernechtrot) if the sections are not thoroughly washed prior to and after exposure to the dye solution. (Gridley reticulum stain with nuclear fast red counterstain, ×115) (AFIP Negative No. 73-4916)

Figure 388. *Nuclear Fast Red (Kernechtrot).* This is the same tissue section as depicted in Figure 387 as observed by partial polariscopy. The aluminum sulfate crystals are strongly anisotropic. (Gridley reticulum stain with nuclear fast red counterstain, partial polariscopy, ×115) (AFIP Negative No. 73-4915)

Figure 389. *Nuclear Fast Red (Kernechtrot).* This is the same tissue section as depicted in Figure 387. However, the field of view is different. Numerous aluminum sulphate crystals, of varied size, are scattered in clumps over the section. Prolonged washing of the tissue section in tap water both before and after application of the counterstain will prevent such artifacts from being present in the finished tissue section. They can be avoided by examining the tissue section microscopically after washing subsequent to dehydration of the counterstained tissue section. If present at the time of this examination, washing of the tissue section should be repeated prior to proceeding further in the preparation of the tissue section. (Gridley reticulum stain with nuclear fast red counterstain, ×80) (AFIP Negative No. 73-4904)

Figure 390. *Nuclear Fast Red (Kernechtrot).* This is the same tissue section and field of view as depicted in Figure 389 as observed by partial polariscopy. If the staining microscope is equipped for polariscopy, it is easier to detect such precipitates during the staining procedure. The aluminum sulphate crystals are more readily detected as being above the focal plane of the tissue section per se than when viewed by conventional bright field microscopy. (Gridley reticulum stain with nuclear fast red counterstain, partial polariscopy, ×80) (AFIP Negative No. 73-4897)

Figure 391. *Oil Red O.* The usual procedure in the staining of frozen-fixed tissue sections with oil red O consists of preparing a working solution of the colorant by taking 12 ml of supersaturated oil red O (2 gms) in isopropyl alcohol (500 ml) and adding distilled water q.s. 20 ml. After mixing, the working solution is allowed to stand for five minutes and it is then filtered through hard filter paper prior to use. During the actual exposure of tissue sections to the working solution, as soon as a precipitate is seen in the Stender dish, a new working solution should be prepared. The precipitates seen throughout this section (see Color Plate 6, Figure 35) of a specimen of a human cerebrum are aggregates of crystalline oil red O which resulted from exposing the tissue section to a working solution of the colorant which had too high a content of the Sudan colorant. (Oil red O, ×350) (AFIP Negative No. 72-7026)

Figure 392. *Periodic Acid-Schiff Reaction.* Malt diastase solution is used for the digestion and removal of glycogen from tissue sections, particularly in control procedures for the periodic acid-Schiff reaction. It is important that the malt diastase be kept in solution during the entire digestion procedure. If the solution is allowed to dry on the slide, as depicted in this photograph, the anisotropic dried malt diastase will yield a positive oxidative-Schiff (PAS) reaction with the Schiff reagent (see Color Plate 6, Figure 36 and Color Plate 7, Figure 37). It is important to recognize this artifact since it may simulate some types of mucoid cells in tissues that have been subjected to the PAS reaction. (PAS, ×180) (AFIP Negative No. 73-4278)

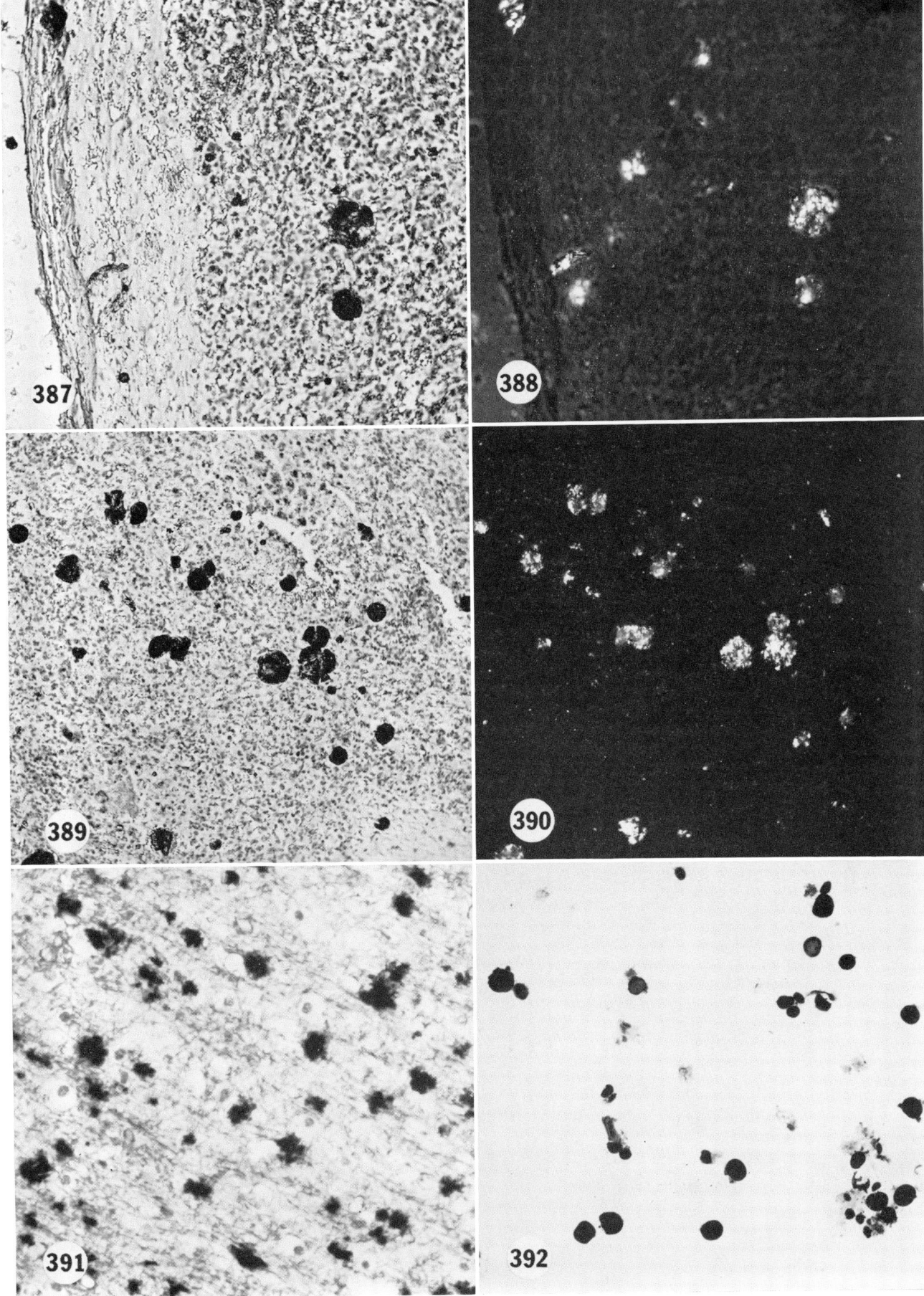

Figure 393. *Rubeanic Acid.* Uzman's rubeanic acid technique is frequently used for the demonstration of copper within tissue sections. The technique was employed with this paraffin-embedded tissue section of a specimen of human liver which had been fixed in Zenker's fluid. Note the numerous mercuric chloride crystals within the field of view. See also Figure 394. (Rubeanic acid, ×150) (AFIP Negative No. 73-4884)

Figure 394. *Rubeanic Acid.* This is a higher magnification of the central portion of the field of view depicted in Figure 393. The mercuric chloride crystals are turned black by some unknown chemical reaction with rubeanic acid (see Color Plate 7, Figure 38). The chromatic effects of mercuric chloride crystals and rubeanic acid should be considered to avoid any possible confusion between copper as observed in cases of Wilson's disease and mercuric chloride crystals resulting from Zenker's fixation. Zenker's fixation should never be used when the need for the demonstration of copper in tissue sections is anticipated. (Rubeanic acid, ×350) (AFIP Negative No. 73-4886)

Figure 395. *Sevier-Munger Silver Method for Neural Tissues.* Granular precipitates of silver are observed in this paraffin-embedded tissue section of a specimen of a carcinoid tumor of a human appendix which was fixed in neutral buffered 10% formalin. In the performance of the method, the slides are exposed to a 20% solution of warm silver nitrate (60°C) for fifteen minutes followed by rinsing in distilled water and subsequent exposure to a working ammoniacal silver solution to which formalin is added. This working solution is quickly poured over the slides and they are allowed to develop for five to thirty minutes until golden brown in color. During this period, the slides must be kept in motion or silver granules will precipitate on the tissue section as shown in this photograph (see Color Plate 7, Figure 39). (Sevier-Munger stain, ×265) (AFIP Negative No. 72-5346)

Figure 396. *Sevier-Munger Silver Method for Neural Tissues.* This is a different field of view of the same tissue section as depicted in Figure 395. The slide was not kept in motion during development with ammoniacal silver solution and silver granules of variable size precipitated on the tissue section. Such artifacts could be mistaken for bacteria or fungi by an inexperienced observer. (Sevier-Munger stain, ×265) (AFIP Negative No. 72-5347)

Figure 397. *Thionin Stain (Mallory's).* This technique is recommended for the metachromatic staining of mucin (Mallory, F. B.: *Pathological Technique.* New York, Hafner Publishing Co., 1938, reprinted 1961, p. 130). The original method specified that a 1% solution of thionin in 25% alcohol should be used. However, the solubility of thionin at 26°C. is 0.25% in either water or alcohol (Lillie, R. D.: *H. J. Conn's Biological Stains.* Baltimore, Williams & Wilkins, 1969, p. 295) and Lillie recommends that a 0.05% solution of thionin in 0.01 M acetate buffer be used for this technique (Lillie, R. D.: *Histopathologic Technic and Practical Histochemistry,* 3rd Edition. New York, McGraw, 1965, p. 508). This paraffin-embedded tissue section of a specimen of a human intestine, fixed in neutral buffered 10% formalin, was stained by means of the original technique using a 1% solution of thionin in 25% alcohol. Thionin dye crystals have precipitated from the dye solution onto the surface of the tissue section. These crystals are above the focal plane of the tissue section per se. (Mallory's thionin stain, ×395) (AFIP Negative No. 72-5661)

Figure 398. *Thionin Stain (Mallory's).* This photograph depicts the same field of view as shown in Figure 397, as viewed by partial polariscopy. The thionin dye crystals are anisotropic and by means of polariscopy they are more clearly depicted as being above the focal plane of the tissue section. (Mallory's thionin stain, partial polariscopy, ×395) (AFIP Negative No. 72-5660)

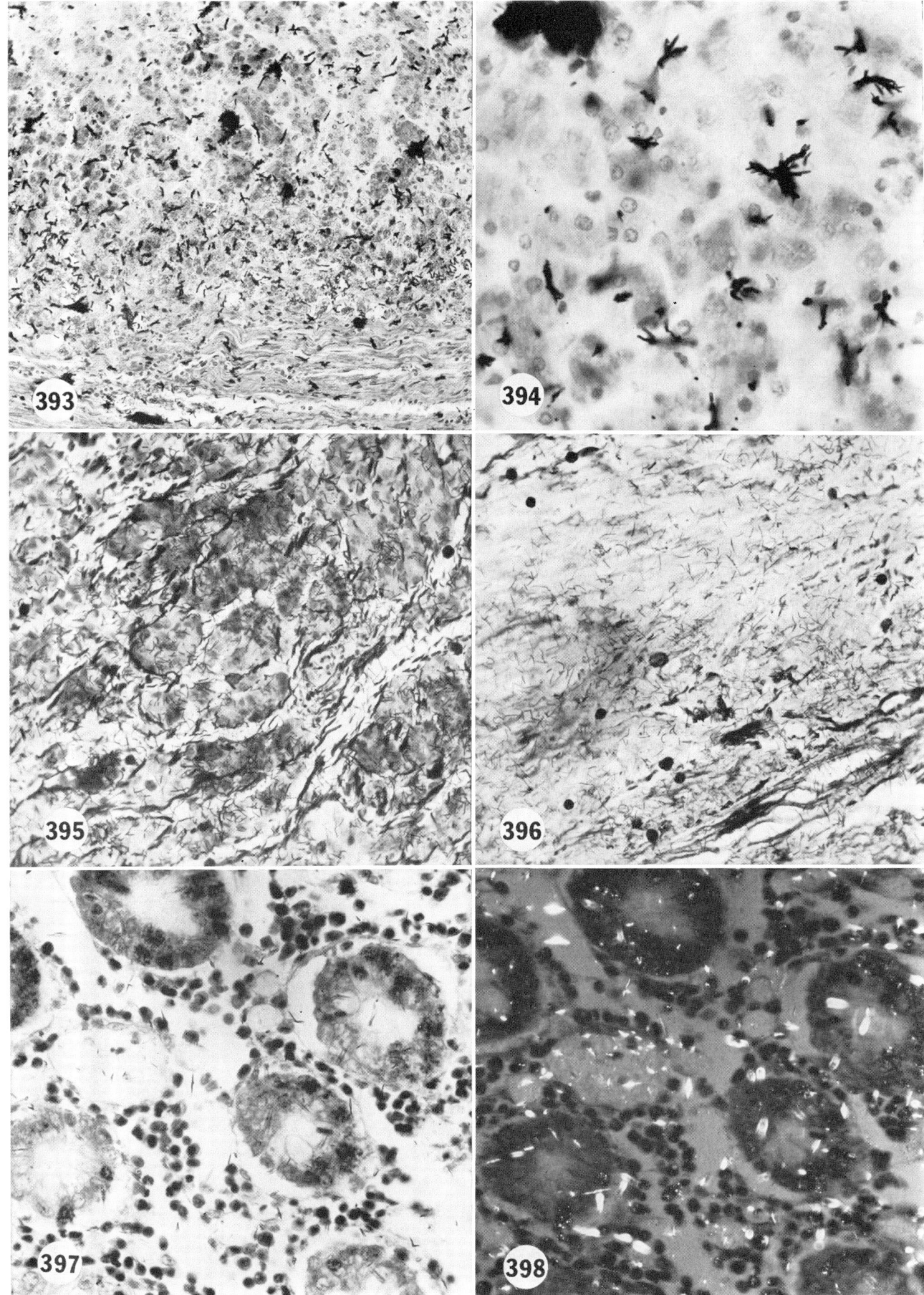

Figure 399. *Trichrome (Masson's)*. It is necessary to mordant formalin-fixed tissue in Bouin's fluid in the Masson trichrome staining procedure. Inadequate mordanting will result in poor staining effects with the Biebrich scarlet acid fuchsin solution. This tissue section of a cross section of human skeletal muscle was prepared from a formalin-fixed specimen which was not adequately mordanted in Bouin's fluid. The light staining areas did not stain properly with the Biebrich scarlet acid fuchsin solution. (Masson's trichrome, ×400) (AFIP Negative No. 74-7446)

Figure 400. *Trichrome (Masson's)*. This is a tissue section of a longitudinal section of human skeletal muscle which was prepared from a formalin-fixed specimen which was not adequately mordanted in Bouin's fluid prior to performing Masson's trichrome staining procedure. The uneven staining is due to inadequate staining with the Biebrich scarlet acid fuchsin solution. (Masson's trichrome, ×400) (AFIP Negative No. 74-7445)

Figure 401. *Walbach's Giemsa Stain*. One of the ingredients of the Walbach's Giemsa stain is glycerin. Tissue sections must be washed well subsequent to exposure to stains that contain glycerin. If glycerin is not washed off of the section completely prior to the application of mounting medium, a beading artifact will appear in the cover-slipped tissue section as depicted in this tissue section of a specimen of a human spinal cord. This artifact resembles the artifact that occurs when moisture accumulates in the clearing xylene of various staining procedures (see Figure 416). The beading effect can be seen throughout this photomicrograph. Note that morphologic details of the tissue are difficult to discern because of the artifact. (Walbach's Giemsa, ×615) (AFIP Negative No. 73-4909)

Figure 402. *Walbach's Giemsa Stain*. This is the same tissue section and same field of view as depicted in Figure 401 as observed with the condenser of the microscope being partially closed. The same effect can be achieved by lowering the substage of the microscope. With either a partially closed condenser or lowered substage, the glycerin beads are more clearly seen to be above the focal plane of the tissue section (see Color Plate 7, Figure 40). (Walbach's Giemsa, ×615) (AFIP Negative No. 73-4908)

Figure 403. *Wright's Giemsa Stain*. The wavy linear structures seen throughout this photograph of a portion of a blood smear were suspected of being some unknown parasite, most probably a helminth (see Color Plate 7, Figure 41). The slide was sent to the Armed Forces Institute of Pathology for identification of the suspected parasite. (Wright's Giemsa, ×145) (AFIP Negative No. 74-6328)

Figure 404. *Wright's Giemsa Stain*. This is a higher magnification of a central portion of the field depicted in Figure 403. Note that the linear structures do appear to resemble a parasitic organism. On close scrutiny, one can see what appears to be internal staining of the structures. Such intensely stained areas are suggestive of the staining of the digestive tract of a helminth. (Wright's Giemsa, ×530) (AFIP Negative No. 74-6329)

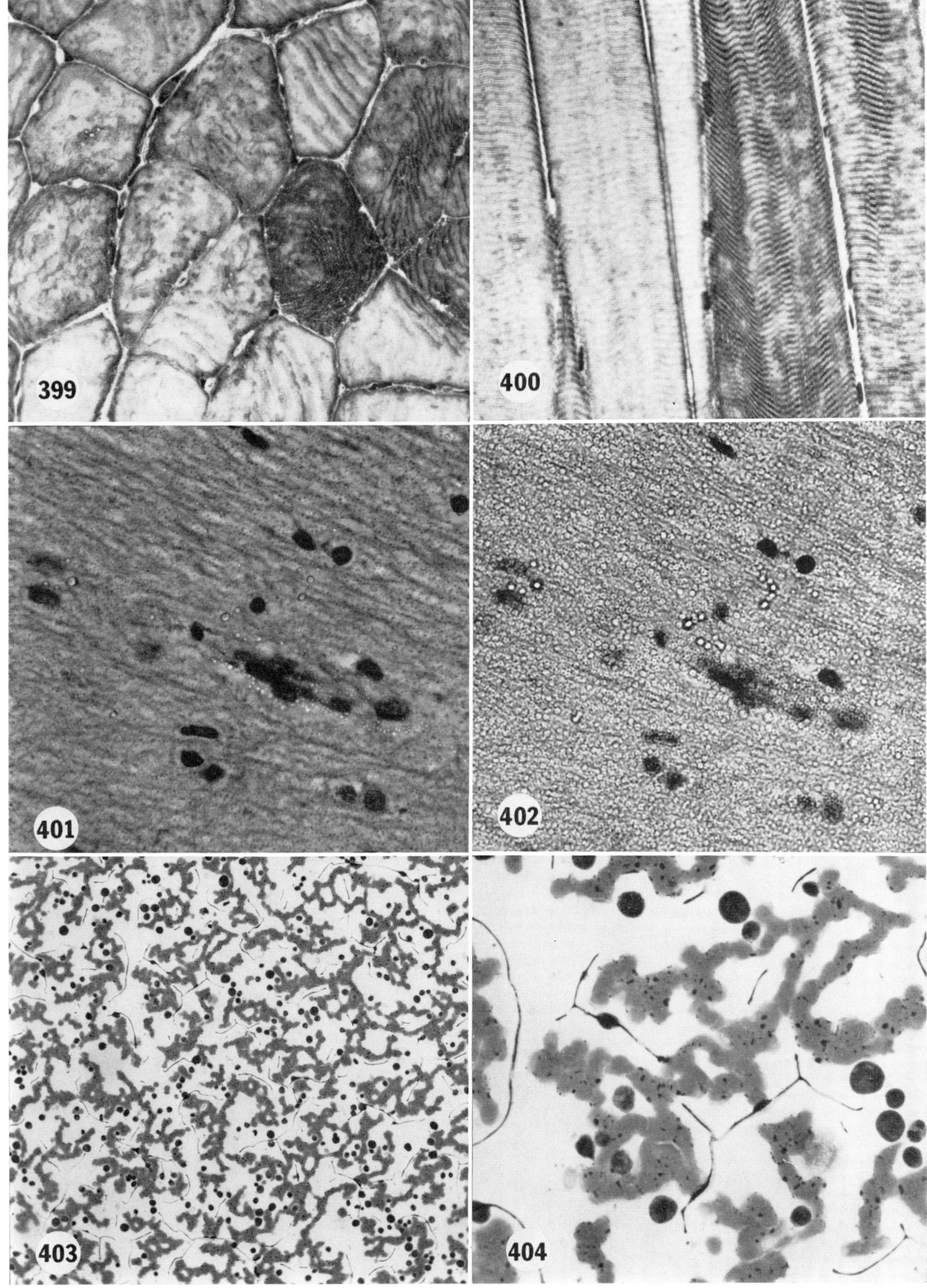

Figure 405. *Wright's Giemsa Stain.* This photograph was taken from a portion of the periphery of the same blood smear depicted in Figures 403 and 404. The linear structures which resembled a parasitic organism when viewed in more central areas of the blood smear (Figures 403 and 404) were identified as wrinkles of the dried plasma film when viewed at the periphery of the blood smear. (Wright's Giemsa, ×210) (AFIP Negative No. 74-6330)

Figure 406. *Wright's Giemsa Stain.* This photograph was taken from a portion of the periphery of the same blood smear depicted in Figures 403 through 405 and clearly depicts the wrinkles of the dried plasma film which were mistaken for parasitic organisms in the more central portions of the smear. The dark staining which resembled the digestive tract of a helminth in the artifacts depicted in Figure 404 resulted from the double staining of both surfaces of the wrinkles within the dried plasma film. (Wright's Giemsa, ×210) (AFIP Negative No. 74-6331)

Figure 407. *Effects of Prolonged Storage of Specimens on Staining.* The tissue specimen of animal skin from which this paraffin-embedded tissue section was prepared was stored in neutral buffered 10% formalin for ten years prior to being processed and embedded. Note the light staining reaction due to prolonged storage as wet tissue. (Mayer's hematoxylin and eosin, ×395) (AFIP Negative No. 68-2851)

Figure 408. *Effect of Prolonged Storage of Specimens on Staining.* This stained, paraffin-embedded tissue section of a specimen of animal skin was prepared immediately after fixation. It was subsequently stored in a slide file cabinet for ten years. By comparing this figure with Figures 409 through 411, one can readily detect the fading of the stains which occurred during this period. Usually, basophilic fading is minimal in stained tissue sections subjected to prolonged periods of file storage. This particular slide was removed from the file numerous times during the ten-year period. (Mayer's hematoxylin and eosin, ×395) (AFIP Negative No. 68-2847)

Figure 409. *Effect of Prolonged Storage of Specimens on Staining.* This paraffin-embedded tissue section of a specimen of animal skin was prepared immediately after fixation. It was subsequently stored in the undecerated and unstained state in a slide file cabinet for a period of ten years. At the end of this period, it was removed from the cabinet, decerated, and stained. Note that the staining quality of the section was not adversely affected by this prolonged period of storage in the unstained state. (Mayer's hematoxylin and eosin, ×395) (AFIP Negative No. 68-2849)

Figure 410. *Effect of Prolonged Storage of Specimens on Staining.* This stained, paraffin-embedded tissue section of a specimen of animal skin was prepared immediately after fixation. It was subsequently stored in a slide file cabinet for ten years. At the end of this period, it was removed from the cabinet, destained, and restained. The staining results compare favorably to those obtained with unstained tissue sections (Figure 409) or tissue sections which were freshly prepared from a block of paraffin-embedded tissue (Figure 411) which were stored for similar periods of time. Usually, no deleterious effect on the nuclear chromatin, which adversely affects its staining characteristics, occurs in stained tissue sections stored for up to ten years in a slide file cabinet. (Mayer's hematoxylin and eosin, ×395) (AFIP Negative No. 68-2848)

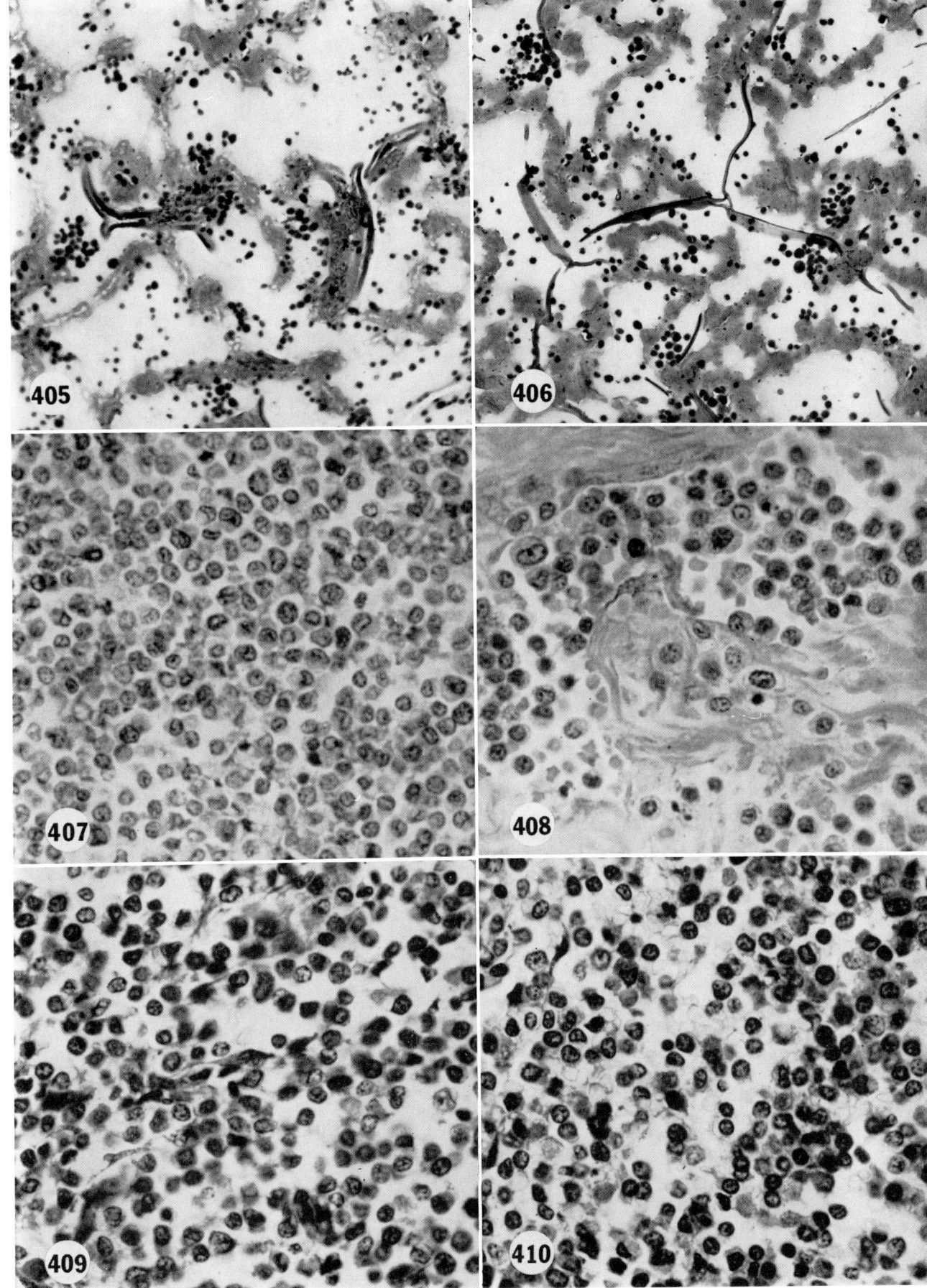

Figure 411. *Effect of Prolonged Storage of Specimens on Staining.* This tissue section was prepared from the same block of paraffin-embedded tissue as the tissue sections depicted in Figures 407 through 410. The tissue section was prepared and stained after the block of embedded tissue had been in storage for a period of ten years. Only slight differences in staining quality are noted when this tissue section is compared with unstained tissue sections (Figure 409) or stained tissue sections (Figure 408) subjected to similar storage conditions. These differences are limited to a slightly increased intensity of cytoplasmic staining and a slightly decreased intensity of the staining of nuclear chromatin. (Mayer's hematoxylin and eosin, ×395) (AFIP Negative No. 68-2851)

Figure 412. *Effect of Prolonged Storage of Specimens on Straining.* The diagnosis for the tissue sections depicted in Figures 407 through 411 is mastocytoma. The tissue sections depicted previously in Figures 407 through 411 and subsequently in Figures 413 through 415 were all prepared from the same specimen of skin tissue from a dog. This photograph and those of Figures 413 through 415 illustrate the influence of prolonged storage of wet tissue, embedded tissue and tissue sections on the results achieved with Walbach's Giemsa stain for the demonstration of mast cells. The tissue specimen from which this tissue section was prepared was stored in neutral buffered 10% formalin for ten years prior to being processed and embedded. Compare with Figure 406 and note that the tinctorial quality of the stain is very light as compared to that observed with stained (Figure 413) and unstained (Figure 414) tissue sections and embedded tissue (Figure 415) stored for a period of ten years. Mast cell granules could be demonstrated in only a few of the mast cells compared to Figures 413 through 415. (Walbach's Giesma stain, ×395) (AFIP Negative No. 68-2859)

Figure 413. *Effect of Prolonged Storage of Specimens on Staining.* This stained, paraffin-embedded tissue section of a mastocytoma was prepared immediately after fixation. It was subsequently stored in a slide file cabinet for ten years. When compared with a similar tissue section prepared after storage of the same wet tissue specimen for ten years (Figure 412) the tinctorial quality of the Giemsa stain is excellent and compares favorably with the results achieved with unstained tissue sections (Figure 414) or freshly prepared sections from embedded tissue (Figure 415) which had been stored for ten years. The purple-stained mast cell granules were easily detected throughout the tissue section when examined microscopically. The various staining effects characteristic of a good Giemsa stain were also evident microscopically. (Walbach's Giemsa stain, ×395) (AFIP Negative No. 68-2855)

Figure 414. *Effect of Prolonged Storage of Specimens on Staining.* This paraffin-embedded tissue section of a mastocytoma was prepared immediately after fixation. It was subsequently stored in the undecerated and unstained state in a slide file cabinet for a period of ten years. At the end of this period, it was removed from the cabinet, decerated, and stained with Walbach's Giemsa stain. When compared with a similar tissue section prepared after storage of the same wet tissue specimen for ten years (Figure 412), the tinctorial quality of the Giemsa stain is excellent and compares favorably with the results achieved with stained tissue sections (Figure 413) or freshly prepared sections from embedded tissue (Figure 415) which had been stored for ten years. The mast cell granules were stained very well. These results demonstrated that file storage of unstained slides for extended periods of time usually produces acceptable staining results. (Walbach's Giemsa stain, ×395) (AFIP Negative No. 68-2856)

Figure 415. *Effect of Prolonged Storage on Embedded Tissue.* This stained, paraffin-embedded tissue section of a mastocytoma was prepared from the same block of paraffin-embedded tissue as the tissue sections depicted in Figures 407 through 414. The tissue section was prepared and stained with Walbach's Giemsa stain after the block of embedded tissue had been in storage for a period of ten years. When compared with a similar tissue section prepared after storage of the same wet tissue specimen for ten years (Figure 412), the tinctorial quality of the Giemsa stain is excellent and compares favorably with the results achieved with stained (Figure 413) or unstained (Figure 414) tissue sections which had been stored for ten years. These results demonstrate that tissue is well preserved when embedded in paraffin and stored in this state for extended periods of time. However, if tissue sections were prepared at the time the specimen was originally embedded, good preservation of the embedded tissue during storage is only possible if the faced-off surface of the block is sealed properly subsequent to sectioning. This is readily accomplished by dipping the faced-off surface of the block into molten paraffin, or by gently touching the faced-off surface of the block with a spatula which has been heated over a Bunsen burner for a sufficient period of time so that it is warm enough to melt the paraffin but not hot enough to burn the tissue. (Walbach's Giemsa stain, ×395) (AFIP Negative No. 68-2857)

Figure 416. *Clearing.* In most staining schedules, after the application of the counterstain, the stained tissue section is dehydrated by passing it through a series of ethyl alcohol solutions of ascending alcohol concentrations. Finally, the tissue section is cleared with xylene prior to being coverslipped. Unless the xylene is frequently replaced in the staining train, alcohol and water droplets will be retained within the stained tissue section and when it is coverslipped the section will look like this paraffin-embedded tissue section of a specimen of human liver which has been fixed in neutral buffered 10% formalin. This artifact is seen best if one lowers the microscope substage (see Color Plate 7, Figure 42). Such artifacts may be corrected by removal of the coverslip, extraction of the mounting medium with xylene followed by dehydration in fresh solutions of alcohol. Fresh xylene is employed after dehydration and finally the tissue section is recoverslipped. (Hematoxylin, ×400)

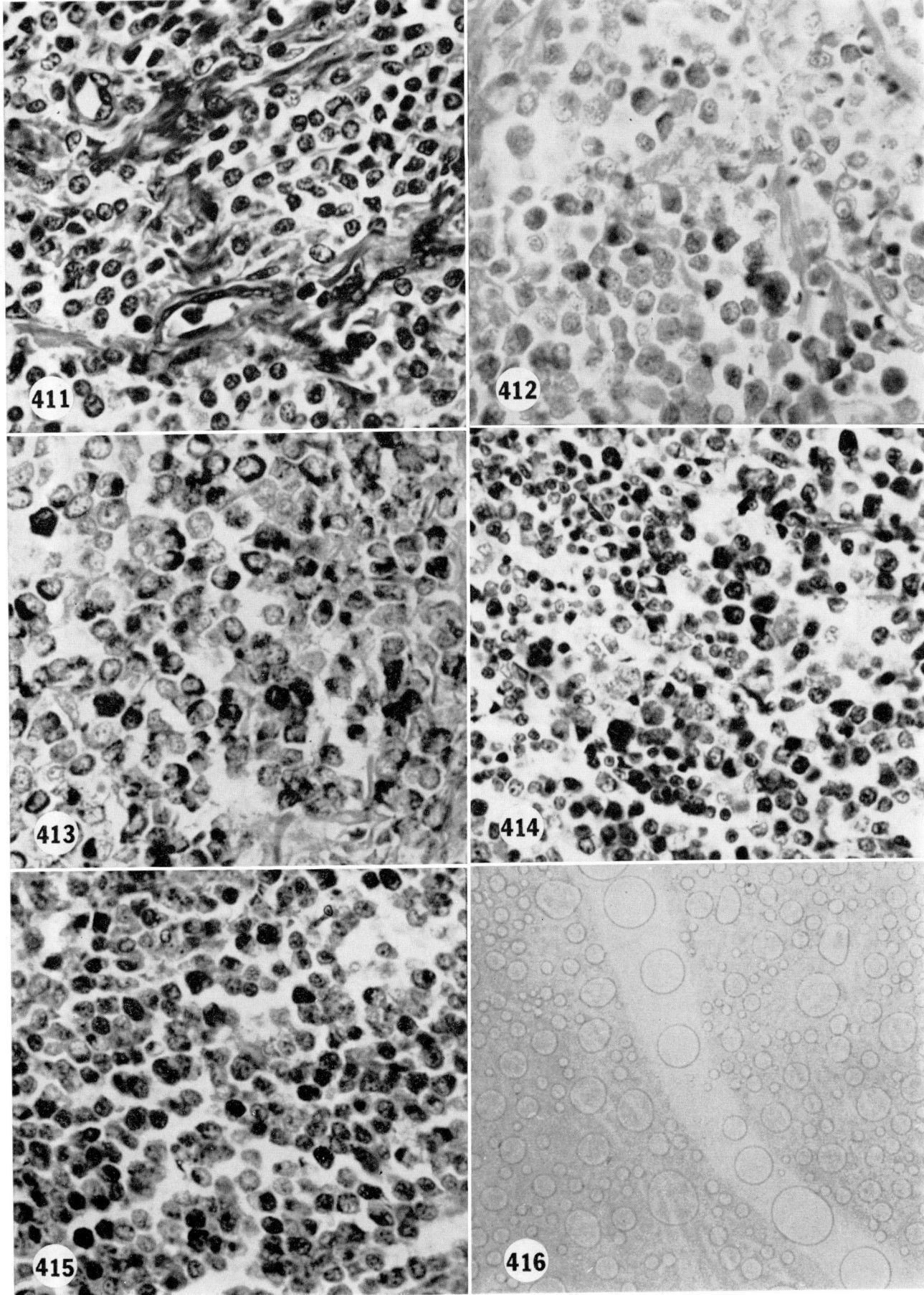

Figure 417. *Clearing.* If a stained and dehydrated tissue section is exposed to xylene for an excessive period of time, it will become dried out prior to being coverslipped. When such a tissue section is finally examined with a microscope, it will look like parched earth as depicted by this fissured paraffin-embedded tissue section of a specimen of human liver, fixed in neutral buffered 10% formalin, which had been overexposed to xylene subsequent to being stained. (Hematoxylin, ×350)

Figure 418. *Clearing.* This is a duplicate tissue section from the same specimen as depicted in Figure 417. It is not divided by fissures because it was not overexposed to xylene. In the routine schedule for Harris' hematoxylin and eosin staining procedure according to S. W. Thompson (*Selected Histochemical and Histopathological Methods.* Springfield, Thomas, 1966, p. 765) two exposures to xylene, each of five minutes duration, are prescribed for the clearing of stained and dehydrated tissue sections. (Harris' H&E, ×350)

Figure 419. *Storage of Microscopic Tissue Sections.* Artifacts may result from the manner in which a finished tissue section is handled long after its preparation. Here three duplicate paraffin-embedded tissue sections from the same embedded specimen (see Color Plate 8, Figure 43) were cut, stained, and coverslipped in an identical manner. The slide depicted at the bottom of the photograph was stored in a covered slide box at room temperature for eighteen days. The slide depicted at the upper right of the photograph was stored in a similar box held at 60°C for eighteen days. Macroscopically and microscopically, there is no detectable difference between these two tissue sections. The tissue section seen at the upper left of the photograph was placed on a windowsill and exposed to sunlight during the daylight hours for a period of eighteen days. The stain has faded to the extent that, microscopically, it appears to be unstained. An artifact may be produced in a prize slide simply by leaving it uncovered on a desk exposed to sunlight for several hours a day for a few days. (H&E, ×3)

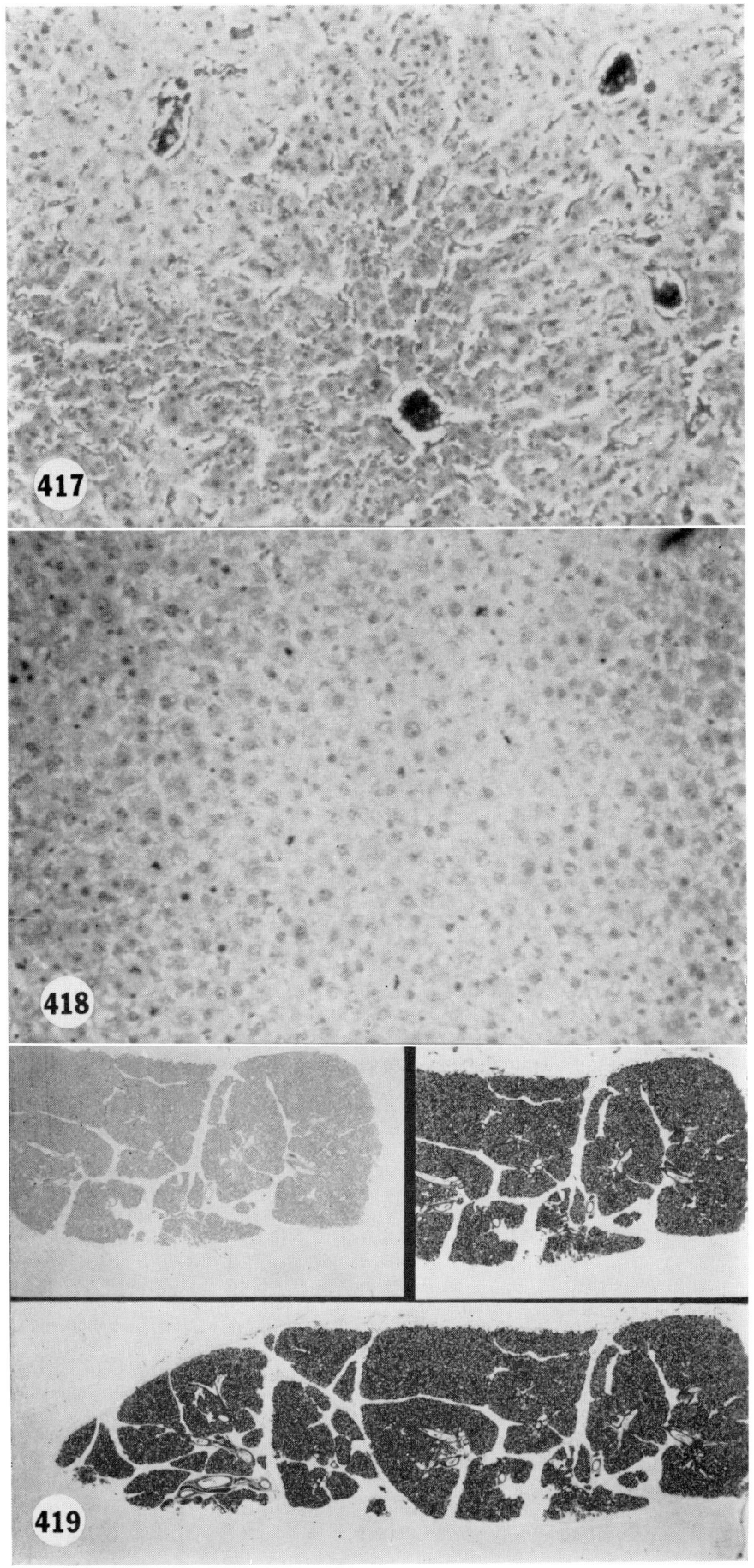

IX

Artifacts Resulting from Coverslipping Procedures

INTRODUCTION

ALL OF THE ARTIFACTS which may be observed in microscopic tissue sections that are the result of coverslipping procedures are caused by faulty or inappropriate laboratory techniques. Examples of such coverslipping artifacts included in this chapter are:

    Contamination of surface of slides with cigarette, cigar, or pipe ashes or lint fibers
    Contamination of mounting medium
    Use of coverslips that are too small
    Faulty positioning of the coverslip
    Use of glass coverslip substitutes
    Entrapment of air during coverslipping
    Use of medium of thick viscosity
    Use of too much mounting medium

Figure 420. *Cigarette Ashes.* The cigarette ash artifact is difficult to differentiate from pencil graphite on microscope slides which have a frosted end for pencil labeling. Histotechnologists should not smoke while performing laboratory procedures. (H&E, ×150) (AFIP Negative No. 73-2493)

Figure 421. *Cigarette Ashes.* This is a higher magnification of a portion of the field of view depicted in Figure 420. The type of deposition of cigarette ashes depicted in this photomicrograph of an unstained glass microscope slide is frequently seen on tissue sections when cigarette ashes are inadvertently dropped on the slides by careless histotechnologists. (Unstained, ×305) (AFIP Negative No. 73-2496)

Figure 422. *Lint Fibers.* Fine lint fibers from gauze or other cloth materials used in the histopathology laboratory are frequently deposited on stained tissue sections at the time of coverslipping (see Figure 424). As depicted in this photomicrograph of a paraffin-embedded tissue section of a specimen of the lung of a human being, such lint fibers are difficult or impossible to detect with routine bright field microscopy. (H&E, ×50) (AFIP Negative No. 72-18040)

Figure 423. *Lint Fibers.* This is the same tissue section and the same field of view as depicted in Figure 422 as observed by partial polariscopy. The lint fiber is strongly anisotropic (see Color Plate 8, Figure 44). (H&E, partial polariscopy, ×50) (AFIP Negative No. 72-18039)

Figure 424. *Lint Fibers.* Although precleaned coverslips and glass microscope slides are available commercially, many laboratories prefer to clean their own coverslips and slides. Regardless of the favorite cleaning procedure used by various laboratories, the final steps in the cleaning procedure usually consist of immersing the coverslips or slides in alcohol, acid alcohol, or a 1% aqueous solution of acetic acid followed by polishing each piece with a soft cloth. The artifact depicted here consists of a fragment of fine linen thread which was left as a residue on a coverslip at the time it was cleaned (see Color Plate 8, Figure 45). The tissue section is from the spinal cord of a goat. The artifact seen within the meninges was originally mistaken by several observers for a nematode. (H&E, ×125) (Contributed by Dr. J. R. M. Innes)

Figure 425. *Contamination of Mounting Medium.* Mounting medium can become contaminated in a variety of ways. If the air in the working area where mounting medium is applied to stained tissue sections is laden with dust particles, the exposed medium on the surface of the slide can readily become contaminated prior to application of the coverslip. Mounting medium was applied to this paraffin-embedded, stained tissue section of a specimen of a kidney of a rat in an environment in which the air was laden with minute carbon particles. The dark granular specks seen in the mounting medium overlaying this tissue section are carbon particles from the exhaust of a forced air heating system which supplied heat to the laboratory. Air filters should be used on such heating systems at the point where the air exhausts into the work area. The contaminants in the mounting medium are above the focal plane of the tissue section per se. (H&E, ×70) (Contributed by Dr. W. L. Wooding)

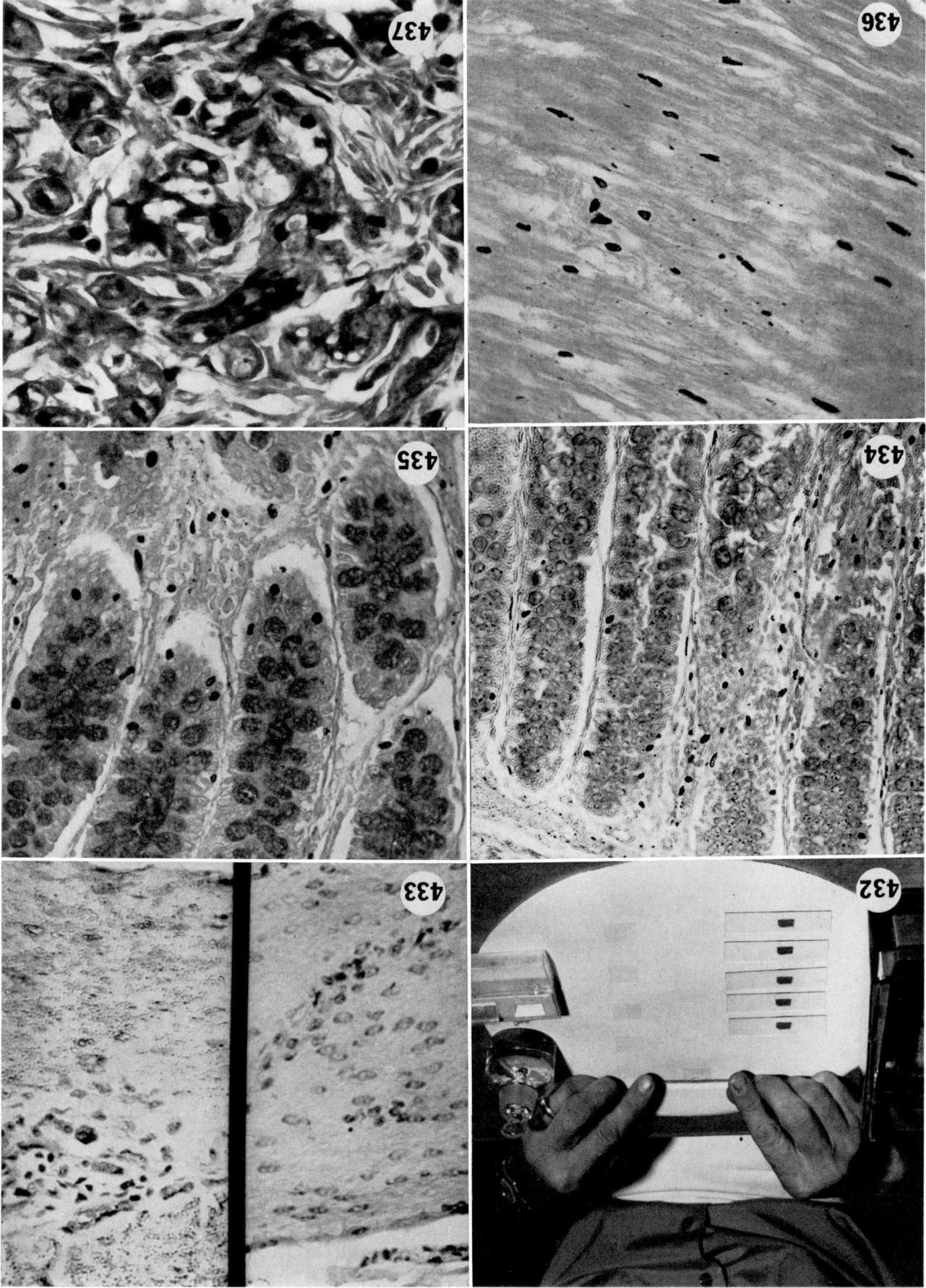

Figure 438. *Entrapped Air.* If the xylene is allowed to evaporate prior to the application of mounting medium, air within the interstitial spaces of the tissue section will be entrapped beneath the mounting medium. These tiny bubbles of entrapped air will impart a glassine, stippled appearance to the coverslipped tissue section as depicted in this paraffin-embedded tissue section of a specimen of the human small intestine which was fixed in neutral buffered 10% formalin. Compare to Figure 446. (H&E, ×70) (AFIP Negative No. 72-3894)

Figure 439. *Entrapped Air.* This photomicrograph is a higher magnification of a portion of the field depicted in Figure 438 which more clearly demonstrates the glassine, stippled appearance produced by the air bubbles which are present in the interstitial spaces of this improperly coverslipped tissue section. Evaporation of the xylene also resulted in dehydration with resultant shrinkage of the peripheral area of the tissue sections (compare with Figure 447). (H&E, ×195) (AFIP Negative No. 72-4057)

Figure 440. *Entrapped Air.* This is a paraffin-embedded tissue section of a specimen of human kidney fixed in neutral buffered 10% formalin which has been allowed to become dry after being removed from xylene prior to the application of mounting medium (see Figures 438 and 439). The stippled glassine appearance of the tissue section is due to minute air bubbles entrapped in the interstitial spaces of the tissue section beneath the mounting medium. (H&E, ×100) (AFIP Negative No. 71-11706)

Figure 441. *Entrapped Air.* This is a photomicrograph of the same tissue section depicted in Figure 440. The glassine stippling becomes more apparent if the substage of the microscope is lowered. (H&E, ×100) (AFIP Negative No. 71-11705)

Figure 442. *Entrapped Air.* This is a microautoradiograph of a paraffin-embedded tissue section of a specimen of the adrenal gland of a dog prepared by the film stripping technique. After development of the film strip, the tissue section was stained with hematoxylin and mounted in Permount synthetic mounting medium. The cohesion between Permount and the film strip is unsatisfactory. The darkened area overlying the tissue section is not a positive reaction of the isotope within the tissue and the silver halide of the film strip. The darkened area is simply entrapped, minute air bubbles within the interstitial spaces of the tissue section. The mounting medium was removed from the film strip tissue section preparation, the preparation subsequently rehydrated and mounted in Paragon® aqueous mounting medium and the artifact did not reoccur. (Hematoxylin, ×125) (Contributed by Mrs. J. R. Matthews)

Figure 443. *Crystals within Mounting Media.* Mounting media may roughly be divided into three main types: resinous, aqueous, and oil media. Resinous mounting media may be composed of either natural or synthetic resins or in some instances combinations of natural and synthetic components. Many of the resinous mounting media have a tendency to crystalize if exposed to air for prolonged periods of time. In particular, crystals frequently form about the neck of stock bottles of resinous mounting media which are closed by metal screw caps. This can be minimized if the neck of the bottle and inner surface of the screw cap are wiped dry after each opening of the stock bottle. Crystals which form as described can fall into the medium contained within the stock bottle or contaminate the medium if it is poured from the bottle. The crystal observed overlaying the paraffin-embedded tissue section of a specimen of kidney from a rat, depicted in this photomicrograph, is crystallized synthetic resin mounting medium which had contaminated the stock bottle containing the medium. It is seen as an anisotropic crystal above the focal plane of the tissue section per se. (H&E, partial polariscopy, ×170) (Contributed by Mr. L. E. Schellhammer)

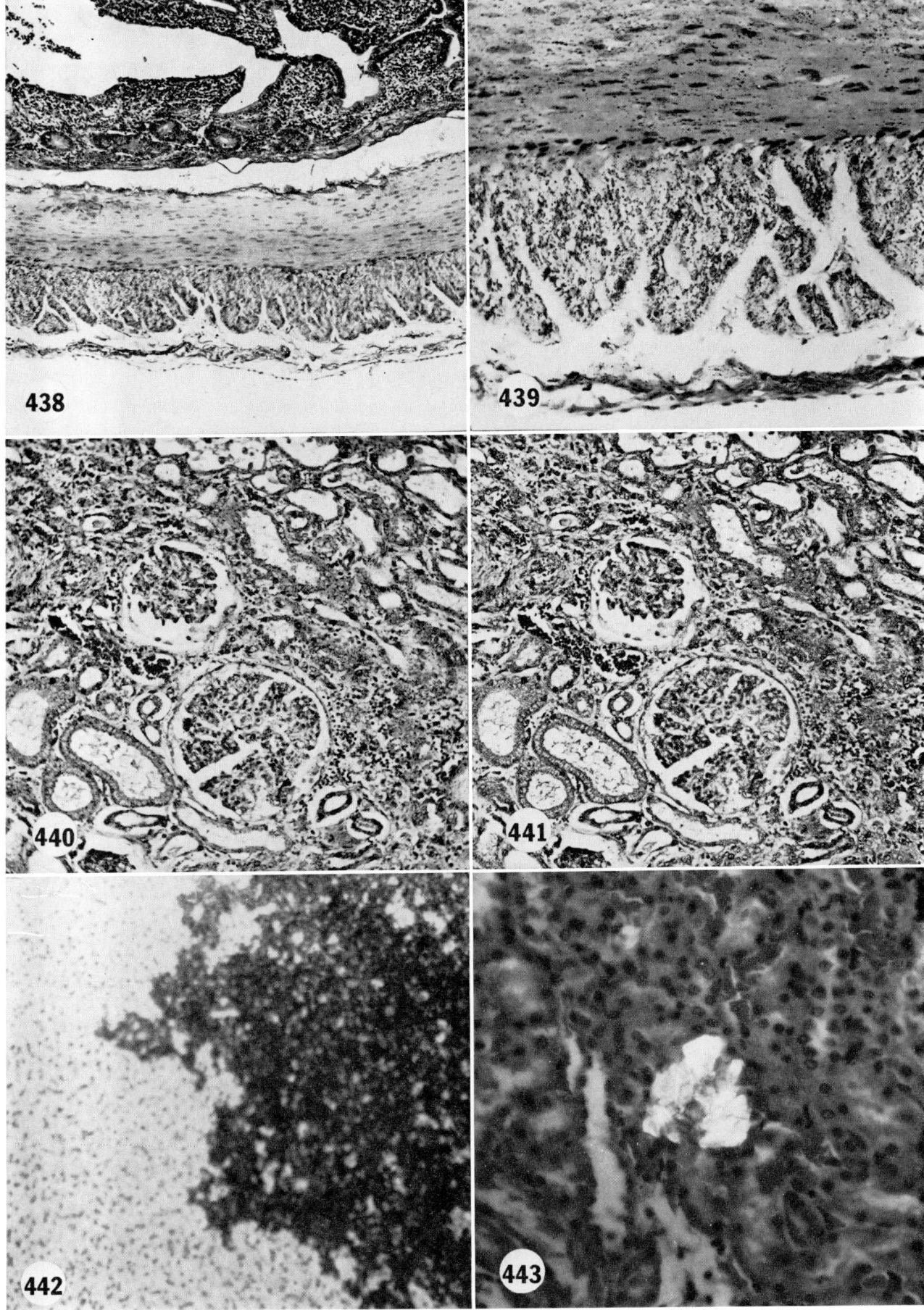

Figure 444. *Mounting Media.* The final step in the preparation of microscopic tissue sections consists of the application of mounting medium to the tissue section and the placing of a coverslip over the tissue section. Mounting media tend to become more viscous as their solvent phase evaporates. One may periodically check the suitability of the mounting media by drawing a 5 ml quantity into a clean glass pipette as shown in this photograph. Holding the pipette in a vertical position, the 5 ml sample of mounting medium is allowed to freely drain from the pipette. The commonly used mounting medium should drain from the pipette in a time interval of seven to nine seconds provided the viscosity is suitable for use in mounting of tissue sections: Balsam/7 seconds; Gum Damar/9 seconds; Histoclad®/8 seconds; Permount/8 seconds. (AFIP Negative No. 66-7992)

Figure 445. *Mounting Media.* If the mounting medium is too viscous, one may inadvertently apply an excessive quantity of mounting medium to a tissue section. More frequently, one may apply too much mounting medium simply because of sloppy technique. As shown in these duplicate paraffin-embedded tissue sections of a specimen of human liver, fixed in neutral buffered 10% formalin, an excess of mounting medium elevates the coverslip. This produces a slight haze over the tissue section when observed under high-power objectives. Mounting medium was correctly applied to the tissue section shown at the left. An excessive quantity of mounting medium was applied to the tissue section shown at the right side of the figure. (H&E, ×500) (AFIP Negative No. 67-2644)

Figure 446. *Proper Technique.* The tissue section depicted in this photomicrograph is a duplicate which was prepared from the same specimen of paraffin-embedded tissue depicted in Figure 438. The mounting medium was applied while the section was still moist with xylene and then it was immediately coverslipped. There are no entrapped air bubbles within the tissue section of this properly coverslipped specimen. (H&E, ×65) (AFIP Negative No. 72-3895)

Figure 447. *Proper Technique.* This photomicrograph is a higher magnification of a portion of the field depicted in Figure 446 which is provided for comparison with Figure 439. (H&E, ×195) (AFIP Negative No. 72-4058)

Figure 448. *Proper Technique.* The tissue section depicted in this photomicrograph was cut from the same block of paraffin-embedded tissue as the tissue section depicted in Figures 440 and 441. There is no glassine stippling of the tissue section due to the fact that the mounting medium was applied while the tissue section was still wet with xylene which precluded the entrapment of air within the interstitial spaces of the section. (H&E, ×100) (AFIP Negative No. 71-11703)

Figure 449. *Abopon Crystals.* Abopon mounting medium is used for mounting tissue sections which have been stained with crystal violet for the demonstration of amyloid. Commercial preparations of abopon are supersaturated solutions and may crystallize out of solution or solidify with changes in temperature. The clear crystalline material seen above the focal plane of this paraffin-embedded tissue section of a specimen of the cornea of a human eye is dried (crystallized) abopon mounting medium. *Note:* Abopon is no longer available commercially. The abopon artifact will continue to be a problem until laboratory supplies are exhausted. (Lieb's crystal violet stain, ×35) (AFIP Negative No. 73-4279)

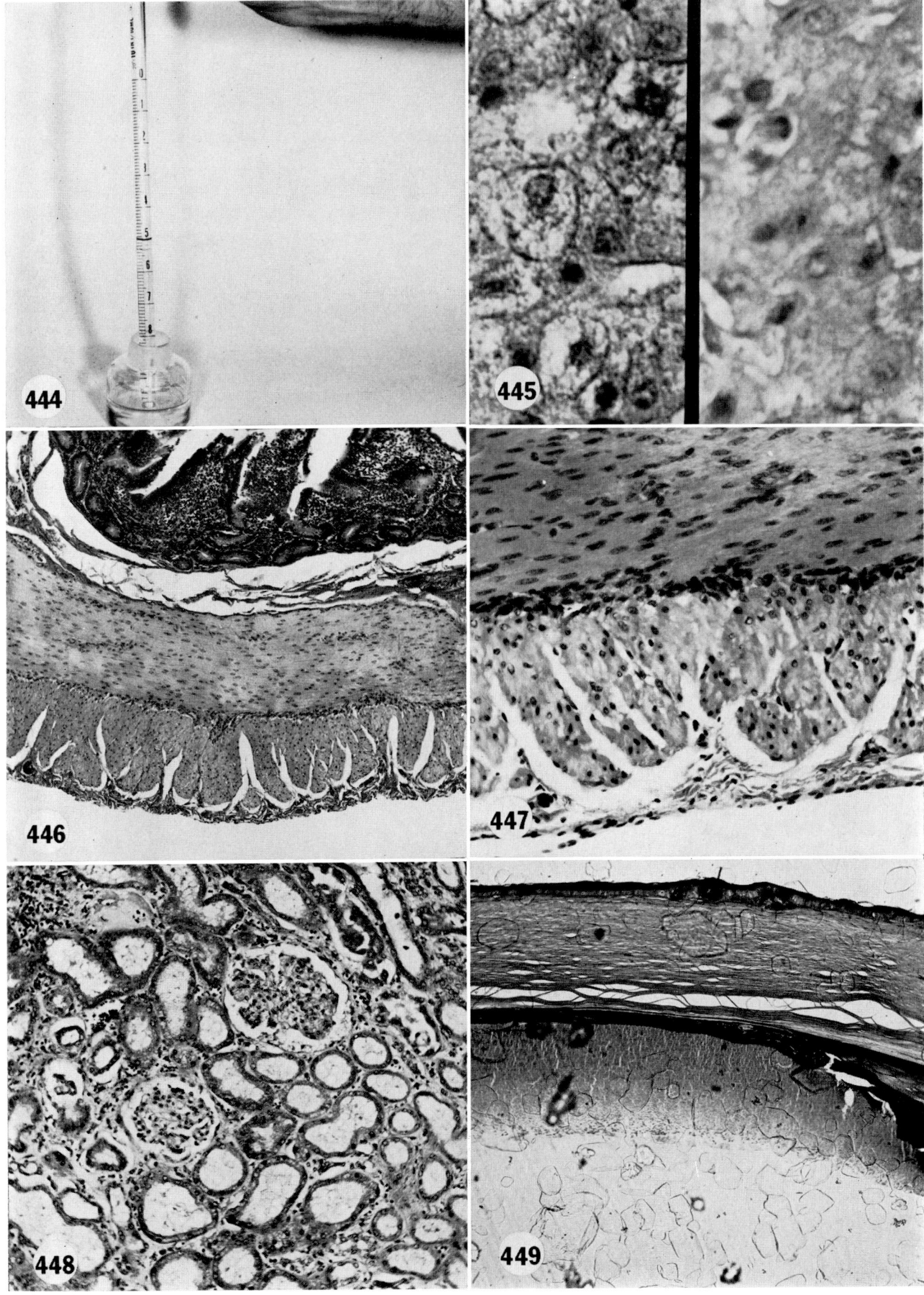

Figure 450. *Abopon Crystals*. This is the same tissue section and field of view as depicted in Figure 449 as observed by partial polariscopy. Note the bizarre forms of the anisotropic abopon crystals. If the mounting medium within the stock bottle is solidified or crystallized, add a few milliliters of distilled water to the container and warm gently over a waterbath while stirring the medium until the crystals dissolve. (Lieb's crystal violet stain, ×35) (AFIP Negative No. 73-4280)

Figure 451. *Abopon*. This tissue section of a specimen of human kidney tissue is mounted with an aqueous mounting medium (abopon). Under bright field microscopy no artifact is observed. Compare with Figure 452. (Lieb's crystal violet stain, ×115) (AFIP Negative No. 73-3268)

Figure 452. *Abopon*. This is the same field of view as depicted in Figure 451 as observed by partial polariscopy. In tissue sections which are mounted with an aqueous mounting medium such as abopon, nuclei are frequently observed to be anisotropic. (Lieb's crystal violet stain, partial polariscopy, ×115) (AFIP Negative No. 73-326)

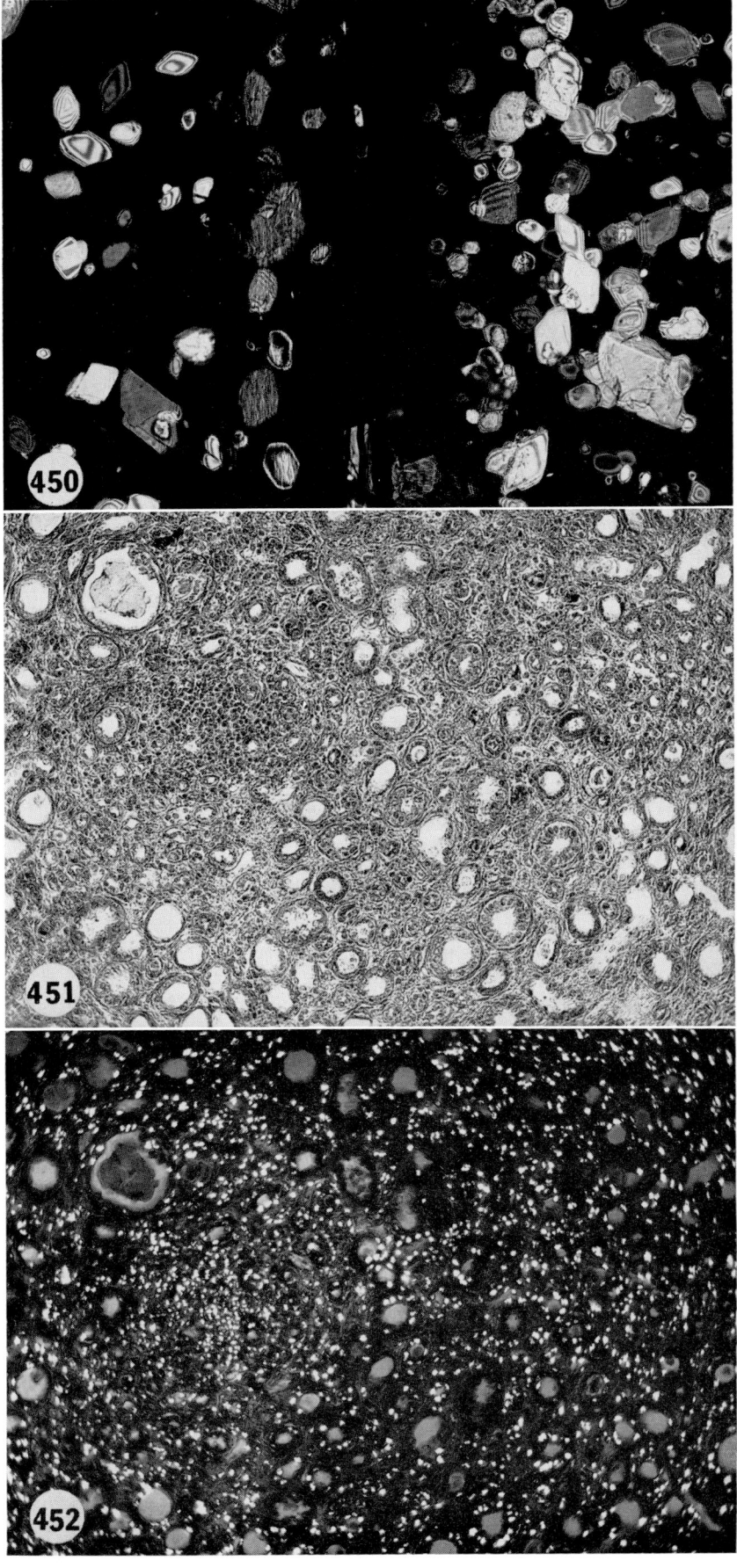

Index

A

Abopon mounting medium (*see also* Mounting, medium)
  anisotropism of nuclei in stained tissue sections, 174, 175
  crystals, 172-175
  use of, 172
Acetic acid, 34-36, 48, 54, 164
  glacial, 36
  role in formation of acid hematin pigments, 54
Acetone (*see* Fixatives)
Acetylphosphatides, effect of Zenker's fixation on, 44
Achromatic staining, 140, 141
Acid, 108, 126, 164 (*see also* specific acids)
  -alcohol, 108, 126, 164
  hematin pigment (*see* Hematin)
Acid-fast, 100, 101, 110, 111, 134, 135, 146, 147
  bacteria (*see* Bacteria)
  Fite-Faraco stain, 100, 101, 134, 135
  Kinyon's stain, 110, 111, 146, 147
Acidophilia, 36, 37, 104, 105, 112, 113, 140, 141, 144, 145
  of epithelial cells, 104, 105
  of gelatin contaminants on tissue sections, 112, 113
  of inclusion bodies, 144, 145
  produced by omission of bluing of hematoxylin stained tissue sections, 140, 141
  produced by Zenker's overfixation, 36, 37
Adenosine triphosphatase, 58
Adhesive (*see* Mounting, adhesive)
Adipose tissue (*see* Tissue)
Adrenal glands (*see* Tissue)
Aerosol spray (*see* Dichlorotetrafluoromethane)
Air, 86, 87, 100, 116-119, 164, 165, 168-172
  beneath tissue sections on microscope slides, 116, 117
  contamination of tissue sections by particulate matter in, 164, 165
  drying of mounted tissue sections by, 118, 119
  entrapped around tissue specimen during embedding, 86, 87, 100
  entrapped within tissue section during coverslipping, 168-172
  filters for, 164
  resembling crystalline material within tissue section, 168, 169
  resembling fungi within tissue section, 168, 169
  resembling silver halide crystals within tissue section, 170, 171
Albumin (*see* Mounting, adhesive)
Alcian blue staining of sites of calcification, 58 (*see also* Stains)
Alcohol, 14, 36, 48, 108, 122, 128, 150, 158, 164
  as a fixative (*see* Fixatives)
  dehydration of stained tissue sections with, 158
  effect on acid mucopolysaccharides, 122
  effect on colloidal iron stain, 122
  effect on tissue specimens, 48, 49
  isopropyl, 150
  use in aldehyde-fuchsin staining procedure, 128
  use in oil red O procedure, 150
Aldehyde-fuchsin stain, 56, 57, 122, 123, 128-131 (*see also* Stains)
  contamination of tissue sections with crystals of, 128-131
  demonstration of acid mucopolysaccharides, 128
  demonstration of aldehyde groups, 128
  demonstration of cystine, 128
  demonstration of elastic tissue, 128
  demonstration of Paget cells, 56, 57, 122, 123
  demonstration of sulfuric acid groups, 128
  effect of unbuffered acid formalin fixation on, 56, 57
  faulty technique, 128-131
  method, 128
Aldehydes, 42, 44, 108, 109, 128
  as oxidation product of polysaccharides, 108
  demonstration by aldehyde-fuchsin stain, 128
  demonstration by Gomori's methenamine silver stain, 108, 109
  demonstration by periodic acid-Schiff reaction, 108, 109
  effect of Zenker's fixation on, 42, 44
Alizarin blue S stain, 130, 131 (*see also* Stains)
  demonstration of copper, 130
  effect of Zenker's fixation on, 130, 131
  reaction with mercurial sublimate crystals, 130, 131
Alum (*see* Mordant)
Aluminum, 134, 148, 150, 151
  -ammonium sulfate as a mordant for hematoxylin, 134
  -chloride in the preparation of carmine stock solution, 148
  -potassium sulfate as a mordant for hematoxylin, 134
  -sulfate crystals on tissue sections stained with nuclear fast red, 150, 151
5-Aminoacridine hydrochloride, 122 (*see also* Fixatives)
Ammonia, 140, 152
  -silver solution, 152
  -water for bluing of tissue sections stained with hematoxylin, 140
Ammonium hydroxide, 42-44, 46, 47, 102, 103
  use in the hydration of the surface of embedded tissue specimens, 102, 103
  use in the identification of mercurial sublimate crystals, 42-44, 46, 47
  use in the identification of urea polymer crystals, 44, 46, 47
Amphoteric dye, 134 (*see also* Hematein)
Amyloid, 132, 133, 172-175
  anisotropism of, 132, 133

demonstration with Congo red stain, 132, 133
demonstration with crystal violet stain, 172-175
Angle, 92
  at which the specimen surface meets the microtome knife, 92
  of cutting clearance of the microtome knife, 92
Anhydrous fixatives, 48 (*see also* Fixatives)
Anionic tissue components, 108, 109, 134
Anisotropism (*see* Polariscopy)
Antemortem procedures, 3-11
Aorta (*see* Tissue)
Appendix, carcinoid tumor of, 152, 153 (*see also* Tissue)
Aqueous mounting medium, 170, 172-175 (*see also* Mounting, medium)
Argyrophilia, 42, 43, 52, 53, 124, 125
  of acid formalin hematin pigment, 52, 53
  of fungi, 42
  of mercurial sublimate crystals, 42, 43, 124, 125
  of protozoan parasites, 42
Artery (*see* Tissue)
Ashes, 114, 115, 164, 165 (*see also* Contamination)
Autolysis, 24-29, 48

B

Bacilli (*see* Bacteria)
Bacteria, 24, 25, 100, 101, 110, 111, 134, 146, 147, 152, 153
  acid-fast, 100, 101, 110, 111, 134, 146, 147
  acid-fast, lepra bacilli, 100, 101, 134
  acid-fast, pathogenic, 100, 101, 146, 147
  acid-fast, simulated by waterbath contaminants, 110, 111
  acid-fast, tubercle bacilli, 146, 147
  coccoid, 110, 111
  contamination of gelatin solutions by, 110, 111
  contamination of tissue flotation waterbath by, 110, 111
  contamination of tissue sections by, 100, 101
  displacement within tissue section, 100, 101
  pathogenic, 110
  rod-shaped, 110, 111
  saprophytic, 24, 25
  simulated by silver precipitates, 152, 153
  transfer from tissue section to mounting medium, 100
  transfer from tissue section to other tissue sections, 100
  transfer from tissue section to tissue flotation waterbath, 100
Baker's formalin-calcium (*see* Formalin)
Balsam mounting medium (*see* Mounting, medium)
Barium, 28, 29
  anisotropism, 28, 29
  contamination of fixatives by, 28
Basophilia, 18, 19, 24, 36, 37, 58, 59, 66, 67, 88, 89, 108, 109, 112, 113, 138-141, 156, 157
  effect of omission of bluing of hematoxylin stained tissue sections on, 140, 141
  effect of prolonged storage of stained tissue sections on, 156, 157
  effect of Zenker's fixation on, 36, 37
  fading of, 156
  of calcium deposits, 58, 59
  of gelatin contaminants on tissue sections, 112, 113
  of molds, 108, 109
  of plasticized paraffin in tissue sections, 88, 89
  of tissue components, 138, 139
  restoration of, 36, 37
Beading artifact in stained tissue sections, 154, 155
Berlin iron reaction (*see* Prussian blue reaction)
Best's carmine stain, 130, 131 (*see also* Stains)
Biebrich scarlet acid fuchsin solution (*see* Masson's trichrome)
Biopsy (*see* Tissue)
Bleaching of stained tissue sections, 160, 161, 166, 167
Blood smears, 148, 149, 154-157
  deposition of nuclear fast red crystals on, 148, 149
  linear structures in, 148, 149, 154-157
  stained with nuclear fast red, 148, 149
  stained with Wright's Giemsa stain, 154-157
  wrinkles in, 154-157
Bloody paraffin-embedded tissue specimens, 102, 103
Bluing of hematoxylin stained tissue sections, 140-143
Blunt microtome knife (*see* Knife)
Bodian's silver protein reaction, 130-133 (*see also* Stains)
Bone, 16, 17, 30, 31, 70, 71, 80-83, 92 (*see also* Tissue)
  cutting clearance angle of microtome knife for, 92
  decalcified, 80, 81
  fragments as contaminants of tissue specimens, 16, 17, 30, 31, 70, 71
  marrow, 80-83
  undecalcified, 16, 17
Bouin's fluid, 48, 49, 122, 123 (*see also* Fixatives)
  as a mordant (*see* Masson's trichrome)
  effect of residues in embedded tissue, 48, 49, *122, 123*
  effect on acid mucopolysaccharides, 122, 123
  effect on colloidal iron stain, 122, 123
  faulty formulation of, 48
  formulation of, 48
  role in the formation of acid hematin pigment in tissues, 48, 49
Brain (*see* Tissue)
Breakdown of hematoxylin dye solutions, 138, 139, 144, 145
Brown and Brenn stain (*see* Stains)
Brownish tint of stained tissue sections, 140, 141, 168, 169
Bubbles, 24, 25, 86, 87, 100, 116, 117, 168-173
  beneath tissue section on flotation waterbath, 116
  beneath tissue section on microscope slide, 116, 117
  of air in stained tissue sections, 168-173
  of air surrounding embedded tissue specimen, 86, 87, 100
  of gas in gross tissue specimens, 24, 25
Burn (*see* Dehydration)
Burned tissue, 82, 83, 86-89
  appearance, 82, 86, 87
  causes, 82, 83, 86-89
  demonstration in stained tissue sections, 82, 83, 86, 87
Burns due to mercurial sublimate crystals (*see* Mercurial sublimate)

C

Calcification, 58 (*see also* Pseudocalcification)
Calcium, 38, 58-61, 124, 125
  -acetate, 58, 59
  -carbonate, 58-61
  -chloride, 58, 60
  deposition simulated by mercurial sublimate crystals, 38, 124, 125
  removed by fixation in unbuffered acid formalin, 54, 56, 57
Carbon particles, 6, 7, 164, 165 (*see also* Contamination)
Carcinoid tumor, 152, 153
Cardiac (*see* Heart)
Carmine stain (*see* Best's carmine stain; Mayer's mucicarmine stain)

Carnoy's fluid, 122, 126, 127 (*see also* Fixatives)
　effect of delayed fixation on staining, 126, 127
　effect on acid mucopolysaccharides, 122
　effect on colloidal iron stain, 122
Casts, renal tubular, 52, 53
Cationic, 108, 109, 134
　dye-lake, 134
　tissue components, 108, 109
Celloidin embedded tissue (*see* Embedded tissue)
Cells, 98, 99, 150, 151 (*see also* specific cells)
　compression during microtomy, 98, 99
　simulated by dried malt diastase on tissue section, 150, 151
Cerebrum, 150, 151
Cetylpyridinium chloride, 122 (*see also* Fixatives)
Chemical dehydration (*see* Dehydration)
Chilling, 92, 102
　of specimen surface of microtome knife prior to microtomy, 102
　of specimen surface of tissue block prior to microtomy, 92, 102
Chloroform, 36, 64
Chromatin, lack of staining, 28, 29, 34-37 (*see also* Nuclear)
Cigar ashes, 114 (*see also* Contamination)
Cigarette ashes, 114, 115, 164, 165 (*see also* Contamination)
Clearing, 64, 65, 76-78, 82, 88, 118, 119, 158-161
　of tissue sections during staining procedures, 118, 119, 158-161
　of tissue specimens during processing procedures, 64, 65, 76-78, 82, 88
Cleavage of tissue sections, 20, 21, 92, 93, 100, 101
Clumping of cytoplasm, 26, 27
Coagulation of tissue protein, 4, 5, 48, 49, 88, 89
Coating of glass microscope slides prior to mounting of tissue sections, 110, 112, 114
Collagen (*see* Tissue)
Collapse of peripheral cells in tissue sections, 48, 49
Colloidal iron stain, 44, 58, 122, 123 (*see also* Stains)
　demonstration of acid mucopolysaccharides, 122, 123
　demonstration of sites of calcification, 58
　effect of Bouin's fixation on, 122, 123
　effect of Zenker's fixation on, 44

fixatives recommended for, 122, 123
reaction with mercurial sublimate crystals, 44
Colored pencil pigment in tissue sections, 72, 73
Compression of tissue sections, 88, 89, 92-101
Condensation of tissue components, 20, 21, 24-27, 32-35 (*see also* Dehydration)
Congo red stain (*see* Stains)
Connective tissue, 18, 19, 100, 101 (*see also* Tissue)
　freezing of, 18, 19
　tumor, 100, 101
Contamination, 4, 5, 14, 15, 24, 25, 28-31, 58-61, 66-73, 92, 100, 104, 105, 108-115, 126, 130-139, 144-155, 158, 159, 164, 165, 170-175
　during the clearing of stained tissue sections, 154, 158, 159
　during the collection of tissue specimens, 4, 5, 14, 15
　during the coverslipping of tissue sections, 164, 165, 170-175
　during the deceration of tissue sections, 134, 135
　during the fixation of tissue specimens, 24, 25, 28-31, 58-61, 144-147
　during the flotation of tissue sections on a waterbath, 100, 110-115
　during the macrosectioning of gross specimens, 70-73
　during the marking of gross specimens, 72, 73
　during the microtomy of tissue sections, 92, 93, 100, 101, 104, 105
　during the mounting of tissue sections, 100, 114, 115, 164, 165, 170, 172, 174
　during the paraffin infiltration of tissue specimens, 70, 71
　during the post fixation washing of tissue specimens, 66-69
　during the processing of tissue specimens, 70, 71, 126
　during the staining of tissue sections, 130-139, 146-155, 158, 159
Copper, 54, 55, 122-125, 130, 131, 152, 153
　demonstration with alizarin blue S stain, 130, 131
　demonstration with p-dimethylamino-benzylidene rhodanine stain, 122-125
　demonstration with rhodanine stain, 122-125
　demonstration with rubeanic acid technique, 54, 55, 152, 153
　preserved by fixation in neutral buffered formalin, 124, 125

removed by fixation in unbuffered acid formalin, 54, 55, 122, 123
removed by fixation in Zenker's fluid, 124, 125, 130, 131, 152, 153
Corrugations across tissue section, 96, 97
Counterstains (*see* specific stain)
Coverslipping, 114, 115, 154, 158, 159, *163-175*
　contamination of tissue sections during, 114, 115, 154, 158, 159, 164, 165, 170-175
　entrapment of air beneath mounting medium during, 168-172
　faulty technique, 166-172
　method, 166-170
　of microautoradiographs, 170, 171
　positioning of coverslip during, 166, 167
Coverslips, 164-167
　cleaning of, 164
　contamination of, 164, 165
　faulty positioning of, 166, 167
　glass, 164, 165
　improperly sealed, 166, 167
　size of, 166, 167
　substitutes for, 166, 167
Cracking of tissue sections, 8-11, 20, 21, 88, 89, 94-97, 118, 119
　due to antemortem procedures, 8-10
　due to embedding procedures, 88, 89
　due to flotation of tissue section, 118, 119
　due to infiltration procedures, 118
　due to microtomy procedures, 88, 94-97
　due to necropsy procedures, 20, 21
　due to processing procedures, 118
　due to staining procedures, 118, 119
Cracks (*see* Cracking)
Crenation of cells, 56, 57
Cresyl echt violet (*see* Stains)
Crevices surrounding embedded tissue specimens, 100
Crumbling of embedded tissue specimens, 30, 31
Cryostats, 92
Crystal violet (*see* Stains)
Crystallinity of paraffin, 76
Crystals, 4, 5, 14, 15, 18, 20, 24, 28, 29, 36-55, 58-61, 64-69, 72, 73, 76, 124, 125, 128-137, 146-153, 168-175
　Abopon, 172-175
　acid hematin, 48-55, 146, 147
　aldehyde-fuchsin, 128-131
　alum, 134-137
　aluminum sulfate, 150, 151
　barium, 28, 29
　calcium carbonate, 58-61
　Congo red dye, 132, 133

179

cresyl echt violet dye, 132, 133
crystal violet dye, 132, 133
hematein, 136, 137
ice, 18, 20, 24
mercurial sublimate, 36-47, 64-67, 124, 125, 130, 131, 152, 153
mercuric chloride (*see* mercurial sublimate)
nuclear fast red dye, 148, 149
oil red O, 150, 151
paraffin, 76
resinous mounting medium, 170, 171
silver halide, 170
silver nitrate, 72, 73
simulated by entrapped air within stained tissue sections, 168, 169
starch, 4, 5, 14, 15, 68, 69
talcum powder, 4, 5, 14, 15, 68, 69
thionine dye, 152, 153
urea polymers, 44-47
Curved tissue sections, 88, 96
Cystine, 128
Cytoplasm, 142-145

D

Dandruff, 104, 105, 114
Debris, tissue, 70, 71, 104, 105, 112-115
 during flotation of tissue sections, 112-115
 during macrosectioning of tissue specimens, 70, 71
 during microtomy, 104, 105
 during paraffin infiltration, 70, 71
 during tissue processing, 70, 71
Decalcification of bone, 80, 82
Deceration of tissue sections, 88, 89, 118, 126-130, 134, 135
 adverse effects of residues in solvent used for, 126, 127
 during the staining procedure for paraffin embedded tissue sections, 118, *126*
 inadequate, 88, 89, 126-130
 method for tissue sections to be stained by Fite-Faraco stain, 134
Degalantha stain for urates (*see* Stains)
Degeneration, 26, 27, 120, 123
 hepatolenticular, 122, 123
 of tissue components, 26, 27
Degradation of hematoxylin dye solution, 138, 139
Dehydration, 6-9, 18-21, 24, 25, 38, 39, 48, 49, 74-78, 82, 83, 86-89, 92, 93, 100-102, 118, 158
 chemical, 6, 7, 48, 49
 due to exposure of tissue specimens to air during processing, 74, 75
 due to freezing, 18-21, 24, 25, 82, 92, 93
 due to Zenker's overfixation, 38, 39

during the embedding of tissue specimens, 86-89, 102
during the microtomy of tissue sections, 92, 93
during the processing of tissue specimens, 74-78, 102
during the staining of tissue sections, 118
excessive, 74-77, 82, 83, 102
inadequate, during tissue processing, 76-78
of tissue sections after staining, 158
thermal, 4-7, 82, 83, 86-89, 102
Delayed fixation (*see* Fixation)
Denaturization of tissue protein, 48, 64, 65
Deoxyribonuclease, 58
Deoxyribonucleic acid, 34
Derangement of tissue specimen, 24
Destaining of tissue sections, 126, 156, 157, 166
Development of silver stains, 152
Diastase, 42-45, 48, 49, 150, 151 (*see also* Digestion)
 contamination of tissue section with, 150, 151
 digestion of glycogen with, 42-45, 48, 49, 150, 151
Dichlorotetrafluoromethane, 72, 100, 101
 artifacts produced by use of, 100, 101
 use of, 92, 100, 101
Dichromate (*see* Mordant and Potassium)
Differentiation of hematoxylin stained tissue sections, 142-145
Diffusion of stains, 48, 49, 122, 123, 130, 131, 166, 167
 in substitutes for glass coverslips, 166, 167
 in tissue sections, 48, 49, 122, 123, 130, 131
Digestion, 24, 25, 42-45, 48, 49, 150, 151
 enzymatic of glycogen, 42-45, 48, 49, 150, 151
 enzymatic of tissue due to inadequate fixation, 24, 25
 with diastase, 42-45, 48, 49, 150, 151
Dimethylaminobenzylidene-p rhodanine stain (*see* Rhodanine)
Disorientation of tissue components, 88, 89, 98, 99
Displacement, 20, 21, 36, 37, 80, 81, 100, 101
 nuclear, 20, 21, 36, 37
 of bacteria in tissue sections, 100, 101
 of bone marrow in tissue sections, 80, 81

of pigment in tissue sections, 100
Dissociation of tissue components, 24-27, 36, 37
Distortion, 16, 17, 48, 49, 78-81, 88, 94-99
 of leukocytes, 48, 49
 of tissue sections, 16, 17, 78-81, 94-99
 pin cushion, due to excessive hardness of tissue embedding medium, 88
Double staining, 114-117, 154-157
 of blood smears, 154-157
 of tissue sections, 114-117
Dry, 102, 103, 160, 161
 paraffin embedded tissue specimens, 102, 103
 tissue sections due to overexposure to xylene during clearing, 160, 161
Drying, 118, 119, 166-171
 of stained tissue sections after clearing in xylene, 168, 169
 of stained tissue sections due to faulty coverslipping, 166, 167, 170, 171
 of tissue sections after mounting from tissue flotation waterbath, 118, 119
Dull microtome knife (*see* Knife)
Dust particles, contamination of tissue sections, 164
Dye-lake, 134

E

Elastic fibers, 4, 5, 128
Elongation of nuclear material, 14, 15
Embedded tissue, 4-9, 14-21, 24-31, 33-40, 42-55, 58-61, 64, 65, 68-83, 86-89, 92-105, 110-117, 122-153, 156-161, 164-173
 celloidin, 60, 61, 82, 83
 effect of crevices around tissue specimen in, 100, 101
 effect of delay in preparation of stained tissue sections from, 48, 49, 122, 123, 158, 159
 effect of entrapped air around tissue specimen in, 86, 87, 100
 effect of excessive hardness of embedding medium of, 88, 89
 effect of excessive heat of embedding medium during preparation of, 86-89
 effect of residues of clearing fluids in, 76, 77, 88
 effect of residues of picric acid in, 48, 49, 122, 123
 effect of residues of processing fluids in, 76, 77, 88
 hydration prior to microtomy of, 102, 103

microtomy of, 86, 92 (*see also* Microtomy)
paraffin, 4-9, 14-21, 24-31, 34-40, 42-55, 58, 59, 64, 65, 68-83, 86-89, 92-105, 110-117, 122-153, 156-161, 164-173
plasticized paraffin, 88, 89, 128, 129
rough cutting of, 70, 79, 80, 102
sealing of surface for storage of, 158, 159
soft areas in, 80
spongy areas in, 80
staining of tissue sections after prolonged storage of, 158, 159
storage of, 158, 159
vibration during microtomy of, 74, 75, 86, 88, 89
Embedding of tissue specimens, 30, *85-89*, 102, 103
excessive dehydration of areas of hemorrhage during, 102, 103
of multiple tissues, 86-89
orientation of tissue specimens during, 86
techniques, 86, 87
Enzymes, preservation with formalin-calcium chloride, 58 (*see also* specific enzyme)
Eosin, 134, 135, 140-145 (*see also* Stains)
agitation of slides during staining with, 134, 144
as a counterstain, 134, 135, 142-145
demonstration of acidophilic inclusion bodies with, 144, 145
ethyl, 134
faulty staining with, 134, 135, 144, 145
overstaining with, 140, 141, 144, 145
precipitation of flakes of unfiltered dye on tissue sections, 134, 135
solubilities in alcohol, 134
-Y, 134
Eosinophilia, 36, 37, 104, 105
Epididymis (*see* Tissue)
Epithelial cells, 104, 105, 114, 115
Erythrocytes, 28, 29, 36, 38, 39, 48-55, 82, 83
anisotropism of, 36, 38, 39
autolysis of, 28, 29
crystallization of, 36, 38, 39
effect of exposure to excessively hot paraffin during infiltration of, 82, 83
effect of Zenker's fixation on, 36, 38, 39
lysis by alcohol fixation of, 48, 49
role in formation of acid formalin hematin pigment, 50-55
Esterases, preservation of, 58
Eye, 30, 31, 78, 79, 144, 145 (*see also* Tissue)

contamination during fixation of, 30, 31, 144, 145
inadequate paraffin infiltration of, 78, 79

F

Fading of stained tissue sections, 122, 123, 140-143, 156, 157, 160, 161, 166, 167
due to exposure to sunlight, 160, 161
due to failure to blue hematoxylin stained tissue sections, 140, 141
due to faulty coverslipping, 166, 167
due to prolonged storage of stained tissue sections, 156, 157
stained with Mayer's hematoxylin, 142, 143
stained with the rhodanine method for copper, 122, 123
Failure, 44, 54-57, 88, 89, 118, 122-125, 138-141
of aldehyde-fuchsin staining, 56, 57, 122, 123
of colloidal iron staining, 44, 122, 123
of hematoxylin staining, 138-141
of the rhodanine stain for copper, 122-125
of the rubeanic acid stain for copper, 54, 55
of tissue ribbons to form during microtomy, 88, 89
of tissue sections to adhere to glass microscope slides, 118
of tissue sections to remain on slides during staining, 118, 119
of tissue sections to stain, 88, 89
Fat cells, 54, 55
Feulgen reaction, 44
Fibroma, 100, 101
Film stripping technique for microautoradiography, 170, 171
Filters, 66, 67, 112, 164
for air, 164
for water, 66, 67, 112
Fissures in tissue sections, causes of, 92, 93, 100, 101, 160, 161
Fite-Faraco stain, 134, 135 (*see also* Stains)
Fixation, *22-61*, 64, 65, 78, 122-127, 130, 131, 144, 145, 156, 157
adequate, 28, 29, 54, 56, 57, 64
comparative effects on nuclear morphology of, 32-37
contamination of tissue specimens during, 24, 25, 28-31, 58-61, 144, 145
delayed, 24, 25, 56, 57, 124-127
duration of, 26-29, 36, 37, 48, 56, 57, 60, 122
effect on results of staining procedures due to, 44, 54-57, *122-127*, 130, 131, 156, 157
excessive, 36-39, 54-57, 122, 123
faulty, 24-29, 36-39, 44, 45, 58-61, 64, 65
freezing of tissue specimens during, 24
inadequate, 24-29, 36, 37, 64, 65, 78
procedures for, 22-61
specimen size for, 26-29, 48, 60
with neutral buffered versus unbuffered formalin, 54-57, 122, 123
Fixative, 26-31, 44, 48, 54-57, 60, 122-125, 130, 131, 144
container for, 28, 30, 31, 144
recommendations for acid mucopolysaccharides, 44, 122
recommendations for aldehyde-fuchsin stain, 56, 57, 122, 123
recommendations for colloidal iron stain, 44, 122, 123
recommendations for copper in tissue specimens, 54, 55, 122-125, 130, 131
volume, 26-29, 48, 60
Fixatives, 26-50, 52, 54, 56-61, 64-79, 88, 89, 112, 113, 122-141, 146-149, 152, 153, 156-161, 170-173
acetone and acetic acid, 54
acetone and formic acid, 54
alcohol, absolute ethyl, 32, 33, *48, 49*, 122
alcohol and acetic acid, 54
alcohol and formic acid, 54
aminoacridine, 5-hydrochloride, 122
Bouin's fluid, 32-35, 48, 49, 56, 57, 122, 123
Carnoy's fluid, 36, 37, 122, 126, 127
cetylpyridinium chloride, 122
formaldehyde, methanol-free, 34, 35
formalin, acid (*see* formalin, unbuffered)
formalin, alcoholic, 48, 54
formalin and calcium acetate, 58, 59
formalin and calcium chloride, 58-61
formalin, neutral buffered, 26-35, 44-49, 54, 56, 57, 64-79, 88, 89, 112, 113, 122-141, 146-149, 152, 153, 156-161, 170-173
formalin, unbuffered, 32, 33, 50, 52, 54, 56, 57, 122-125
formol-calcium, 32, 33
formol-saline, 32-35
glutaraldehyde, 34, 35
paraformaldehyde, 34, 35
Zenker's acetic fluid, 126, 127
Zenker's fluid, 36-48, 64-66, 124, 125, 130, 131, 152, 153
Zenker's formol fluid, 126, 127
Flattening of tissue sections, 110, 111, 114, 116, 118

Flotation of tissue sections, 70, 78, 100, 110-119
　air bubbles beneath tissue sections during, 116, 117
　air drying of mounted tissue sections after, 118, 119
　contamination of tissue sections during, 70, 112-115
　contamination of water in waterbath during, 100, 110-115
　effect of excessively hot water in waterbath during, 78, 118
　effect of inadequate temperature of waterbath during, 118
　use of distilled water for, 112, 114
　use of filtered water for, 112
　use of tap water for, 112
　waterbath used for, 110, 111, 118, 119
　wrinkling of tissue sections during, 116-118
Fluorinated hydrocarbons, 92, 93, 100, 101
　artifacts produced by use of, 92, 93, 100, 101
　use of, 92, 100, 101
Formaldehyde, 32-35, 48 (*see also* Fixatives; Hematin)
Formalin, 44-52, 54, 56-61, 64-67, 122, 123, 156-159 (*see also* Fixatives)
　alcoholic, 48, 54
　denaturization of tissue components by, 64, 65
　effect on staining reactions of prolonged storage of tissue in, 156-159
　effect on tissue glycogen, 48, 49
　mercurial sublimate crystals in tissue fixed in, 64-67
　neutral buffered versus unbuffered acid formalin fixation, 54, 56, 57, 122, 123
　pigment (*see* Hematin)
　role in urea polymer formation in Zenker's fixed tissue, 44-47
　unbuffered, effect on aldehyde-fuchsin staining reaction, 56, 57, 122, 123
　unbuffered, effect on calcium, 54, 56, 57
　unbuffered, effect on copper, 54, 55, 122, 123
　unbuffered, effect on heme, 50
　unbuffered, effect on hemoglobin, 50, 54
　unbuffered, effect on iron, 54
　unbuffered, effect on minerals, 56
　unbuffered, effect on pigments, 56
　unbuffered, role in formation of hematin pigments, 50, 52, 54
　with calcium acetate, 58
　with calcium chloride, 58-60

Formic acid, role in formation of hematin pigments, 50, 54
Formol, calcium or saline (*see* Fixatives)
Fracture, 80, 81, 92, 93
　lines in tissue sections, 92, 93
　of bone trabeculae, 80, 81
Fragmentation of tissue sections due to dull microtome knife, 94, 95
Fragments of tissue as contaminants of tissue sections, 112, 113
Freezing, 48 (*see also* Dehydration)
　-drying technique, 48
　-substitution technique, 48
Frozen tissue sections, 26, 100, 150, 151
Fungi, 42, 108, 109, 146-149, 152, 153, 168, 169
　pathogenic, 108
　simulated by acid formalin hematin pigment, 146, 147
　simulated by entrapped air within stained tissue sections, 168, 169
　simulated by mercurial sublimate crystals, 42
　simulated by mold contaminants of glass microscope slides, 108, 109
　simulated by silver granules, 152, 153
　simulated by undissolved fused carmine dye, 148, 149
　staining reactions for, 108, 109, 146, 147, 168

G

Gastrointestinal tract (*see* Tissue)
Gauze, surgical, in tissue specimens, 8, 9
Gelatin, 110-113 (*see also* Mounting, adhesive; Mounting, medium)
　contamination by bacteria, 110, 111
　contamination of tissue sections by, 112, 113
Giemsa stain, 44, 68 (*see also* Stains; Walbach's; Wright's)
　reaction with mercurial sublimate crystals, 44
　reaction with starch particles, 68
　reaction with talcum powder particles, 68
Glandular tissue (*see* Tissue)
Glass coverslips and microscope slides, 104, 105, 108-111, 114, 115, 164, 165
　cleaning of, 108, 164
　contamination of, 104, 105, 108-111, 114, 115, 164, 165
　glazed appearance of, 108
Glassine effect due to entrapment of air in tissue section, 168-173
Glia, demonstration by phosphotungstic acid hematoxylin, 144, 145

Glucosaminidase, N-acetyl-beta, preservation, 58
Glucuronidase, beta, preservation, 58
Glutaraldehyde (*see* Fixatives)
Glycerin(e) (*see* Mounting, medium)
Glycogen, 42-45, 48, 49, 130, 131, 150, 151
　cellular distribution of, 48
　demonstration within tissue sections, 48, 49, 130, 131
　diastase digestion of, 42-45, 48, 49, 150, 151
　effects of fixation on, 48, 49
　solubility in trichloroacetic acid, 48
　solubility in water, 48
Gomori's stains (*see* Aldehyde-fuchsin stain; Prussian blue reaction; Methenamine silver nitrate stain)
Gridley's stains (*see* Stains)
Grocott's stain (*see* Methenamine silver nitrate stain; Stains)
Gross tissue specimens, 14, 30, 31, 66-69, 71-73 (*see also* Contamination; Macrosectioning)
　marking of, 71-73
　washing of, 14, 30, 31, 66-69
Gum damar, 172

H

Hair, 14-17, 30, 31, 86, 92 (*see also* Tissue)
　attached to skin, orientation for microtomy, 86
　contamination of edge of microtome knife by, 92
　contamination of tissue specimens with, 14-17, 30, 31
Hale's colloidal iron stain (*see* Colloidal iron stain)
Halo surrounding embedded tissue specimens, 76
Harris' hematoxylin, 138, 139, 144, 145 (*see also* Stains)
　differentiation of, 144, 145
　effect of overstaining with eosin counterstain, 144, 145
　optimal staining with, 138, 139
Haze over tissue section, 172, 173
Heart, effect of inadequate paraffin infiltration, 78, 79 (*see also* Tissue)
Heat (*see* Dehydration)
Helminth, simulated by wrinkles in blood smears, 154-157
Hematein, 134, 136-139
　as an amphoteric dye, 134
　as a cationic dye-lake, 134
　crystals in tissue sections, 136, 137
　oxidation products of, 134, 136, 138, 139
Hematin pigment, 48-55, 146, 147
　anisotropism of, 48-55, 146, 147
　argyrophilia of, 52, 53, 146, 147

distribution within tissue sections, 48-55, 146, 147
formation in acetic acid-acetone fixed tissue, 54
formation in acetic acid-alcohol fixed tissue, 54
formation in Bouin's fixed tissue, 48, 49
formation in formic acid-acetone fixed tissue, 54
formation in formic acid-alcohol fixed tissue, 54
formation in unbuffered, acid formalin fixed tissue, 50, 52
isotropism when stained with methenamine silver nitrate, 146, 147
microscopic characteristics of, 54
preformed in neutral buffered formalin fixed tissues, 48, 49, 52
removal from tissue sections, 48, *52*
simulation of pathogenic organisms in tissue sections stained with silver, 146, 147
Hematoxylin, 130, 131, 134-143 (*see also* Harris' hematoxylin; Hematoxylin and eosin; Mayer's hematoxylin; Phosphotungstic acid hematoxylin; Stains)
bluing of tissue section following staining with, 140-143
breakdown of dye solution, 138, 139
counterstained with Best's carmine stain, 130, 131
counterstained with the periodic acid-Schiff reaction, 136, 137
diminished staining quality of, 138, 139
dye, 134, 135
faulty formulation of, 138
hematein content of, 134, 136, 138
mordants for, 134, 138
oxidation products of, 134, 136
surface oxidant artifacts due to, 138, 139
Hematoxylin and eosin, 24, 25, 40-45, 56, 57, 66-69, 82, 83, 86-89, 108, 109, 112, 113, 126-130, 144, 145 (*see also* Stains)
differentiation of, 112
effect of delayed fixation on staining with, 24, 25, 56, 57, 124-127
effect of inadequate deceration on staining with, 88, 89, 126-130
staining of anionic tissue components with, 108, 109
staining of burned tissue with, 82, 83, 86, 87
staining of cationic tissue components with, 108, 109
staining of fungi by, 108, 109
staining of gelatin contaminants of tissue sections by, 112, 113

staining of mercurial sublimate crystals by, 40-45
staining of slime on tissue sections by, 66, 67
staining of starch particles on tissue sections by, 68, 69
staining of talcum powder particles on tissue sections by, 68, 69
uneven staining with the eosin counterstain, 144, 145
Heme, role in formation of acid formalin hematin pigments, 50
Hemoglobin, role in the formation of acid hematin pigments, 48, 50, 54
Hemorrhage, 50-53, 102, 103
acid formalin hematin pigment formed in sites of, 50-53
excessive drying of sites within tissue specimens of, 102
hydration of sites within embedded tissue, 102, 103
shattering of sites within tissue sections during microtomy, 102, 103
Hemosiderin, 30, 48, 68
Hepatitis, acute toxic, 24
Hepatocytes, separation of, 24, 26, 36, 37
Hepatolenticular degeneration, 54, 55, 122, 123, 152, 153
Histoclad mounting medium, 172
Holes in tissue sections, causes for, 16, 17, 80, 81, 102, 103
Honing of microtome knives (*see* Knife, microtome)
Hyaluronic acid, effect of Zenker's fixation, 44
Hydration, 102, 103, 118
of the face of embedded tissue prior to microtomy, 102, 103
of tissue sections during the staining procedure, 118
Hydrolysis of polysaccharides by acid, 108, 109
Hydrophilia of components of embedded tissue, 76, 102, 103
Hydrophobia of components of embedded tissue, 102, 103
Hyperacidophilia of tissue sections, 4, 5, 36, 37

I

Ice, 18, 20, 24, 102
crystals in tissue specimens, 18, 20, 24
use in chilling of specimen surface of embedded tissue block, 102
use in chilling of specimen surface of microtome knife, 102
Inclusion bodies in tissue sections, 144, 145

India ink as a contaminant in tissue sections, 72-75
Infiltration of tissue specimens with paraffin, 64, 70, 76-83, 118
adverse effect of excessive temperature of paraffin during, 82, 83
adverse effect of inadequate dehydration of tissue prior to, 76-78, 118
contamination of tissue specimen during, 70, 71, 76, 77
faulty technique during, 78-81, 118
Intestine, inadequate paraffin infiltration, 78, 79 (*see also* Tissue)
Iodine, 36, *38,* 39, 42-44
alcoholic, use with Zenker's fixed tissue, 36, *38,* 39, 42, 43
Gram's, use for removal of mercurial sublimate burns in tissue sections, 44
Lugol's, use for removal of mercurial sublimate burns in tissue sections, 44
Iron, 30, 31, 54, 66-69, 112, 113, 144, 145, 148, 149
contamination of fixatives with, 30, 31, 144, 145
contamination of tissue flotation waterbath with, 112, 113
contamination of tissue sections with, 112, 113, 144, 145
contamination of tissue specimens during post-fixation washing with, 112, 113
contamination of water with, 66-69, 112
demonstration in blood smears of, 148, 149
demonstration in tissue sections of, 30, 31, 68, 69, 144, 145
demonstration in water of, 66, 67
pathologic deposition removed by unbuffered acid formalin fixation, 54
simulation of hemosiderin by, 68, 69, 144, 145
Isotope, 170
Isotropism, 66, 146, 147

K

Kernechtrot stain (*see* Nuclear fast red stain)
Kidney, 78, 79, 132, 133 (*see also* Tissue)
amyloid in the, 132, 133
inadequate paraffin infiltration of the, 78, 79
Kinyon's acid-fast stain, 110, 111, 146, 147 (*see also* Stains)
demonstration of acid-fast bacteria with, 110, 111, 146, 147
demonstration of contaminants which

simulate acid-fast bacteria with, 110, 111
use of methylene blue counterstain with, 146, 147
Knife, microtome, 16, 17, 30, 74, 78, 86, 88, 92-102, 104, 116
artifacts in tissue sections due to a blunt edge of the, 94-101
artifacts in tissue sections due to a dull edge of the, 94-101
artifacts in tissue sections due to a sharp edge of the, 92, 93, 102
bending of the, 100
bevel rounding of the, 96
chilling of the specimen surface of the, 102
contamination of the cutting edge of the, 92
contamination of the specimen surface of the, 104
corrugations across the tissue section produced by the, 96, 97
curving of the edge of the, 96
cutting clearance angle of the, 92
damage to the edge of the, 16, 30, 88, 96
feather edge of the, 100
honing of the, 96
lines in the tissue section produced by the, 16, 17
sharpening technique for, 94-96
stropping technique for, 96
test for sharpness of, 96
vibration of during microtomy, 16, 74, 86, 92, 100
Knife, thermal, 4-7

L

Leaching of the stain from tissue sections, 166, 167
Leder's stain, effect of inadequate deceration of tissue section, 128, 129 (*see also* Stains)
Lendrum's stain (*see* Stains)
Lens, hand, use in embedding of tissue specimens, 30
Leprosy, 100, 101, 134
Leptospirosis, 24, 26
Leukocytes, effect of alcohol fixation, 48
Lieb's crystal violet stain, demonstration of amyloid, 172-175 (*see also* Stains)
Light green stain, 146, 147, 156-159 (*see also* Stains)
as a counterstain, 146, 147
staining of tissue sections prepared after prolonged storage of tissue in neutral buffered formalin, 156-159

Lint fibers, 92, 164, 165
contamination of the edge of the microtome knife with, 92
contamination of tissue sections with, 164, 165
Lipid, 100, 101, 126
demonstration in tissue sections of, 100
simulated by residue of fluorinated hydrocarbons, 100, 101
use with solvent in deceration of tissue sections, 126
Lithium carbonate, 140
Liver (*see* Tissue)
Loss of tissue sections during the staining procedure, 118, 119
Luna-Parker stain (*see* Stains)
Luna's reaction for mercuric chloride crystals, 42-44, 46, 47
Lung (*see* Tissue)
Lymph node (*see* Tissue)
Lysol, 6, 7

M

Macrosawing of bone, 70, 71
Macrosectioning of tissue specimens, 68-71
Mallory's method for iron (*see* Prussian blue reaction)
Mallory's thionine stain (*see* Stains, thionine)
Marble chips (*see* Calcium, carbonate)
Marking of gross tissue specimens, 71-73
Masson's trichrome stain, 154, 155, 168, 169 (*see also* Stains)
chromatic effect of entrapped air within tissue sections stained by, 168, 169
technique for, 154, 155
Mast cells, 158, 159
Mastocytoma, 158, 159
Mayer's hematoxylin stain, 142, 143, 156-159 (*see also* Stains)
Mayer's mucicarmine stain, 148, 149, 168, 169 (*see also* Stains)
Meninges (*see* Tissue)
Mercurial sublimate, 36-47, 64-67, 124, 125, 130, 131, 152, 153
burns in tissue caused by, 42-45
crystals, anisotropism of, 38-41, 44-47, 64, 65
crystals, argyrophilia of, 42, 43, 124, 125
crystals, forms of within tissue sections, 38-47, 64, 65, 130, 131
crystals in formalin fixed tissue, 64-67
crystals, reaction with alizarin blue S stain, 130, 131
crystals, reaction with ammonium hydroxide, 42-44, 46, 47

crystals, reaction with rhodanine stain, 124, 125
crystals, reaction with rubeanic acid stain, 152, 153
crystals, reaction with von Kossa stain, 124, 125
crystals, removal from tissue specimens/sections, 36-39, 42-45
crystals, simulation of calcium deposits within tissue sections by, 38, 124, 125
crystals, simulation of fungi within tissue sections by, 42
crystals, simulation of protozoan parasites within tissue sections by, 42
crystals, staining characteristics of, 40-44, 124, 125, 152, 153
crystals, unstained within tissue sections, 40, 41
fixatives (*see* Zenker's fluid)
hardening of tissue by, 36
Mercuric chloride (*see* Mercurial sublimate)
Mesentery (*see* Tissue)
Metachromatic dye, 132
Metal, 30, 31, 144, 145
contamination of fixatives by, 30, 31, 144, 145
in unfiltered water, 30
Methenamine silver nitrate stain, 42, 43, 108, 109, 146, 147 (*see also* Stains)
demonstration of argyrophilic tissue components with, 146
light green counterstain with, 146, 147
reduced by acid formalin hematin pigment, 146, 147
reduced by aldehydes, 108, 109
reduced by fungi, 108, 109, 146, 147
reduced by hydrolyzed polysaccharides, 108
reduced by mercurial sublimate crystals, 42, 43
reduced by non-aldehyde reducing substances, 108, 109
reduced by *Pneumocystis carinii*, 146, 147
stock solution of, 146
Methylene blue stain (*see* Kinyon's acid-fast stain; Stains)
Microautoradiographs, 170, 171
Microscope, dissecting, 30
Microscopy, 108, 112, 130, 132, 136, 138, 146, 148, 150, 152, 154, 164, 165, 168-173
lowering of substage condenser to detect beading artifact, 154
lowering of substage condenser to

detect entrapped air in tissue section, 168-171
partial closure of substage condenser to detect beading artifact, 154
use in the detection of contaminants above the focal plane of the tissue section, 108, 112, 130, 132, 136, 138, 146, 148, 150, 152, 154, 164, 165, 170-173
use in the detection of contaminants below the focal plane of the tissue section, 108, 112
use in the detection of contaminants in the focal plane of the tissue section, 108, 112, 130, 132, 136

Microtome, 86, 92, 100 (*see also* Knife)
clinical, 92
effect of loose screw on knife holder of, 86, 92, 100
effect of loose screw on specimen chuck of, 86, 92, 100

Microtomy, 8-11, 20, 21, 88, 89, *91-105* (*see also* Knife)
alternate thick and thin zones in tissue sections caused by, 98-101
cellular alterations caused by, 98, 99
chilling of specimen surface of tissue block prior to, 92, 100, 101
cleavage of tissue sections during, 92
compression of tissue sections during, 92-101
contamination of knife edge during, 92, 93
contamination of knife specimen surface during, 104, 105
cracks in tissue sections caused by, 8-11, 20, 21, 88, 89, 94-97
curved tissue sections during, 88, 89
cutting clearance angle of knife for, 92
disorientation of soft tissue components in tissue sections caused by, 98, 99
displacement of bacteria in tissue section during, 100, 101
displacement of pigment in tissue section during, 100
distorted tissue sections caused by, 94-99
effect of loose microtome knife during, 74, 86, 92, 100
effect of loose specimen chuck during, 74, 86, 92, 100
fissures in tissue sections caused by, 92, 93
orientation of tissue block for, 86, 92
pin point distortion of tissue sections caused by, 88, 89
ribbons fail to form during, 88, 89, *98*

rolled up tissue sections during, 88, 89
shattered tissue sections caused by, 94-99
shrinkage of tissue sections caused by, 98-101
tissue sections adhere to the block on upstroke during, 98
venetian blind effect in tissue sections caused by, 92, 93

Mildew contamination of glass microscope slides, 108, 109
Minerals, 56, 66, 68, 112
in tissue specimens, effect of fixation, 56
in water used to wash tissue specimens, 66, 68, 112
Moisture content of tissue specimens, 18
Mold contamination of glass microscope slides, 108, 109
Mordants, 60, 134-139, 154
alum, 134-139
anisotropism of, 136, 137
as a pigment in tissue sections, 134, 135
contamination of tissue sections with, 134, 135
crystals of, 134-137
hematoxylin surface oxidant artifacts caused by, 138, 139
recrystalization of, 134, 135
use with hematoxylin, 134, 135
Bouin's fluid for Masson's trichrome stain, 154
dichromate-calcium for formalin-calcium fixed tissue specimens, 60
Moth-eaten effect observed in tissue sections, 76, 77, 80, 81, 102, 103
Mounting adhesive, 110-114, 118, 119
albumin, 114
gelatin, 110-114
tissue section fails to adhere to glass microscope slide due to faulty use of, 118, 119
Mounting medium, 100, 101, 118, 154, 155, 164-175
Abopon, 172-175
application to tissue sections of, 172, 173
aqueous, 170
balsam, 172
contamination of, 100, 101, 164, 165, 170, 172, 174
crystallization of, 170-175
effect of clearing of stained tissue sections on, 118
effect of deceration of tissue sections on, 118
effect of dehydration of tissue sections during staining on, 118

effect of drying of tissue sections after clearing in xylene on, 168-171
effect of entrapped air in tissue section on, 168-171
effect of faulty coverslipping on, 166-172
effect of glycerin residues in tissue section on, 154, 155
effect of hydration of tissue section during staining on, 118
effect of improper positioning of coverslip on, 166, 167
gum damar, 172
glycerin(e), 100, 154, 155
Histoclad, 172
oil, 170
Paragon, 170
Permount, 170, 172
resins, 170, 172
viscosity of, 172, 173
Mounting of tissue sections on glass microscope slides, 70, 76, *107-119*
Mucicarmine stain, 148, 149
Mucin, 88, 89, 128, 129, 148, 149
Mayer's mucicarmine stain for, 148, 149
of epithelial origin, 148
simulation by residues of plasticized paraffin in tissue sections, 88, 89, 128, 129
Mucocytes, 88, 89, 128, 129
Mucoid cells simulated by dried malt diastase on tissue sections, 150, 151
Mucoid material, 24
Mucopolysaccharides (*see* Mucosaccharides)
Mucosaccharides, 44, 58, 122, 123, 128-131, 148, 149 (*see also* Polysaccharides)
aldehyde-fuchsin stain for, 128-131
associated with sites of calcification, 58
colloidal iron stain for, 44, 122, 123
effect of Bouin's fixative on, 122, 123
effect of Zenker's fixative on, 44
fixatives recommended for, 44, 122, 123
Mayer's mucicarmine stain for, 148, 149
Mucosubstances (*see* Mucosaccharides)
Multiple embedding procedures, 86-89
Muscle (*see* Tissue)
Mutilation of tissue specimens during embedding and microtomy, 86, 87
Mycelial forms, prevention during fixation, 60
Myelin, 60, 61
Myocardium (*see* Heart)

N

Necropsy procedures, *13-21,* 30
Negri body, 144, 145
Neoplastic tissue, 100, 101, 124-127, 132, 133, 152, 153 (*see also* Carcinoid; Fibroma; Mastocytoma; Sarcoma)
Nerve cells, 132, 133, 144, 145
Nerve fibers, 130-133, 144, 145, 152, 153
Neuron (*see* Nerve cells)
Nicks in edge of microtome knife (*see* Knife)
Nissl substance, 132, 133
Nuclear alteration, 28, 29, 36, 37, 126, 127
Nuclear chromatin, 26-29, 32-37, 124-127, 138, 139, 156-159
Nuclear fast red stain (*see* Stains)
Nuclear material, 14, 15
Nuclear shrinkage, 32-37, 126, 127
Nuclear swelling, 36, 37
Nuclei, 126, 127, 130, 131, 140-143, 174, 175
   anisotropism, in aqueous mounted tissue sections, of, 174, 175
   brownish color, in hematoxylin stained tissue sections, of, 140, 141
   failure to retain hematoxylin of, 140, 141
   lack of chromatic difference *vs* cytoplasm of, 142, 143
   light staining with hematoxylin of, 140, 141
   pyknosis due to delayed fixation of, 126, 127
   staining with Best's carmine of, 130, 131
Nucleoli, 26, 27
Nucleotidase, 5', preservation, 58

O

Oil, 100, 101, 134, 135, 150, 151, 170
   as a mounting medium, 170
   -like residue on surface of tissue sections, 100, 101
   red O stain (*see* Stains)
   residues on tissue sections from deceration for Fite-Faraco stain in, 134, 135
Organelles, cellular, simulated by crystal violet crystals, 132, 133
Orientation of tissue specimens during embedding and microtomy, 14, 86, 92, 93
Overexpansion of tissue sections on waterbath, 78, 79, 118, 119
Overexposure of tissue sections during clearing in xylene, 160, 161
Overfixation of tissue specimens with Zenker's fluid, 36-39
Overprocessing of tissue specimens, 74, 75
Overstaining of tissue sections, 140-142, 144-147
Over-Zenkerization, 36-39
Oviduct (*see* Tissue)
Oxidase, monamine, preservation, 58
Oxidation, 30, 31, 134, 136, 138, 144
   of hematein, 134, 136, 138
   of hematoxylin, 134, 136, 138
   of metal covers of fixative containers, 30, 31, 144
   of mordants, 138
   of phosphotungstic acid hematoxylin, 144

P

Paget cells, 56, 57, 122, 123
Pancreas (*see* Tissue)
Paraffin, 64, 68, 70, 71, 76, 82, 83, 88, 89, 114, 116, 126-129 (*see also* Deceration; Embedded tissue; Plasticized paraffin)
   excessive hardness, *vs* embedded tissue, of, 88, 89, 114, 116
   excessive softness, *vs* embedded tissue, of, 116
   excessive temperature, effect on tissue, of, 82, 83
   hydrophobia of, 76
   infiltration with, 64, 68, 70, 71, 76
   residues in lipid solvent used for deceration of, 126
   residues in stained tissue sections of, 126-129
Paraformaldehyde (*see* Fixatives)
Paragon, 170
Paraplast, 128, 129 (*see also* Plasticized paraffin)
Parasites simulated by wrinkles in blood smears, 154-157
Parathyroid (*see* Tissue)
Parched earth effect observed in tissue sections, 8-11, 118, 119, 160, 161
Pericardium (*see* Tissue)
Periodic acid oxidation of aldehydes, 108
Periodic acid-Schiff reaction, 42-44, 48, 49, 68, 108, 109, 136, 137, 150, 151, 166, 167 (*see also* Stains)
   diffusion of Schiff's reagent into glass coverslip substitutes after the, 166, 167
   of aldehydes, 108, 109
   of dried malt diastase, 150, 151
   of fungi, 108, 109
   of glycogen, 48, 49, 150
   of mercurial sublimate burns in embedded tissue, 42-44
   of mildew contaminants on glass microscope slides, 108, 109
   of mold contaminants on glass microscope slides, 108, 109
   of polysaccharides, 108, 109
   of starch, 68
   of talcum powder, 68
   preceded by malt diastase digestion, 150, 151
   with a hematoxylin counterstain, 136, 137
Perl's iron reaction (*see* Prussian blue reaction)
Permount, 170, 172
Phloxine (*see* Stains)
Phosphatase, acid and alkaline, preservation, 58
Phospholipids, 60
Phosphotungstic acid hematoxylin (*see* Stains)
Picric acid, 34, 35, *48,* 122, 123
   effect in embedded tissue of, 48, 122, 123
   removal from tissue sections of, 48, 122
Pigment, 56, 100, 134, 135, 168, 169 (*see also* Color pencil; Hematin; Hemosiderin; India ink; Iron)
   displacement within tissue section of, 100
   effect of fixation with unbuffered acid formalin on, 56
   simulated by air entrapped within tissue sections, 168, 169
   simulated by alum crystals in tissue sections, 134, 135
   transfer from tissue sections to mounting medium of, 100
   transfer from tissue sections to other tissue sections of, 100
   transfer from tissue sections to water-bath of, 100
Pipe ashes (*see* Ashes)
Pituitary gland (*see* Tissue)
Plant material observed within tissue sections, 14, 15
Plasmal reaction of Feulgen (*see* Feulgen reaction)
Plasmalogen, 44
Plasticized paraffin, 88, 89, 128, 129
   simulation of mucin in tissue sections by, 88, 89, 128, 129
   staining with cationic dyes of, 88, 89, 128
Pneumocystis corinii, 52, 53, 146, 147
   argyrophilia of, 52, 53, 146, 147
   confusion with acid formalin hematin pigment of, 52, 53, 146, 147
   isotropism of, 146, 147
Polariscopy, 4, 5, 8-11, 14-16, 24, 28, 29, 38-41, 44-55, 58-61, 68, 69, 72, 73, 126-129, 132, 133, 146-153, 164, 165, 170, 171, 174, 175

demonstration of amyloid stained with Congo red by, 132, 133
detection of alum crystals in tissue sections by, 150, 151
detection of crystallized mounting medium on tissue sections by, 170, 171, 174, 175
detection of dried malt diastase on tissue sections by, 150
detection of lint fibers on tissue sections by, 164, 165
detection of paraffin residues in stained tissue sections by, 126-129
detection of precipitates of recrystallized dyes on tissue sections by, 132, 133, 136, 137, 148, 149, 152, 153
distinguishing acid formalin hematin pigment from argyrophilic tissue components by, 146, 147
Polysaccharides, 108, 109
Potassium dichromate, effect on rhodanine stain for copper, 124, 125
Precipitates, 128-137, 148-153 (*see also* Contamination; Crystals; Debris; Residues)
of aldehyde-fuchsin on stained tissue sections, 128-131
of alum crystals on stained tissue sections, 134-137
of aluminum sulfate crystals on stained tissue sections, 150, 151
of Best's carmine stain on stained tissue sections, 130, 131
of Congo red dye on stained tissue sections, 132, 133
of cresyl echt violet on stained tissue sections, 132, 133
of crystal violet on stained tissue sections, 132, 133
of dried malt diastase on stained tissue sections, 150, 151
of eosin flakes on stained tissue sections, 134, 135
of hematein crystals on stained tissue sections, 136, 137
of nuclear fast red on stained blood smears, 148, 149
of oil red O on stained tissue sections, 150, 151
of silver on stained tissue sections, 130, 131, 152, 153
of thionine dye on stained tissue sections, 152, 153
of undissolved fused carmine dye on stained tissue sections, 148, 149
Pressure effects observed in tissue sections, 14, 15
Processing of tissue specimens, 30, *63-83*, 102, 103, 118, 126, 127

Processor for tissue specimens, 66, 74, 75
automatic, 74, 75
inadequately filled solution containers of, 74, 75
vacuum, 66
Prolonged fixation, 36-39
Protein, 48 (*see also* Coagulation)
Protozoan parasites simulated by mercurial sublimate crystals, 42
Prussian blue reaction for iron (*see* Stains)
Pseudocalcification observed in tissue sections, 58-61
Punched out areas in tissue sections, 60, 61 (*see also* Holes in tissue sections)
Pyknosis, 126, 127

Q

Quick-freeze spray (*see* Aerosol spray)

R

Rabies, 144
Razor, artifacts produced when substituted for microtome knife, 100
Reembedding procedures, 30, 118
Refrigeration, 56, 57, 124-127, 146
adverse effect on unfixed tissue specimens of, 56, 57, 124-127
of methenamine silver nitrate stock solution, 146
Rehydration of embedded tissue specimens, 88, 89
Reprocessing procedures, 78
Residues, 48, 49, 76, 77, 80, 88, 100, 101, 114, 115, 122, 123, 126-129, 134-137, 146-155, 158, 159, 164, 165, 170-175 (*see also* Contamination; Crystals; Debris; Mercurial sublimate; Precipitates)
in embedded tissue specimens, 48, 49, 76, 77, 80, 88, 114, 115, 122, 123, 164, 165
of alcohol in stained tissue sections, 158, 159
of alcohol in xylene used for clearing stained tissue sections, 158, 159
of clearing fluids in embedded tissue specimens, 76, 77, 88
of paraffin in stained tissue sections, 126-129
of paraffin in xylene used for deceration of tissue sections, 126
of picric acid in embedded tissue specimens, 48, 49, 122, 123
of processing fluids in embedded tissue specimens, 80
of processing fluids in xylene used for deceration of tissue sections, 126

of water in stained tissue sections, 158, 159
of water in xylene used for clearing of stained tissue sections, 154, 158, 159
of water in xylene used for deceration of tissue sections, 126
on blood smears, 148, 149
on embedded tissue specimens, 100
on glass coverslips, 164, 165
on glass microscope slides, 114, 115, 164, 165
on stained tissue sections, 100, 101, 114, 115, 128-131, 134, 135, 146, 147, 150-155, 158, 159, 164, 165, 170-175
Resinous mounting media, 170-172
Respirator, artificial, 8-11
Restaining of tissue sections, 126, 156, 157
Reticulum stain (*see* Stains, Gridley reticulum stain)
Rhodanine stain for copper (*see* Stains)
Rolled up tissue sections, 88
Rough-cutting of embedded tissue, 70, 76-78, 92, 100, 101
Rubeanic acid method for copper (*see* Stains)
Rust, as a fixative contaminant, 30, 31, 144, 145

S

Saffron-hematoxylin-phloxine (*see* Stains)
Salivary gland (*see* Tissue)
Sarcoma, reticulum cell, 124-127
Scott's water for bluing of hematoxylin stained tissue sections, 140
Scratches in tissue sections, 74, 75
Scum on surface of working solution of hematoxylin, 138, 139
Separation of tissue observed in tissue sections, 20, 21, 36, 37, 78, 79 (*see also* Cleavage)
Sevier-Munger silver method for neural tissues (*see* Stains)
Sharp, microtome knife (*see* Knife)
Sharpening of microtome knives, 94, 96
Shattering of tissue sections, 4, 5, 16, 17, 94-97, 102, 103, 116, 117
Shrinkage, 26-29, 32-37, 48, 49, 64, 65, 78, 82, 83, 98, 99, 118, 126, 127, 170, 171
of bone marrow, 82, 83
of cells, 26-29, 36, 37, 48, 49
of nuclei, 32-37, 126, 127
of tissue components, 64, 65
of tissue sections, 98, 99, 118, 170, 171
of tissue specimens, 78, 98

187

Silver, 72, 73, 130-133, 146, 170 (*see also* Stains)
  halide crystals, 170
  nitrate, 72, 73, 146
  precipitates on stained tissue sections, 130-133
Skeletal muscle (*see* Tissue, muscle)
Skin (*see* Tissue)
Slides (*see* Glass coverslips and microscope slides)
Slime, contamination of tissue specimens, 66, 67
Smoke (*see* Carbon)
Soaking of the surface of embedded tissue blocks, 74, 76, 78, 80, *102, 103*
Sodium bicarbonate, use in restoration of basophilia, 36
Sodium thiosulfate, use with Zenker's-fixed tissue, 36, *38,* 39, 42-45
Soft areas in embedded tissue specimens, 80
Soft tissue components, disorientation of, 98, 99
Soot (*see* Carbon)
Spinal cord (*see* Tissue)
Spleen (*see* Tissue)
Splitting of tissue sections, 14-17, 30, 31
Spongy areas in embedded tissue specimens, 80
Spraying of glass microscope slides with adhesive medium, 114
Spraying of specimen surface of tissue block prior to microtomy, 92, 100, 101
Spreading of tissue sections on waterbath, 78, 79, 118, 119
Staining, 16, 17, 24, 25, 34, 35, 38, 39, 44, 54-57, 64, 65, 88, 89, 94, 95, *112-161*
  achromatic, 140, 141
  adverse effect of Bouin's fixation on, 44, 122, 123
  adverse effect of contamination of clearing xylene on, 154, 158, 159
  adverse effect of contamination of deceration xylene on, 126
  adverse effect of delayed fixation of tissues on, 24, 25, 56, 57, *124-127*
  adverse effect of inadequate mordanting in Masson's trichrome method on, 154, 155
  adverse effect of omission of bluing after hematoxylin on, 140-143
  adverse effect of position of slide on, 148, 149
  adverse effect of prolonged storage of Bouin's-fixed embedded tissue on, 48, 49, 122, 123
  adverse effect of prolonged storage of stained tissue sections on, 156-159
  adverse effect of prolonged storage of tissue in neutral buffered formalin on, 156-159
  adverse effect of unbuffered formalin fixation on, 54-57, 122, 123
  adverse effect of Zenker's fixation on, 44, 124, 125, 130, 131, 152, 153
  cracking of tissue sections during, 118, 119
  diffusion of dye in tissue section during, 48, 49, 122, 123, 130, 131
  double, 114-117, 154-157
  erratic due to lack of proper drying of tissue section prior to, 118, 119
  failure due to inadequate deceration of tissue section prior to, 88, 89, 126-129
  intensity of, 16, 17, 24, 25, 34, 35, 38, 39, 56, 57, 94, 95, 112-119, 124-127, 138-145, 154-159
  irregular due to inadequate dehydration during processing of tissue prior to, 76, 77
  lack of chromatic difference between nuclei and cytoplasm after, 142, 143
  loss of tissue sections during, 118, 119
  of tissue sections prepared from embedded tissue after prolonged storage, 158, 159
  of undecerated and unstained tissue sections after prolonged storage, 156-159
  procedures, 120-161
  quality of, 48, 134, 135, 138, 139, 142-145
  splotchy (*see* uneven)
  uneven, 64, 65, 88, 89, 118, 119, 126-129, 154, 155
  variable due to degradation of dye solution used for, 138, 139, 144, 145
  variable due to delayed fixation of tissues prior to, 24, 25, 56, 57, 124-127
  variable due to dull knife distortions on tissue section prior to, 94, 95
  variable due to faulty formulation of dye solution used for, 138, 139
  variable due to fragments of tissue overlaying tissue section during, 112, 113
  variable due to tissue section overlaying air bubble during, 116, 117
  variable due to tissue section overlaying tissue debris during, 114, 115
  variable due to wrinkles in tissue sections prior to, 116, 117
Stains, 4-9, 14-21, 24-31, 34-61, 64-83, 86-89, 92-105, 108-119, 122-151, 154-161, 164-175
  alcian blue, 6, 7, 58
  aldehyde-fuchsin, 56, 57, 122, 123, 128-131
  alizarin blue S for copper, 130, 131
  Best's carmine, 130, 131
  Bodian's silver protein, 130, 131
  Brown and Brenn, 110, 111
  colloidal iron, 44, 58, 122, 123
  Congo red, 132, 133
  cresyl echt violet, 132, 133
  crystal violet, 132, 133, 172-175
  Degalantha's for urates, 44
  eosin, 134, 135, 140-145
  Fite-Faraco, 100, 101, 134, 135
  giemsa, 8, 9, 14, 44, 68, 154, 155, 158, 159
  Gomori's aldehyde-fuchsin, 56, 57, 122, 123, 128-131
  Gomori's methenamine silver, 42, 43, 72, 73, 108, 109
  Gridley's fungi, 168, 169
  Gridley's reticulum, 150, 151
  Grocott's methenamine silver, 52, 53
  Hale's colloidal iron, 44, 58, 122, 123
  Harris' hematoxylin, 138, 139, 144, 145, 160, 161
  hematoxylin, 134-143, 158-161, 170, 171
  hematoxylin and eosin, 4-9, 14-21, 24-31, 34-40, 42-61, 64-83, 86-89, 92-105, 108-119, 122-129, 134-145, 156-161, 164-173
  hematoxylin and phloxine, 70, 71
  hematoxylin-phloxine-saffron, 54, 55, 82, 83
  Kinyon's acid-fast, 110, 111, 146, 147
  Leder's 128, 129
  Lendrum's, 92, 93, 100, 101
  Lieb's crystal violet, 172-175
  light green, 146, 147
  Luna-Parker for mercurial sublimate crystals, 40-42
  Masson's trichrome, 6, 7, 154, 155, 168, 169
  Mayer's hematoxylin, 78, 79, 142, 143, 156-159
  Mayer's mucicarmine, 148, 149, 168, 169
  methenamine silver nitrate, 42, 43, 52, 53, 72, 73, 108, 109, 146, 147
  methylene blue, 146, 147
  mucicarmine, 148, 149, 168, 169
  nuclear fast red, 44, 68, 69, 74, 75, 148-151
  oil red O, 150, 151
  periodic acid-Schiff, 14, 42-44, 48,

49, 68, 69, 108, 109, 136, 137, 150, 151, 166, 167
phloxine-eosin, 78, 79
phosphotungstic acid hematoxylin, 144, 145
Prussian blue for iron, 30, 31, 66-69, 74, 75, 112, 113, 144, 145, 148, 149
rhodanine for copper, 122-125
rubeanic acid for copper, 54, 55, 152, 153
Sevier-Munger silver, 152, 153
thionine, 32-35, 132, 133, 152, 153
Van Gieson's elastica, 6, 7
Verhoeff's elastica, 4-7, 82, 83
von Kossa's for calcium salts, 58, 59, 124, 125
Walbach's giemsa, 154, 155, 158, 159
Woelcke's for myelin, 60, 61
Wright's giemsa, 154-157
Starch as a contaminant of tissue sections, 4, 5, 14, 15, 68, 69
  anisotropism of, 4, 5, 14, 15, 68, 69
  staining reactions of, 14, 68, 69
Stippling effect due to entrapped air in tissue section, 168-172
Stomach (*see* Tissue)
Storage, 146, 156-161
  of methenamine silver nitrate stock solution, 146
  of neutral buffered formalin-fixed tissue specimens, 156-159
  of paraffin-embedded tissue specimens, 158, 159
  of stained paraffin-embedded tissue sections, 156-161
  of unstained and undecerated tissue sections, 156-159
Streaks observed across tissue section, 96, 97
Stretching of tissue section overlaying tissue debris, 114, 115
Stropping of microtome knives, 96
Sudan colorants, 150, 151
Sulfuric acid groups, demonstration in tissue sections, 128
Suture material in tissue specimens, 4, 5, 16, 17
Swelling of tissue specimens, 34, 36, 37, 76

T

Talcum powder (*see* Starch as a contaminant of tissue sections)
Tearing of tissue sections, 14
Testes (*see* Tissue)
Thermal dehydration (*see* Dehydration)
Thermal knife, 4-7
Thick and thin zones observed in tissue sections, 16, 17, 98-103 (*see also* Venetian blind effect)

Thionine, solubility in alcohol and water, 152 (*see also* Stains)
Thyroid (*see* Tissue)
Tissue, 4-11, 14-21, 24-33, 36-61, 64-83, 86-89, 92-105, 108-119, 122-149, 152-161, 164-175
  adipose, 20, 21, 54, 55, 68, 69, 112, 113
  adrenal gland, 20, 21, 86-89, 92, 93, 100-103, 170, 171
  aorta, 18, 19
  appendix, 152, 153
  artery, 52, 53, 58, 59, 92, 93, 114, 115
  blood vessels, 48-53, 58, 59, 72, 73, 82, 83, 116, 130, 131
  bone, 16, 17, 30, 31, 70, 71, 80-83, 92
  bone marrow, 54, 55, 70, 71, 80-83
  brain, 8-11, 16, 17, 42, 43, 60, 61, 68-71, 88, 89, 116-119, 128-135, 144, 145
  collagen, 24, 74, 75, 80, 81
  connective, 18, 19, 100, 101
  epididymis, 116, 117
  eye, 30, 31, 70-73, 78, 79, 114, 115, 144, 145, 172-175
  fibrous, 92
  gastrointestinal tract, 88, 89
  glandular, nonspecific, 138, 139
  hard, 92
  heart, 40, 41, 44-47, 58, 59, 64, 65, 70, 71, 78, 79, 118, 119, 124, 125
  intestine, general, 78, 79, 96-99, 132, 133, 136, 137, 144, 145, 152, 153, 168-171
  intestine, large, 78, 79
  intestine, small, 136, 137, 170, 171
  kidney, 18, 19, 28-31, 48-57, 66-69, 76-79, 82, 83, 88, 89, 92, 93, 108, 109, 112, 113, 132, 133, 140, 141, 164, 165, 170, 171, 174, 175
  liver, 14, 15, 18, 19, 24-31, 36-45, 48, 49, 54, 55, 58, 59, 66, 67, 72, 73, 76, 77, 86, 87, 94-97, 102-105, 110, 111, 116, 117, 122-127, 130, 131, 136, 137, 152, 153, 158-161, 172, 173
  lung, 6, 7, 18, 19, 28, 29, 52, 53, 58, 59, 102, 103, 112, 113, 146, 147, 164-167
  lymph node, 26, 27, 56, 57, 92, 93, 96, 97, 100, 101, 134, 135, 148, 149
  mammary gland, 82, 83, 168, 169
  mass, 8, 9
  meninges, 164, 165
  mesentery, 20, 21
  muscle, 4, 5, 42, 43, 66, 67, 72-75, 118, 119, 124, 125, 154, 155
  nerve fibers, 130-133

oviduct, 114, 115
pancreas, 20, 21, 98, 99, 166, 167
parathyroid gland, 20, 21
pericardium, 70, 71
pituitary gland, 68, 69, 94, 95, 116, 117
salivary gland, 128-131
skin, 4-7, 14, 15, 20, 21, 24, 25, 32, 33, 36, 37, 48, 49, 56, 57, 64, 65, 74, 75, 78-81, 86, 87, 98-101, 114, 115, 118, 119, 122, 123, 126-129, 134-137, 142, 143, 146, 147, 156-159
soft, 18, 19, 118, 119, 138-141
spinal cord, 88, 89, 154, 155, 164, 165
spleen, 36-39, 48, 80, 81, 92-95, 114, 115, 138, 139
stomach, 20, 21, 48
testes, 18, 19
thyroid gland, 14, 15, 20, 21
trachea, 14, 15, 136, 137
unstained, 10, 11, 40, 41
uterus, 6, 7, 86, 87, 92, 100, 101, 112, 113
veins, 50-53
Tissue-block, 74, 76, 80, 86, 87, 92, 93, 98, 100, 101, 158, 159
  chilling specimen surface prior to microtomy of the, 92, 93, 100, 101
  crevices around tissue specimen in the, 100
  entrapped air around tissue specimen in the, 86, 87, 100
  halo around tissue specimen in the, 76
  orientation for microtomy of the, 86, 92, 93
  sections adhere on microtome upstroke to the, 98
  soft or spongy areas in the, 80
  storage of, 158, 159
  vibration during microtomy of the, 74, 86, 92, 93, 100
  vibration of tissue specimen within the, 74, 86, 100
Trachea (*see* Tissue)
Trichloroacetic acid, effect on glycogen, 48
Trichrome stain (*see* Masson's trichrome stain; Stains)
Trimming of gross specimens (*see* Macrosectioning)
Tubercle bacilli (*see* Bacteria)
Tubing, plastic and rubber, 66, 67

U

Undecerated tissue sections, storage and its effects on subsequent staining, 156-159
Uneven staining (*see* Staining)
Unfixed tissue, 18-21, 56, 57

adverse effect of freezing on, 18-21
adverse effect of refrigeration on, 56, 57
Unsaturated fatty acids, effect of Zenker's fixation, 44
Unstained tissue sections, 10, 11, 100, 101, 156-159, 164, 165
   effect of storage on subsequent staining of, 156-159
   storage of, 156
Urates, Degalantha's stain, 44
Urea, 44-47
   polymers of, 44-47
   reaction with formalin of, 44, 46
   use in Zenker's fluid of, 44, 46
Uric acid, Degalantha's stain, 44
Uterus (*see* Tissue)
Uzman's rubeanic acid method for copper (*see* Stains, rubeanic acid)

V

Vacuolation of tissue specimens, 4, 5, 18-21, 24, 25, 74, 75, 80-83, 130, 131
Vacuum ovens and tissue processors, 66, 80, 86
Van Gieson's elastica stain (*see* Stains)
Veins (*see* Tissue)
Venetian blind effect observed within tissue sections, 74, 75, 86, 87, 92, 93
Verhoeff's elastica stain (*see* Stains)
Vibration, 74, 86, 92, 93
   of microtome knife, 74, 86, 92, 93
   of tissue block in microtome specimen chuck, 74, 86, 92, 93
   of tissue specimen within paraffin block, 74, 86
Virchow-Robin space, 68, 69, 88, 89, 128, 129
Vogt's method for nerve cell products (*see* Stains, cresyl echt violet)
Von Kossa staining technique (*see* Stains)

W

Walbach's giemsa stain (*see* Stains)

Washing of tissue sections, 150, 154, 155
Washing of tissue specimens prior to processing, 14, 30, 31, 66-69, 122, 124
Water, 48, 60, 66-69, 76, 102, 103, 110, 112, 114, 126, 140, 142, 158, 159 (*see also* Filter; Flotation; Mounting medium)
   ammonia, 140
   bath, 110
   contamination of clearing xylene with, 158, 159
   contamination of deceration xylene with, 126
   contamination of tissue specimens with, 66-69, 76, 158, 159
   distilled, for tissue flotation waterbath, 112, 114
   effect on glycogen of, 48
   effect on phospholipids of, 60
   filtered, for tissue flotation waterbath, 112
   mineral content of, 66, 68, 112
   Scott's, bluing of hematoxylin stained tissue sections, 140
   softening of embedded tissue prior to microtomy with, 102, 103
   tap, adverse effect of use in tissue flotation waterbath, 112
   tap, bluing of hematoxylin stained tissue sections, 140, 142
   testing for presence of iron in, 66
   tissue components soluble in, 48
Wavy linear structures in blood smears, 154, 155
Wavy zones observed in tissue sections, 16, 17
Wet tissue storage, 36, 44, 46, 48, 60, 156-159
   of alcohol-fixed tissue, 48
   of formalin-calcium-fixed tissue, 60
   of neutral buffered formalin-fixed tissue, 156-159
   of Zenker's-fixed tissue, 36
   of Zenker's urea fluid-fixed tissue, 44, 46
Wilson's disease, 54, 55, 122, 123, 152, 153

Woelcke's stain for myelin (*see* Stains)
Wright's giemsa stain (*see* Stains)
Wrinkled blood smears, 154-157
Wrinkled tissue sections, 76-79, 88, 89, 114-117

X

Xylene, 14, 64, 126, 154, 158-161, 168-172
   contamination with alcohol of, 158, 159
   contamination with paraffin of, 126
   contamination with processing fluids of, 126
   contamination with water of, 126, 154, 158, 159
   effect, during coverslipping, of evaporation of, 168-171
   effect of overexposure, during clearing of stained tissue sections, to, 160, 161
   use in clearing of stained tissue sections of, 154, 158-161
   use in clearing of tissue specimens during processing of, 64
   use in coverslipping procedures of, 168, 170, 172
   use in deceration of tissue sections of, 126

Z

Zenker's fluids, 36-48, 124-127, 130, 131, 152, 153 (*see also* Fixatives; Mercurial sublimate; Overfixation)
   effect on alizarin blue S stain for copper of, 130, 131
   effect on colloidal iron staining procedure of, 44
   effect on rhodanine stain for copper of, 124, 125
   effect on rubeanic acid stain for copper of, 152, 153
   effect on staining reactions of delayed fixation with, 126, 127
   effect on tissue of, 36-48
   fixation procedure with, 36, 38, 124
   with urea, 44-47